Radiology Imaging
Words and Phrases

Diagnostic Imaging
Interventional Radiology
Therapeutic Radiology
Nuclear Medicine
Neuroradiology
Ultrasonography
Computed Tomography
Magnetic Resonance Imaging

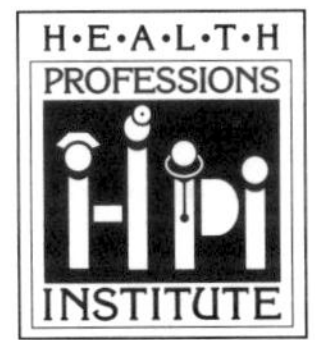

Health Professions Institute • Modesto, California • 1997

Radiology Imaging Words and Phrases

Diagnostic Imaging, Interventional Radiology, Therapeutic Radiology, Nuclear Medicine, Neuroradiology, Ultrasonography, Computed Tomography, Magnetic Resonance Imaging

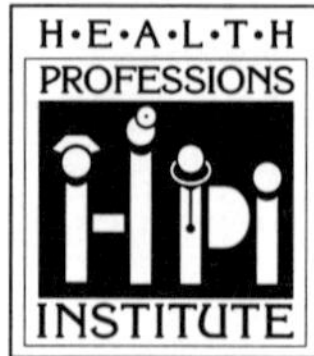

Sally Crenshaw Pitman
Editor & Publisher
Health Professions Institute
P. O. Box 801
Modesto, CA 95353-0801
Phone 209-551-2112
Fax 209-551-0404
E-mail: hpi@ainet.com
Web site: http://www.hpisum.com

Printed by
Parks Printing & Lithography
Modesto, California

ISBN 0-934385-68-8

Last digit is the print number: 9 8 7 6 5 4

To

Bud Parks

Preface

Radiology Imaging Words and Phrases is more than an update of *Radiology Words and Phrases,* second edition, published in 1990. It has been greatly expanded to include over 50,000 entries from diagnostic imaging, interventional radiology, therapeutic radiology, nuclear medicine, neuroradiology, ultrasonography, computed tomography (CT), magnetic resonance imaging (MRI), and hundreds of imaging agents.

Terminology in the field of radiology imaging crosses all body systems and medical specialties, thus challenging us to cover all the bases with a minimum amount of redundancy. With so many new developments in medicine, surgery, and technology in the past six years, it was easy to find new terms and new products.

We tried to limit this quick-reference book to the basic words and phrases widely used in radiology reports, and to new terminology that might appear in imaging reports in the future. Technology advances in radiology have spawned monoclonal antibody-labeled isotopes, giving rise to the radiopathology laboratory. Advances in neuroradiology, microradiology, and holography have made possible the imaging of very small anatomical structures that heretofore could not be imaged using standard radiology techniques. Radiation therapy in combination with monoclonal antibody imaging has made the science of oncology more precise. Thus, the reader will note the addition of relevant pathology terms in this edition.

This book is by no means an exhaustive list of words and phrases in the radiology imaging specialties. We've culled words and phrases from hundreds of transcripts of radiology imaging dictation, references and textbooks, scholarly journals in all specialties, and have taken liberal advantage of the educational material available on the Internet.

Physicians and other healthcare professionals who dictate patient health records often refer to radiology imaging diagnostic and therapeutic studies. We hope that this book will be useful for medical transcriptionists in all specialties, not just those who work exclusively in radiology imaging departments.

Research and editing for this book were done primarily by Linda Campbell and Kathy Cameron, with proofreading assistance provided by Vera Pyle and John H. Dirckx, M.D. My warmest gratitude to all.

Sally Crenshaw Pitman
Editor & Publisher

How to Use This Book

The words and phrases in this book are alphabetized letter by letter of all words in the entry, ignoring punctuation marks and words or letters in parentheses. The possessive form ('s) is omitted from eponyms for ease in alphabetizing. Numbers are alphabetized as if written out, with the exception of subscripts and superscripts which are ignored.

Eponyms may be located alphabetically as well as under the nouns they modify. For example, *Cholebrin imaging agent* is found alphabetically under the C's as well as under the main entry *imaging agent*. *Technetium* is found in the T's as well as under *imaging agent*, which includes a list of nearly a thousand imaging agents. Under alternate terms such as *contrast medium, isotope, radioisotope,* and *radionuclide*, there is a *see imaging agent* reference.

Names of various radiology imaging studies have been combined under the broad category *imaging,* while names of various kinds of technology used in radiology imaging are listed under the broad term *system.*

Many anatomical terms are found in the book, but no attempt was made to be comprehensive. Rather, we refer readers to our recent *Laboratory/Pathology Words and Phrases* (1996), which includes tables of arteries, bones, muscles, nerves, and veins, with both English and Latin forms in tabular form for quick reference.

Main entries with a lengthy list of subentries include the following:

artery	node
bone	scanner
catheter	shunt
deformity	sign
fracture	stenosis
imaging	system
imaging agent	technique
lesion	ultrasound
ligament	vein
muscle	view

A, a

AA (ascending aorta)
AAA (abdominal aortic aneurysm)
Abbott artery
ABC (aneurysmal bone cyst)
abdomen
  acute
  acute surgical
  boat-shaped
  distended
  nondistended
  postlymphangiography
  postsurgical
  scaphoid
  surgical
abdominal abscess
abdominal aneurysm
abdominal aorta
abdominal aorta thrombosis
abdominal aortic aneurysm (AAA)
abdominal aortic coarctation
abdominal aortography
abdominal carcinosis
abdominal circumference (AC)
abdominal contents
abdominal distention
abdominal iron deposition
abdominal mass

abdominal paracentesis, ultrasonic
    guidance for
abdominal pregnancy
abdominal situs inversus
abdominal vascular accident
abdominis rectus muscle
abdominopelvic mass
abducens (or abducent) nucleus
abducens nerve (sixth cranial nerve)
abduction fracture
abduction stress test
abductor muscle of little finger
abductor muscle of little toe
abductor digiti quinti (ADQ) muscle
abductor hallucis muscle
abductor pollicis brevis (APB)
    muscle
abductor pollicis longus (APL)
    muscle
abductovalgus, hallux
aberrant
aberrations, intersegmental
ABGd imaging agent
ABI (ankle/brachial index)
ablation
    percutaneous radiofrequency
    radiofrequency (RF)

ablation *(cont.)*
  saline-enhanced RF tissue
  stereotactic or stereotaxic
  surgical
  thermal
  total
  ultrasound-guided percutaneous
    interstitial laser
ablative laser therapy
abnormality
  accumulation
  acral
  arch of aorta
  augmentation
  bony
  bulbar
  cranial nerve
  cytoarchitectonic
  definitive
  fetal
  figure-of-eight
  focal
  frontal plane growth
  functional
  gestational sac
  gray matter
  obstructive
  perfusion
  restrictive
  screening-detected
  soft tissue
  torsional
  tracer
  ultrastructural
  white matter
  vasculature
  vessel wall
aboral direction
Abrikosov tumor
abrupt vessel closure
abruptio placentae (abruption of
  placenta)

abscess (pl. abscesses)
  abdominal
  actinomycotic brain
  acute
  amebic liver
  anaerobic lung
  appendiceal
  arthrifluent
  Aspergillus cerebral
  bone
  brain
  Brodie
  Brodie metaphyseal
  cerebral
  collar-button
  cuff
  daughter
  deep interloop
  deep pelvic
  encapsulated brain
  enteroperitoneal
  epidural
  extradural
  frontal
  gallbladder wall
  growth plate
  hepatic
  horseshoe (in the hand)
  interloop
  intermesenteric
  intersphincteric
  intra-abdominal
  intradural
  intrahepatic
  intramesenteric
  intraosseous
  intraperitoneal
  ischiorectal
  liver
  lung
  metaphyseal
  midpalmar

abscess *(cont.)*
Paget
pancreatic
paracolic
pararectal
pararenal
perianal
periappendiceal
pericecal
pericolic
pericolonic
perinephric
perirectal
phoenix
postoperative
Pott
psoas
pyogenic liver
rectal
retroperitoneal
retroperitoneal-iliopsoas
serous
spinal epidural (SEA)
splenic
subaponeurotic
subdiaphragmatic
subdural
subgaleal
subhepatic
subperiosteal
subphrenic
subungual
suture
thecal
thenar space
tubo-ovarian
absence of uptake
absence seizure
absent aortic knob
absolute artery dimensions
absolute emission probability
absolute-peak efficiency calibration

absolute scotomata
absorbed dose per unit
absorbed dose range
absorber
absorptiometry
double photon (DPA)
dual x-ray
single photon (SPA)
single-energy x-ray (SXA)
x-ray
absorption
actinide
bony
impaired
linear
lysosomal (of cartilage in
rheumatoid arthritis)
absorption cavity
absorption coefficient
absorption of radionuclide
abstraction
abut, abutted
abutment
abutting
AC (abdominal circumference)
AC (acromioclavicular) joint separation
AC (anterior commissure)
AC-PC (anterior commissure-
posterior commissure)
AC-PC line
AC-PC plane
ACA (anterior cerebral artery)
ACA (anterior choroidal artery)
ACAD (atherosclerotic carotid artery
disease)
acalculous cholecystitis
acanthopelvis
ACAT (automated computed axial
tomography)
ACB (asymptomatic carotid bruit)
accelerated acute rejection
accelerated fractionation

accelerated hyperfractionated
   radiotherapy
accelerated peristalsis
acceleration time
accelerator
   alpha particle
   Bevatron
   dual-energy
   electron linear
   linear
   medical linear
   particle
   Philips linear
   Siemens Mevatron 74 linear
accelerator mass spectrometry (AMS)
accentuation of markings
access, vascular
accessory atlantoaxial ligament
accessory bones
accessory lobe
accessory organ
accident
   cardiovascular
   cerebrovascular (CVA)
   vascular
accidental correction
Accu-Flo CSF reservoir
Accu-Flo ventricular catheter
accumulation, abnormal tracer
accumulation of air in interlobar
   spaces
accumulation of gas
ACE fixed-wire balloon catheter
ACE inhibition scintigraphy
ace of spades sign on angiogram
acetabular bone
acetabular cup
acetabular depth to femoral head
   diameter (AD/FHD)
acetabular fossa
acetabular labrum
acetabular notch

acetabular osteolysis
acetabular roof
acetabuli, os
acetabulum (pl. acetabula)
   deep-shelled
   dysplastic
acetazolamide (Diamox) challenge test
acetazolamide-enhanced SPECT
acetylcholine receptor antibody
   (AChRab)
ACF (anterior cervical fusion)
ACG (apexcardiogram, apexcardiography)
ACh (acetylcholine) receptor
achalasia
   classic
   cricopharyngeal
   pelvirectal
   sphincteral
   ureteral
   vigorous
Achiever balloon dilatation catheter
Achilles bulge sign
Achilles bursa
Achilles+ ultrasound bone densitometer
Achilles tendon (tendo Achillis)
achillodynia
achlorhydria, gastric
achlorhydric
acholic stool
achondroplasia
achondroplastic dwarfism
AChR (acetylcholine receptor)
   antibody
AChRab (acetylcholine receptor
   antibody)
acid
   DTPA (diethylenetriamine
     pentaacetic)
   low-dose folinic
acidophilic pituitary tumor

Ackerman criteria for osteomyelitis
Ackrad balloon-bearing catheter
ACL (anterior cruciate ligament)
ACM (automated cardiac flow measurement) ultrasound technology
ACMI ulcer measuring device
ACoA (anterior communicating artery)
Acoma scanner
acoprosis
acoprous
acoustic backscatter characteristics of blood
acoustic impedance
acoustic interface
acoustic nerve
acoustic nerve tumor
acoustic neurinoma
acoustic neuroma
acoustic quantification, left ventricular ejection fraction
acoustical shadowing (in ultrasonography)
acoustic window
acquired disease
acquired toxoplasmosis
acquired tracheobronchomalacia
acquired unilateral hyperlucent lung
acquired ventricular septal defect (AVSD)
acquisition
    data
    ECT
    image
    multisection multirepetition
    multislice
    sequential image
    spirometric
    volume
acquisition technique
acquisition time
ACR teleradiology standard
acral abnormality

Acrel ganglion
acro-osteosclerosis
acropectorovertebral dysplasia
acrocephalosyndactyly
acromegaly
acromial angle
acromial bone
acromioclavicular (AC) joint
acromiocoracoid ligament
acromiohumeral interval (AHI)
acropachy
acrosyndactyly
ACS (Advanced Cardiovascular Systems)
    ACS Endura coronary dilation catheter
    ACS JL4 (Judkins left 4) French catheter
    ACS Mini catheter
    ACS Multilink coronary stent
    ACS RX coronary dilatation catheter
    ACS SULP II balloon
ACTH (adrenocorticotrophic hormone) antibody
    ACTH independent hyperplasia
    ACTH-producing pituitary adenoma
    ACTH-producing pituitary tumor
actinomycosis, retroperitoneal
actinomycotic brain abscess
active biplanar MR imaging guidance
active emptying fraction (left atrium)
Acuson computed sonography
Acuson linear array transducer
Acuson 128EP imager
Acuson 128XP ultrasound system
Acuson transvaginal sonography
acutance, image edge profile
acute abdominal series
acute avulsion fracture
acute cholecystitis

acute coronary insufficiency
acute myocardial infarction (AMI)
acute phase gene expression
acute renal failure (ARF)
AD (Alzheimer disease)
AD (aortic diameter)
adactyly (adactylia)
adamantinoma
Adamkiewicz (also Adamkiewitz)
   Adamkiewicz artery
ADC (analog-to-digital) conversion
   quantization error
Addison point
adduct
adduction fracture
adduction to neutral
adductor canal
adductor hiatus
adductor magnus
adductor sweep of thumb
adductor tubercle
adductus
   metatarsus (MTA)
   true metatarsus (TMA)
adenocarcinoma
   annular
   colloid
   exophytic
   giant cell
   infiltrating
   metastatic
   papillary
   scirrhous
   ulcerating
adenohypophysial
adenohypophysis
adenoma
   acidophilic
   acinous
   ACTH-producing pituitary
   basophilic
   bile duct (BDA)

adenoma *(cont.)*
   bronchial
   chromophobic
   colonic
   cutaneous
   eosinophilic
   gallbladder
   glycoprotein-secreting
   gonadotropin-secreting
   hepatic
   hepatocellular (HCA)
   intraspinal
   liver cell
   moderately differentiated
   mucinous
   null cell
   papillary
   parotid pleomorphic
   pituitary
   poorly differentiated
   prolactin-secreting
   sebaceum
   sessile
   suprasellar
   toxic
   tubular
   tubulovillous
   undifferentiated
   villoglandular
   villous
   well-differentiated
adenomatoid malformation
adenomatosis
adenomatous hyperplasia
adenomatous polyposis coli
adenomyomatosis
adenomyosis
   diffuse
   uterine
adenopapillomatosis, gastric
adenopathy
Adenoscan contrast medium

adenosine echocardiography
adenovirus, enteric
AD/FHD (acetabular depth to femoral
 head diameter)
adherent thrombus
adhesed
adhesion
adhesive
ADI (atlanto-dens interval)
adiabatic demagnetization
adiabatic fast passage
adiabatic off-resonance spin-locking
adiabatic RF (radiofrequency) pulses
adiabatic slice-selective RF pulses
adiadochokinesia
adipose ligament
adipose tissue
adiposogenital dystrophy
aditus pelvis
adjacent voxels
adjuvant radiation therapy
adjuvant therapy
adnexa (*not* adnexae)
adnexal masses
adolescent hallux valgus
adolescent idiopathic scoliosis (AIS)
ADQ (abductor digiti quinti) muscle
ADR ultrasound
adrenal cortical adenoma
adrenal gland
adrenal hyperandrogenism
adrenal hyperplasia
adrenal imaging MIBG (metaiodobenzylguanidine)
adrenal medulla
adrenal medullary hyperplasia
adrenal scintiscanning
adrenal tuberculosis
adrenogenital syndrome
ADR Ultramark 4 ultrasound
adult respiratory distress syndrome
 (ARDS)

advanced cortical disease
Advanced NMR Systems scanner
adventitia
adventitious bursa
adynamic ileus
AE (above-elbow) amputation
AE1, AE3 antibody
AEG (acute erosive gastritis)
AER (apical ectodermal ridge)
aerate, aerated
aeration
aerophagia
aerosol ventilation study
aerosolized Tc-DTPA evaluation
aerosolized Tc-PYP
AF (arcuate fasciculus)
A-FAIR (arrhythmia-insensitive flow-
 sensitive alternating inversion
 recovery) imaging
afferent digital nerve
afferent loop
afferent view
affix, affixed
AFP (alpha-fetoprotein) test
afterloader
 ^{192}I high-dose-rate remote
 remote
afterloading, high-dose-rate
AG (angular gyrus)
aganglionic segment of colon
AGC (anatomically graduated
 component)
age
 bone
 chronologic
 gestational
 menstrual
AGE (acute gastroenteritis)
AGE (angle of greatest extension)
agenesis
 corpus callosum
 lung

agenesis (*cont.*)
  renal
  sacral
agenetic fracture
agent (see *imaging agent*)
AGF (angle of greatest flexion)
Agfa CR system
Agfa Medical scanner
Agfa PACS system
aglutition
agonist muscle groups
agyria
AHI (acromiohumeral interval)
AHO (acute hematogenous
    osteomyelitis)
AICA (anterior inferior cerebellar
    artery)
AICA (anterior inferior cerebral
    artery)
AICA ("i'-ka") (anterior inferior
    communicating artery)
Aicardi syndrome
AICS (artery of inferior cavernous
    sinus)
AIDS dementia complex (ADC)
AI 5200 diagnostic ultrasound system
air
  bowel loop
  colonic
  free
  intracranial
  intramural colonic
  intraorbital
  intraperitoneal
  pleural cavity
  subcutaneous
air-block syndrome
air bolus
air bronchogram
air cavity
air cisternography
air column, corrugated

air-conditioner lung
air contrast barium enema
air cyst
air cystogram
air density
air embolism
air enema
air enema fluoroscopic imaging
air exchange
air-filled lungs
air-fluid level
air gap
air hunger
air inflation
air insufflation
air interface on x-ray
air leak
airless lung
airlessness, alveolar
air luminogram
air myelogram
air plethysmography
air pocket
air sac
air space
  apical
  terminal
air-space consolidation
air-space disease
air-space opacity
air-tissue interface
air trapping, localized
airway fluoroscopy
airway narrowing
airway obstruction
airway opening
airway pressure
airways disease, reversible
airways tuberculosis
airway trees
AIS (adolescent idiopathic scoliosis)
Aitken classification of epiphyseal
    fracture

AJC (ankle joint complex)
Ajmalin liver injury
AK (above-knee) amputation (AKA)
Akerlund deformity
akinetic posterior wall
akinetic segmental wall motion
ala (pl. alae)
   nasal
   sacral
ala cerebelli
ala magna
Alagille syndrome
Alanson amputation
alar bone
alar ligament
Albers-Schönberg (Schoenberg)
   disease
Albers-Schönberg marble bones
Albright-McCune-Sternberg syndrome
Albunex ultrasound imaging agent
Alcock canal
alcohol embolization
alcoholic cirrhosis of liver
alcoholic liver disease (ALD)
ALD (alcoholic liver disease)
aldosteronoma
Alexander disease
algorithm
   annealing
   bioeffects
   clustering
   cone-beam reconstruction
   contour-following
   correlation (CR)
   decryption
   defuzzification
   DIP
   document-recognition
   dual lookup table
   dynamic range control (DRC)
   edge-enhanced error diffusion
   edge-enhancing
   encryption

algorithm *(cont.)*
   Feldkamp
   fringe thinning
   histogram equalization
   image restoration
   interpolation
   iterative
   JPEG (joint photographic experts
     group)
   K-means clustering
   least-squares (LS)
   lossy
   mapping
   maximum-likelihood
   memory-intensive
   mensuration
   MIP (maximum intensity
     projection)
   neural evaluation
   pixel-oriented
   quantizer-design
   Ramesh and Pramod
   reconstruction
   SSD (shaded-surface display)
   3D elastic subtraction
   wavelet scalar quantization (WSQ)
   word segmentation
   z-interpolation
alias artifact
aliasing (wrap-around ghosting)
   artifact
aliasing phenomenon in Doppler studies
aliasing, temporal
alien hand sign
alignment
   anatomic
   angular
   field
   fracture fragment
   integrity and
   rotational
   torsional

alignment *(cont.)*
  transverse-plane
  vertebral body
alignment and registration of 3D
  images
alimentary canal
alimentary system
alimentary tract
alkaline reflux gastritis
ALL (anterior longitudinal ligament)
Allis sign
Allman classification of acromioclavicular injury
allocortex
allodynia
alloesthesia
allogenic marrow transplantation
allogenous bone graft
alloy
  cobalt-chromium
  stainless steel
  Ti-Nidium
  Ti6A14V
  Wood
All-Tronics scanner
Aloka color Doppler imaging
Aloka echocardiograph machine
Aloka linear scanner
Aloka sector scanner
Aloka SSD ultrasound system
AL-1 catheter
Alouette amputation
Alpers disease
alphafetoprotein level
alpha index
alpha motor neuron
alpha particle bombardment
alpha particle emitter
ALS (amyotrophic lateral sclerosis),
  carcinomatous
alta, patella
alteration in blood-brain barrier

alterations
  bilateral
  hemodynamic
alternator, film
altitudinal anopsia
altitudinal hemianopsia
alveolar bone fracture
alveolar clouding
alveolar consolidative process
alveolar edema
alveolar infiltrate
alveolar opacities
alveolar rhabdomyosarcoma
alveolar sarcoid
alveolus (pl. alveoli)
Alzate catheter
Alzheimer disease (AD)
Alzheimer neurofibrillary degeneration
Alzheimer-type, senile dementia
  (SDAT)
AMA-Fab scintigraphy
amaurosis
  central
  cerebral
  uremic
amaurosis fugax
ambient air
ambient cistern
ambifixation
ambilevosity
ambilevous
amblyaphia
ambulant
ambulatory equilibrium angiocardiography
AME (American Medical Electronics)
AME (Austin Medical Equipment)
amebiasis (see *amoebiasis*)
amebic abscess
ameboma
amelia
amenorrhea

amentia
American Shared-CuraCare scanner
americium (Am) radioactive source
ameroid occluder
AMI 121 contrast medium
AMI 227 contrast medium
amine
    basophilic
    macrolytic
aminopolycarboxylic acid imaging
    agent
Amipaque contrast medium
AML (amyotrophic lateral sclerosis)
Ammon horn (mesial temporal)
    sclerosis
amniocentesis, ultrasonic guidance for
amniography
amniotic fluid
amniotic sac
A-mode echocardiography
A-mode encephalography
A-mode ultrasound
amorphous collection of contrast
Amoss sign
amphetamine precursor
Amplatz catheter
amplifier, linear
amplitude image
amplitude limits
ampulla of Vater
ampulla, rectal
ampullary carcinoma
ampulloma
amputation
    above-elbow (AE)
    above-knee (AK, AKA)
    Alanson
    Alouette
    Beclard
    below-knee (BK, BKA)
    Berger interscapular
    Bier

amputation *(cont.)*
    Boyd ankle
    Bunge
    Burgess below-knee
    button toe
    Callander
    Carden
    chop
    Chopart
    Chopart hindfoot
    circular supracondylar
    closed flap
    complete
    congenital
    digital
    femoral head
    fingertip
    fish-mouth
    forearm
    forefoot digital
    forequarter
    Gritti-Stokes distal thigh
    guillotine
    Hey
    hindquarter
    incomplete
    index ray
    interinnominoabdominal
    interphalangeal
    interscapular
    interscapulothoracic
    Jaboulay
    Kirk distal thigh
    Le Fort
    Lisfranc
    midthigh
    nonreplantable
    one-stage
    Pirogoff
    ray
    replantable

amputation *(cont.)*
  supramalleolar open
  Syme
  Syme ankle disarticulation
  Teale
  toe
  transcarpal
  transcondylar
  translumbar
  transmetatarsal (TMA)
  traumatic
  two-stage
  Vladimiroff-Mikulicz
amputation neuroma
amputation stump
AMS (accelerator mass spectrometry)
AMT-25-enhanced MR images
amygdala of cerebellum
amygdalofugal pathway
amygdaloid area
amygdaloid nuclear complex
amyloid disease
amyloidoma
amyostatic syndrome
amyotonia congenita
amyotrophic lateral sclerosis (ALS)
anal atresia
anal bulging
anal column
anal crypt
anal dilatation
anal endosonography
anal fissure
anal protrusion
anal stricture
anal verge
analog (see *analogue*)
analog-to-digital (ADC) conversion
  quantization error
analog-to-digital converter
analogous

analogue (analog)
  adenosine
  dysprosium
  L-arginine
  tamoxifen
analysis
  activation
  biomechanical
  cephalometric
  Cerenkov scintillation
  clinicopathological
  diagnostic efficacy
  digital frequency
  discriminant
  duplex ultrasound
  eigenvector
  electro-oculographic
  fission track (of urine)
  flow cytometry DNA
  folding-potential
  footprint
  fractal
  gamma spectrometric
  kinetic parameter
  late effect
  liquid scintillation
  multi-elemental neuron activation
  neutron activation
  nuclide
  phase
  pole figure texture
  power spectral (PSA)
  prospective
  pulse height spectral
  range-gated Doppler spectral flow
  residual stress
  risk
  Sassouni
  signal
  sonographic feature
  stepwise regression
  teboroxime resting washout (TRW)

analysis *(cont.)*
  thin film
  total body neutron activation
    (TBNAA)
  volumetric
anaplastic astrocytoma
anaplastic glioma
anastomosis (pl. anastomoses)
    (anatomical or surgical)
  aorta-to-vein
  aortic
  aorticopulmonary or aorto-
    pulmonary
  arterio-arterial
  arteriolovenularis
  arteriovenous
  ascending aorta to pulmonary
    artery
  beveled
  bidirectional cavopulmonary
  Billroth II
  cavopulmonary
  cobra-head
  coiling of
  colocolic
  diamond
  diamond-shaped
  dilatation of
  distal
  embryonic
  end-to-end
  end-to-side portacaval
  extradural
  extrapericardial
  glomeriform arteriovenous
  heterocladic
  homocladic
  ileorectal
  intercavernous
  intercoronary
  internal mammary artery to
    coronary artery

anastomosis *(cont.)*
  intradural
  intrapericardial
  laser-assisted microvascular
    (LAMA)
  left pulmonary artery to
    descending aorta
  LIMA (left internal mammary
    artery)
  mesocaval
  microvascular
  outflow
  portacaval
  portosystemic
  precapillary
  proximal
  pyeloileocutaneous
  right atrium to pulmonary artery
  right internal mammary artery
  right pulmonary artery to
    ascending aorta
  right subclavian to pulmonary
    artery
  Roux-en-Y
  side-to-end
  side-to-side
  simple arteriovenous
  splenorenal
  superior vena cava to distal right
    pulmonary artery
  superior vena cava to pulmonary
    artery
  systemic to pulmonary artery
  tendon
  terminoterminal
  tracheal
  transureteroureteral
  ureteroileocutaneous
  ureteroureteral
  vascular
anastomotic defect
anastomotic disruption

anastomotic leakage
anastomotic pseudoaneurysm
anastomotic site
anastomotic stoma
anastomotic stricture
anatomic alignment
anatomic distribution
anatomic landmarks
anatomic moment erratum
anatomic neck
anatomic position
anatomic snuffbox
anatomic variability
anatomic variant
anatomical dead space
anatomical snuffbox
anatomically dominant
anatomy
  anomalous
  distorted
  left-dominant coronary
  medullary venous
  right-dominant coronary
  Saltzman
  sectional
  segmental
anconeal fossa (also anconal fossa)
anconeus
anconoid
ancyroid cavity (also ankyroid)
Anderson-Hutchins tibial fracture
android pelvis
anechoic area
anechoic center
anechoic fluid collection
anencephaly
anesthesia
anesthetic
aneurysm
  abdominal
  abdominal aortic (AAA)
  acquired

aneurysm *(cont.)*
  ampullary
  aortic
  aortic arch
  aortic sinus
  aortic sinusal
  aortoiliac
  arterial
  arteriosclerotic
  arteriovenous
  arteriovenous pulmonary
  ascending
  ascending aortic
  aspergillotic
  atherosclerotic
  atrial septal
  axillary
  bacterial
  basilar artery
  berry
  berry intracranial
  bland aortic
  brachiocephalic arterial
  brain
  bulge of
  bulging
  calcified wall of
  cardiac
  carotid artery
  cavernous carotid
  cavernous sinus
  cavity of
  cerebral
  circle of Willis
  circumscript
  cirsoid
  clinoid
  clip ligation of
  clipping of
  coating of
  coiling of
  compound

aneurysm *(cont.)*
  congenital
  congenital aortic sinus
  congenital arteriosclerotic
  congenital cerebral
  contained leak of aortic
  coronary artery
  coronary vessel
  cranial
  cylindroid
  de novo
  debulking of
  descending thoracic
  dilatation of
  dissecting
  dissecting abdominal
  dissecting aortic
  dissecting intracranial
  distal aortic arch
  dome of
  ductal
  ectatic
  embolic
  extracerebral
  extracranial
  false
  feeding artery of
  fundus of
  fusiform
  giant
  great cerebral vein of Galen
  hematoma of
  hemorrhage of
  hernial
  hunterian ligation of
  imperforate
  infected
  infrarenal abdominal aortic
  innominate
  internal carotid artery
  intracerebral
  intracranial

aneurysm *(cont.)*
  intramural coronary artery
  isthmus
  juxtarenal
  juxtarenal aortic
  late false
  lateral
  left ventricular
  luetic aortic
  M1 segment
  miliary
  mixed
  mural
  mycotic
  mycotic intracranial
  mycotic suprarenal
  neck of
  neoplastic
  nodular
  orbital
  pararenal aortic
  pelvic
  phthisis of
  PICA (posterior inferior cerebellar
    artery)
  popliteal
  posterior communicating artery
  postinfarction ventricular
  precursor sign to rupture of
  prerupture of
  pulmonary arteriovenous
  pulmonary artery compression
    ascending aorta
  pulmonary artery mycotic
  racemose
  rebleeding of
  renal
  renal artery
  reruption of
  ruptured
  ruptured atherosclerotic
  ruptured intracranial

angiography *(cont.)*
  celiac
  cerebral
  cine
  computed tomographic (CTA)
  computerized tomographic hepatic
    (CTHA)
  contrast
  coronary
  cystic duct
  diagnostic
  digital subtraction (DSA)
  digital subtraction cerebral
  digital subtraction pulmonary
  digital subtraction rotational
  directional color (DCA)
  dobutamine thallium
  DSA (digital subtraction)
  dynamic tagging MR
  ECG-synchronized digital subtraction
  elastic subtraction spiral CT
  electrocardiogram-synchronized
    digital subtraction
  Epistar subtraction
  equilibrium radionuclide
  first-pass nuclide rest and exercise
  first-pass radionuclide exercise
  fluorescein
  FluoroPlus
  four-vessel cerebral
  gated blood pool
  gated equilibrium radionuclide
  gated nuclear
  gated radionuclide
  IDIS (intraoperative digital
    subtraction)
  indocyanine green
  innominate
  intercostal artery
  internal carotid
  intra-arterial digital subtraction
    (IADSA)

angiography *(cont.)*
  intra-arterial DSA (digital
    subtraction)
  intravenous DSA (digital subtraction)
  intravenous fluorescein (IVFA)
  Judkins coronary
  left ventricular
  magnetic resonance (MRA)
  mesenteric
  nonselective
  nontriggered phase-contrast MR
  pancreatic
  phase-contrast
  postangioplasty
  postembolization
  postoperative
  post-tourniquet occlusion
  preoperative
  PTCA coronary
  pulmonary
  pulmonary artery wedge
  pulmonary vein wedge
  pulmonary wedge
  radionuclide (RNA)
  renal
  rest and exercise gated nuclear
  RI (resistive index)
  segmented k-space time-of-flight
    MR
  Seldinger
  selective
  selective coronary cine
  selective presaturation MR
  shaded-surface display (SSD) CT
  single plane
  SIR
  sitting-up view
  small angle-double incidence
    (SADIA)
  spinal
  STAR
  stereotactic cerebral

annulus umbilicalis
anococcygeal raphe
anode tube reloading
anomalous insertion
anomalous origin
anomalous pathway
anomalous pulmonary venous
      connection
  partial
  total
anolomous pulmonary venous return
anomalous vein of scimitar syndrome
anomalous vessel
anomaly (pl. anomalies)
  aortic arch
  back-angle
  bell clapper (BCA)
  cardiac
  cloacal
  congenital
  congenital cardiac
  conotruncal congenital
  cranial
  Cruveilhier-Baumgarten
  cutaneous vascular
  Ebstein
  extracardiac
  Freund
  May-Hegglin
  migrational
  multiple congenital (MCA)
  radial ray
  Shone
  Taussig-Bing
  tricuspid valve
  Uhl
  vascular
  vertebral segmentation
  Zahn
anorectal ring
anoxic ischemia
ansa (pl. ansae)

anserinus, pes
antagonist muscle groups
antebrachial fascia
antebrachium
antecolic anastomosis
antecubital approach for cardiac
    catheterization
antecubital fossa
antecubital space
antecubital vein
anteflexion
antegonial angle
antegonial notch
antegrade (forward)
antegrade blood flow
antegrade fast pathway
antegrade filling of vessels
antegrade flow
antegrade imaging
antegrade perfusion
antegrade pyelography
antegrade refractory period
antegrade urography
anterior cardiac vein
anterior cerebellar artery syndrome
anterior colliculus
anterior column of spine
anterior commissure
anterior communicating artery
anterior compartment syndrome
anterior coronary plexus (of heart)
anterior corpus
anterior corticospinal tract
anterior cruciate ligament (ACL)
anterior cusp
anterior descending artery
anterior fascicular block
anterior feet view
anterior fibular ligament
anterior gray column of cord
anterior head region
anterior horns of spinal cord

anterior hypothalamus
anterior inferior cerebellar artery
   (AICA)
anterior inferior cerebral artery
   (AICA)
anterior inferior communicating artery
   (AICA)
anterior inferior iliac spine
anterior intercostal artery
anterior interhemispheric cistern
anterior interhemispheric fissure
anterior internodal pathway
anterior internodal tract of Bachman
anterior interventricular groove
anterior leaflet prolapse
anterior lobe
anterior maxillary spine
anterior mediastinum
anterior motion of posterior mitral
   valve leaflet
anterior papillary muscle
anterior planar image
anterior/posterior (AP)
anterior projection
anterior pulmonary plexus
anterior semilunar valve
anterior septal myocardial infarction
anterior spinal artery
anterior spinocerebellar tract
anterior spinothalamic tract
anterior superior iliac spine (ASIS)
anterior talar dome
anterior talofibular ligament
anterior tibial artery
anterior tibial compartment
anterior tibiofibular ligament
anterior tibiotalar ligament
anterior urethra
anterior wall dyskinesis
anterior wall myocardial infarction
anteroapical wall myocardial infarction
anterofundal placenta

anterograde peristalsis
anterolateral wall
anterolateral white matter of cord
anterolisthesis
anteromedial
anteroposterior (AP) (also anterior-
   posterior)
antetorsion, femoral
anteversion
   angle of
   femoral
   Magilligan technique for measuring
   neutral
anteversion determination, Budin-
   Chandler
anteverted
anthracosilicosis
anthrocotic tuberculosis
anthropoid pelvis
anthropometric imaging
anthropometry, 3D surface
anti-AChR (antiacetylcholine receptor)
   antibody
anti-aliasing techniques
antibody (pl. antibodies) (see also
   imaging agent)
   AChR (acetylcholine receptor)
   ACTH
   AE1
   AE3
   anti-ACh receptor
   anti-AChR (antiacetylcholine
     receptor)
   anticardiolipin (aCL)
   antiglioma monoclonal antibody
   antimyosin
   antimyosin monoclonal (with Fab)
   antinuclear (ANA)
   antiphospholipid
   antistriated muscle
   beta-endorphin
   CAM 5.2

antibody *(cont.)*
   carcinoma-specific monoclonal
   cytokeratin
   EMA (epithelial membrane antigen)
   GFAP (glial fibrillary acidic protein)
   glutinin 1
   growth hormone
   heterophile
   IgM anti-human parvovirus
   ImmuRAID (CEA-Tc 99m)
   indium
   indium-labeled antimyosin
   kinase C
   kinase C antiglioma monoclonal
   lectin
   luteinizing hormone
   lym-1 monoclonal
   Mab-170 monoclonal
   MG (myasthenia gravis)
   monoclonal (MOAB, MoAb)
   neuron-specific enolase (NSE)
   neutralization
   NSE (neuron-specific enolase)
   OKT3 monoclonal
   polyclonal anticardiac myosin
   prealbumin
   precipitating
   prolactin hormone
   RCA (Ricinus communis
     agglutinin 1)
   Re-188 labeled
   7E3 monoclonal antiplatelet
   sheep antidigoxin Fab
   S-100 protein
   SS-A (Ro)
   SS-B (La)
   St. Louis encephalitis
   teichoic acid
   thyrotropin hormone
   UE (*Ulex europaeus*)
   vimentin
   VZ (varicella-zoster)
   whole blood monoclonal

antibody-antigen complex
antibody-conjugated paramagnetic
   liposomes (ACPLs)
antibody-labeled circulating
   granulocytes
antibody labeling
anticardiolipin (aCL) antibody
anticoincidence circuit
antifibrin (T2G1s) antibodies F(ab)2
antifibrin antibody imaging
antifibrin-MoAb imaging agent
antifibrin scintigraphy
antigen
   antiproliferating cell nuclear
   Aspergillus
   autogenous
   CA 15-3
   carcinoembryonic (CEA)
   epithelial membrane (EMA)
   histocompatibility
   HLA-B27
   human leukocyte, B27
   major histocompatability complex
     class II (MHC-2)
   prostate-specific (PSA)
   serum cryptococcal
anti-estrogen radiologic therapy
antigravity muscles
antimesenteric border of distal ileum
antimesenteric fat pad
antimesocolic side of the cecum
antimony
antimotility drug
antimyosin antibodies
antineoplastic therapy
antinuclear antibody (ANA) test
antiphospholipid anticardiolipin
   antibody
antistreptolysin O (ASO) titer
Antoni-A classification of neurinoma
Anton syndrome
antral edema

antral gastritis
antral stasis
antrum
  cardiac
  gastric
  Malacarne
  prepyloric
  pyloric
  retained
  Willus
anulus (see *annulus*)
anus
anvil bone
anvil sign
Ao, AO (aorta)
AO (aortic opening)
AO/AC (aortic valve opening/aortic
  valve closing) ratio
AO classification of ankle fracture
AO-Danis-Weber classification of
  ankle fracture
AOIVM (angiographically occult
  intracranial vascular malformation)
aorta (Ao, AO)
  abdominal
  aneurysmal widening of
  arch of
  ascending (AA)
  bifurcation of
  biventricular origin of
  biventricular transposed
  calcified
  central
  cervical
  coarctation of
  coarcted
  D-malposition of
  descending
  descending thoracic
  dextroposed
  dextropositioned
  double-barreled

aorta *(cont.)*
  draped
  dynamic
  ectasia of abdominal
  ectasia of thoracic
  elongated
  infrarenal
  infrarenal abdominal
  kinked
  L-malposition
  overriding
  pericardial
  porcelain
  preductal coarctation of
  recoarctation of the
  reconstruction of
  retroesophageal
  root of
  sclerosis of
  small feminine
  stenosis of
  supraceliac
  supradiaphragmatic
  terminal
  thoracic
  thoracoabdominal
  tortuous
  transposed
  unwinding of
  ventral
  wide tortuous
  widening of
aorta-iliac-femoral bypass
aorta-renal bypass
aorta-subclavian-carotid bypass
aorta-to-vein anastomosis
aortic allograft
aortic anastomosis
aortic aneurysm
aortic angiography
aortic annular region
aortic annulus

apex of petrous portion of temporal
    bone
APEX 409 camera
APEX 415 camera
apexcardiogram, apexcardiography
    (ACG)
aphagia
aphalangia
aphtha (pl. aphthae)
apical air space on x-ray
apical and subcostal four-chambered
    view
apical cap
apical cap sign
apical capping
apical corn
apical duodenal ulcer
apical four-chamber view
apical granuloma
apical hypoperfusion on thallium scan
apical impulse
apical infiltrate
apical-lateral wall myocardial
    infarction
apical ligament
apical posterior artery
apical posterolateral region of left
    ventricle
apical scar
apical scarring
apical segment
apical short-axis slice
apical surface of heart
apical thinning
apical tissue
apical two-chamber view
apical view
apical wall
apical window
apices (pl. of apex)
apicoabdominal bypass
apicoposterior bronchi

apiculate waveform
aPL (antiphospholipid) antibody
APL (abductor pollicis longus) muscle
aplasia, cerebellar
aplasia of deep veins
APM (anterior papillary muscle)
Apogee CX 200 echo system
Apogee ultrasound device
A point
aponeurosis
    bicipital
    digital
    epicranial
    external oblique
    internal oblique
    palmar
    plantar
    tendon
aponeurotic band
aponeurotic triangle
aponeurotic troika
apophyseal fracture
apophyseal joint
apophysis of Rau
apophysitis
    calcaneal
    iliac
apoplexy
    Broadbent
    cerebellar
    delayed
    pineal
    pituitary
    postpartum pituitary
    posttraumatic (of Bollinger)
    pulmonary
    pulmonary artery
    pulmonary vein
apotentiality, cerebral
APP (average pixel projection)
appearance
    bat wing
    beading of activity

appearance *(cont.)*
  beaten-silver (of the skull)
  beavertail (of balloon profile)
  blade of grass
  cauliflower
  Christmas tree
  cobblestone
  cobra-head
  cobweb
  coiled spring
  collar-button (in colon)
  corkscrew
  cottage loaf
  distortions of image
  drooping lily
  feathery
  flame
  frog-like
  frondlike
  heterogeneous
  homogeneous
  Honda sign
  isodense
  lobulated saccular
  moth-eaten
  onion peel
  signet ring
  spiral
  string-of-beads
  super scan
  target
  trilaminar
  trilayer
  whorled
appendage
  atrial
  cecal
  epiploic
  left atrial (LAA)
  right atrial (RAA)
  truncated atrial
  vermicular

appendage *(cont.)*
  wide-based blunt-ended
    right-sided atrial
appendiceal abscess
appendiceal stump
appendices or appendixes (pl.)
appendicitis, acute
appendicolithiasis
appendicular skeleton
appendix (pl. appendixes, appendices)
  cecal
  ensiform
  epiploic
  filiform
  Morgagni
  paracecal
  preileal
  retrocecal
  retroileal
  subcecal
  vermiform
  xiphoid
appendolithiasis
apple core lesion
applicator, nucletron
application-specific integrated circuit
  (ASIC)
appose
apposing articular surfaces
apposition
  bone-to-bone
  close
  fracture in close
apposition of leaflets
apron
  abdominal
  lead
  quadriceps
APS (air plasma spray) hydroxyapatite
APTC (anteroposterior talocalcaneal)
  angle
apudoma

AquaSens FMS 1000 fluid monitoring
  system
aqueduct
  cerebral
  forking of sylvian
  gliosis of
  mesencephalon
  midbrain
  Monro
  Sylvius
  ventricular
aqueduct compression
aqueduct occlusion
aqueduct stenosis
aqueous scintillator
AR (aortic regurgitation)
AR (atrial rate)
AR 2 diagnostic guiding catheter
arachnodactyly
arachnoid canal
arachnoid cyst
arachnoid granulation
arachnoid of uncus
arachnoid villi
Aran-Duchenne amyotrophy
Arani double loop guiding catheter
Arantius canal
arborescent
arborization of ducts
arborize
arcade
  collateral
  Frohse ligamentous
  mitral
  septal
  Struthers
  superficialis
Arcelin view
arch
  anterior atlas
  anterior metatarsal
  aortic

arch *(cont.)*
  articular
  atlas
  carpal
  cervical aortic
  coracoacromial
  deep
  distal aortic
  double aortic
  flat
  flattened longitudinal (of foot)
  Hapad metatarsal
  hemal
  high
  Hillock
  hypoplastic
  longitudinal (of foot)
  lung
  mid aortic
  mural
  neural vertebral
  palmar arterial
  plantar
  plantar arterial
  posterior metatarsal
  pubic
  right aortic
  right-sided
  Riolan
  subpubic
  superciliary
  superficial palmar arterial
  tarsal
  transverse (of foot)
  transverse aortic
  vertebral
  Zimmerman
  zygomatic
arch and carotid arteriography
Archer syndrome
archicortex
arch index

arching of mitral valve leaflet
architectural alterations of bone
architecture
  bony
  brain
  foot
  hepatic
  intranodal
  lung
  lobular
  network
Arco classification
arcuate artery
arcuate complex
arcuate eminence
arcuate fasciculus (AF)
arcuate fiber involvement
arcuate ligament
arcuate movement
arcuate nucleus
arcuate vessel
ARDS (adult respiratory distress
  syndrome)
area (see also *region*)
  anechoic
  aortic
  arrhythmogenic
  artery
  Bamberger
  body surface (BSA)
  Broca
  Brodmann
  callosal (parolfactory nerve)
  cardiac frontal
  cortical motor
  cross-sectional (CSA)
  denervated
  echo-free
  effective balloon dilated (EBDA)
  Erb
  Haeckerman

area *(cont.)*
  hilar
  hot
  hyperechoic
  hypoechoic
  ischemic
  language
  luminal cross-sectional
  midsternal
  mitral valve (MVA)
  olfactory
  parietal association
  parietotemporal
  perihilar
  peroneal
  premotor
  pulmonic
  rarefied
  sclerotic
  septal
  sonolucent
  stenosis
  subglottic
  suprapubic
  tricuspid
  valve
  watershed (of periventricular
    white matter)
  Wernicke
area-length method for ejection
  fraction
area of abnormal density
area of denudation
area of increased "radiolabeling"
areola
areolar plane
ARF (acute respiratory failure)
argentaffinoma
argon laser
Argyle Medicut R catheter
A ring, esophageal

arm
  abductor lever
  C-
  flail
  Leyla
  linebacker's
  outrigger
  Popeye
Arnold-Chiari (type II) malformation
array
  annular
  convex
  electrode
  high-density
  linear
  linear electrode
  NMRA quadrature detection
  phased
  symmetrical phased
  voxel
array processor (MRI equipment)
arrest
  anoxic
  asystolic cardiac
  bradyarrhythmic cardiac
  cardiac
  cardiopulmonary
  cardiorespiratory
  circulatory
  electrical circulatory
  epiphyseal
  flow
  heart
  hypothermic
  intermittent sinus
  profound hypothermic circulatory
    (PHCA)
  recurrent cardiac
  respiratory
  sinus
  transient sinus
 arrested circulation

arrest reaction
arrhenoblastoma
arrhythmia-insensitive flow-sensitive
  alternating IR
arrhythmogenic area
arrhythmogenic border zone
arrhythmogenic right ventricular
  dysplasia (ARVD) syndrome
arrhythmogenic ventricular activity
  (AVA)
Arrow-Berman balloon angioplasty
  catheter
ArrowFlex sheath
ArrowGard Blue Line catheter
ArrowGard central venous catheter
arrowhead-shaped
Arrow-Howes multilumen catheter
Arrow pulmonary artery catheter
arterial aneurysm
arterial avulsion
arterial blockage
arterial brachiocephalic trunk
arterial calcification
arterial cannula
arterial cannulation
arterial capillary
arterial circulation
arterial cutoff
arterial deficiency pattern
arterial degenerative disease
arterial dilatation and rupture
arterial dissection
arterial flow phase image
arterial graft
arterial hyperemia
arterial intima
arterial lumen
arterial malformation (AM)
arterial obstruction
arterial occlusion
arterial patency
arterial peak systolic pressure

arterial portography
arterial pressure
arterial pulsation artifact
arterial recoil
arterial return
arterial runoff
arterial rupture
arterial sclerosis
arterial segment
arterial sheath
arterial spasm
arterial steal
arterial supply
arterial thrombosis
arterial tonus
arterial topography
arterial tree
arterial varices
arterial wall dynamics
arterial wall thickness
arterialization of venous blood
arterio-arterial anastomosis
arteriocapillary sclerosis
arteriogram
arteriography
   aorta and runoff
   aortofemoral (with run-off views)
   arch and carotid
   balloon occlusion
   biplane pelvic
   biplane quantitative coronary
   brachial
   brachiocephalic
   bronchial
   carotid
   celiac
   cerebral
   cine-
   contrast
   coronary
   CT (computed tomography)
   delayed phase of

arteriography *(cont.)*
   femoral
   four-vessel
   hepatic
   infrahepatic
   intraoperative
   Judkins selective coronary
   left coronary cine-
   longitudinal
   lumbar
   mesenteric
   percutaneous
   percutaneous femoral
   peripheral
   pruned-tree
   pulmonary
   pulmonary artery
   quantitative coronary (QCA)
   renal
   retrograde
   runoff
   selective
   selective cerebral
   selective coronary
   Sones selective coronary
   subclavian
   superior mesenteric
   thrombotic pulmonary (TPA)
   vertebral
   visceral
   wedge
arteriolar sclerosis
arteriole
arterioplasty
arteriorenal
arteriosclerosis
   calcific
   cerebral
   coronary
   generalized
   hyaline
   hypertensive

arteriosclerosis *(cont.)*
  infantile
  intimal
  medial
  Mönckeberg (Moenckeberg)
  obliterative
  peripheral
  presenile
  pulmonary
  senile
arteriosclerosis obliterans (ASO)
arteriosclerotic cardiovascular disease
  (ASCVD)
arteriosclerotic deposits
arteriosclerotic heart disease (ASHD)
arteriosclerotic intracranial aneurysm
arteriosclerotic peripheral vascular
  disease
arteriosclerotic plaque
arteriosclerotic thoracoabdominal
  aortic aneurysm
arteriostenosis
arteriosus, ductus
arteriovenous (AV)
arteriovenous aneurysm
arteriovenous angioma
arteriovenous fistula (AVF)
arteriovenous interhemispheric
  angioma
arteriovenous malformation (AVM)
arteriovenous pressure gradient
arteriovenous varix
artery (pl. arteries)
  A1-A5 segments of anterior cerebral
  Abbott
  abdominal aorta
  aberrant
  aberrant coronary
  aberrant left pulmonary
  Adamkiewicz (Adamkiewitz)
  aneurysm of internal carotid
  aneurysm of posterior
    communicating

artery *(cont.)*
  angular MCA (middle cerebral
    artery)
  anomalous origin of
  anterior cerebral (ACA)
  anterior choroidal (ACA or AChA)
  anterior communicating (ACoA)
  anterior descending branch of
    left coronary
  anterior inferior cerebellar (AICA)
  anterior inferior cerebral (AICA)
  anterior inferior communicating
    (AICA)
  anterior spinal
  anterior spinal canal
  anterior temporal branch of
    posterior cerebral
  aortoiliofemoral
  apical posterior
  arcuate
  ascending frontoparietal (ASFP)
  atrioventricular node
  AV (atrioventricular) nodal
  axillary
  basal perforating
  basilar
  beading of
  bifurcation of anterior
    communicating
  bifurcation of common carotid
  bifurcation of internal carotid
  bifurcation of middle cerebral
  brachial
  brachiocephalic
  branch of
  calcarine
  calcified
  callosomarginal
  cannulated
  carotid
  celiac
  cerebral

artery *(cont.)*
  choroidal branch of internal
    carotid
  choroidal pericallosal
  circumflex (circ, CF, CX)
  circumflex groove
  collateral circulation in
  common carotid (CCA)
  common femoral
  common iliac
  compression of
  C1-C5 segments of internal carotid
  conus
  corduroy
  coronary
  cortical branch of middle cerebral
  costocervical
  course of
  deltoid branch of posterior tibial
  descending septal
  diagonal branch of
  diagonal branch of left anterior
    descending coronary
  diagonal coronary
  dilated
  dissection of
  distal circumflex marginal
  dominant coronary
  dominant left coronary
  dominant right coronary
  dorsal spinal
  Drummond marginal
  dural
  dynamic entrapment of vertebral
  eccentric coronary
  en passage feeder
  epicardial coronary
  external carotid (ECA)
  external iliac
  extracranial vertebral
  extradural
  familial fibromuscular dysplasia of

artery *(cont.)*
  feeder
  femoropopliteal
  first diagonal branch
  first obtuse marginal
  friable
  frontopolar (FPA)
  gastroepiploic
  high left main diagonal
  hilar
  hypogastric
  iliac
  inferior epigastric
  inferior mesenteric
  infragenicular popliteal
  infrageniculate
  innominate
  intercostal
  intermediate coronary
  internal carotid (ICA)
  internal iliac
  internal iliac gluteal
  internal mammary (IMA)
  internal thoracic
  intraacinar pulmonary
  intracavernous internal carotid
  intracranial vertebral
  ipsilateral downstream
  Kugel
  labyrinthine
  LAD (left anterior descending)
  lateral posterior choroidal (LPCh)
  LCA (left coronary)
  LCF or LCX (left circumflex)
  left anterior descending
  left circumflex coronary
  left common femoral
  left coronary (LCA)
  left internal mammary (LIMA)
  left main coronary (LMCA)
  left pulmonary (LPA)
  lenticulostriate

artery *(cont.)*
     leptomeningeal
     LIMA (left internal mammary)
     LMCA (left main coronary)
     M1-M5 segments of middle
        cerebral
     main pulmonary (MPA)
     mainstem coronary
     maintenance of flow in
     mammary
     marginal branch of left circumflex
        coronary
     marginal branch of right coronary
     marginal circumflex
     medial plantar
     medial posterior choroidal (MPCh)
     median sacral
     meningeal
     meningohypophyseal trunk (MHT)
     mesencephalic
     mesenteric
     middle cerebral (MCA)
     middle meningeal
     musculophrenic
     narrowing of
     native coronary
     nodular induration of temporal
     nutrient
     obtuse marginal (OM) coronary
     occipital branch of external carotid
     occlusion of
     ophthalmic
     overriding great
     paramalleolar
     paramedian thalamopeduncular
     parietal MCA
     parieto-occipital branch of
        posterior cerebellar
     patency of
     PDA (posterior descending)
     peduncular segment of superior
        cerebellar

artery *(cont.)*
     perforating
     pericallosal
     peripancreatic
     peroneal
     petrous segment of carotid
     phrenic
     pipestem
     plantar metatarsal
     plaque-containing
     P1-P4 segments of posterior
        cerebral
     pontine
     popliteal
     post-temporal MCA
     posterior cerebral (PCA)
     posterior choroidal
     posterior communicating (PCA)
     posterior descending (PDA)
     posterior descending branch of
        right coronary
     posterior descending coronary
     posterior inferior cerebellar (PICA)
     posterior inferior communicating
        (PICA)
     posterior intercostal
     posterior parietal
     posterior spinal
     posterior temporal
     posterior tibial
     posterolateral spinal (PLSA)
     precommunicating segment of
        anterior cerebral
     primitive trigeminal (PTA)
     profunda femoris
     proximal anterior descending
     proximal digital
     proximal left anterior descending
     proximal popliteal
     pulmonary (PA)
     radial digital
     radicular

artery *(cont.)*
  radiculomedullary
  radiculospinal
  ramus intermedius
  ramus medialis
  recurrent (of Heubner)
  renal
  reperfused
  resilient
  retinal
  retroesophageal right subclavian
  right coronary (RCA)
  right femoral
  right inferior epigastric
  right internal iliac
  right pulmonary (RPA)
  right ventricular branch of right
    coronary
  scalp branch of external carotid
  segmental branch of vertebral
  septal perforator
  SFA (superficial femoral)
  sinoatrial node
  sinus nodal
  splenial branch of posterior
    cerebral
  splenic
  stenotic coronary
  subclavian
  subcostal
  superficial femoral (SFA)
  superficial temporal (STA)
  superior cerebellar (SCA)
  superior epigastric
  superior genicular
  superior intercostal
  superior mesenteric
  superior thyroid
  supraclinoid carotid
  takeoff of
  temporal
  thalamocaudate

artery *(cont.)*
  thalamogeniculate
  thalamoperforating
  thyrocervical trunk of subclavian
  thyroid
  trifurcation of middle cerebral
  truncal
  twig of
  ulnar
  ulnar digital
  vertebral
  vertebral basilar
  weakened
artery-vein-nerve bundle
arthrempyesis
arthrifluent abscess
arthritic talonavicular changes
arthritis (pl. arthritides), rheumatoid
  (RA)
arthritis deformans
arthrogram
arthrography
  Brostrom-Gordon
  coronal computed tomographic
    (CCTA)
  CT (computed tomography)
  double-contrast
  Gordon-Brostrom single-contrast
  indirect MR
  joint
  MR
  saline-enhanced MR
  single-contrast
  temporomandibular joint
arthrophyte
arthropyosis
arthroscintigraphy
arthrosis
  crystal-induced
  degenerative
  IRM spiral
arthrosis deformans

artifact *(cont.)*
  corduroy
  crescent
  crinkle
  cross-talk effect
  crown
  CSR fluid flow
  data-clipping detection error
  data spike detection error
  DC (direct current) offset
  developer
  distortion of limitations of image
    reconstruction algorithm
  dog
  double exposure
  double exposure drift
  eddy current
  edge-boundary
  edge misalignment
  edge ringing
  effusion
  end-pressure
  entry slice phenomenon
  equipment
  faulty RF (radiofrequency)
    shielding
  flow effect
  flow-induced
  foreign material
  gaseous oxygen
  geophagia
  ghosting
  Gibbs
  Gibbs phenomenon
  glass eye
  glove phenomenon
  half-moon
  hot spot
  image
  image post-processing errors
  imbalance of phase or gain
  intensifying screen

artifact *(cont.)*
  iron overload
  kink
  kissing-type
  lettering
  linear
  low-attenuation pulsation
  "magic angle" effects
  magnetic susceptibility
  main magnetic field inhomogeneity
  mercury
  mirror image
  mitral regurgitation
    (cineangiography)
  moiré
  moiré fringes
  mosaic
  motion
  movement
  muscle
  overlying attenuation
  pacemaker
  pacing
  paramagnetic
  partial volume effect
  patient motion
  pellet
  phase-encoded motion
  pica
  "pseudofracture"
  quadrature phase detector (QPD)
  radiofrequency (RF) spatial distri-
    bution problem reconstruction
  respiratory motion
  reticulation
  RF (radiofrequency) overflow
  screen craze
  skin crease
  skin fold
  skin lesion
  slice-overlap
  slice profile

artifact *(cont.)*
 stairstep
 stimulated echo
 subcutaneous injection of contrast
 summation shadow
 superimposition
 susceptibility
 swallowing
 swamp-static
 temporal instability
 tree
 truncation
 truncation band
 twinkling
 venetian blind
 voluming
 wheelchair
 wrap-around
 wrap-around ghost (aliasing)
 wrap-around ghosting
 wrinkle
 zebra
 zebra stripes
 zero-fill
 zipper
artifacts mimicking intimal flaps
artifactual
artificial cardiac valve
artificial left ventricular assist device
 (LVAD)
artificial neural network
artificial pneumothorax
Artoscan MRI system
Arvidsson dimension-length method
 for ventricular volume
aryepiglottic fold
arytenoid cartilage
arytenoid sparing
AS (aortic stenosis)
asbestos bodies
asbestos exposure
asbestos-induced pleural fibrosis

asbestos pleural plaques
asbestosis
A-scan ultrasound
ascending aorta (AA)
ascending aorta hypoplasia
ascending aortic aneurysm
ascending colon
ascending contrast phlebography
ascending hypoplasia of aorta
ascending phlebography
ascending tract
ascertain, ascertained
Aschoff-Tawara node
ascites
ascitic fluid
ASCVD (arterio- or atherosclerotic
 cardiovascular disease)
ASD (atrial septal defect)
aseptic myocarditis of newborn
aseptic necrosis
ASFP (ascending frontoparietal) artery
ASH (asymmetric septal hypertrophy)
ASHD (arteriosclerotic heart disease)
Asherson syndrome
Ashhurst fracture classification system
Ashhurst sign
ASIS (anterior superior iliac spine)
ASO (atherosclerosis obliterans)
aspect
 anterior
 anterolateral
 anteroposterior (AP)
 apical
 axial
 dorsal
 dorsilateral
 dorsoplantar
 inferior
 infrapatellar
 lateral
 lordotic
 medial

aspect *(cont.)*
  mediolateral
  posterior
  posterolateral
  proximal
  superior
  superolateral
  ventral
Aspect computer
aspergilloma
aspergillosis
aspergillotic aneurysm
aspergillus bronchiolitis
Aspergillus invasion of the nervous
  system
aspirated debris
aspirated foreign body
aspiration
  air
  blood
  CT-guided
  foreign body
  pulmonary
  tracheal
  transtracheal
  ultrasonic
  ultrasound-guided transthoracic
    needle
aspiration biopsy
aspiration pneumonia
aspiration pneumonitis
aspiration of ova, ultrasonic guidance
  for
aspiration-tulip device for in vitro percutaneous removal of rigid clots
Aspire continuous imaging (CI) system
asplenia
ASPVD (atherosclerotic pulmonary
  vascular disease)
assay
  predictive
  radioisotope clearance

assessment
  activity
  aortoiliac inflow
  invasive
  noninvasive
  quantitative Doppler
  real-time
  regional wall motion
associated sequestrum
association cortex of parietal lobes
asthmatic airways
asthmatic bronchitis
asthmatic crisis
astragalar bone
astragalocalcanean
astragalocrural
astragaloscaphoid bone
astragalotibial
astragalus (talus)
  aviator's
  fracture of
astroblastoma
astrocytic gliosis
astrocytic tumor
astrocytoma
astroglial tumor
asymmetric appearance time
asymmetry
  amplitude
  congestive
  facial
  hypertrophic
  interhemispheric
  limb length
  narrowing
  septal
  skull
  thoracic
asymptomatic
asynchronous transfer mode (ATM)
asynchronous ventricular contraction
asyndetic communication

asynergic myocardium
asynergy
   infarct-localized
   left ventricular
   regional
   segmental
asystole
   Beau
   cardiac
   complete atrial and ventricular
   ventricular
asystolic pauses
AT-II (angiotensin II)
atelectasis
   absorption
   acquired
   acute
   acute massive
   apical
   basilar
   bibasilar discoid
   chronic
   compression
   confluent areas of
   congenital
   congestive
   dependent
   disc-like
   discoid
   initial
   lobar
   lobular
   lower pulmonary lobe
   middle pulmonary lobe
   obstructive
   patchy
   peripheral parenchymal
   perpetuation of
   platelike
   platter-like
   primary
   reabsorption

atelectasis *(cont.)*
   relaxation
   resorption
   secondary
   segmental
   slowly developing
   streaks of
   subsegmental bibasilar
   subsegmental lower lobe
   upper pulmonary lobe
atelectatic lung
ATF (anterior talofibular ligament)
atherectomized vessel
atherectomy
   directional
   directional coronary
   percutaneous coronary rotational
     (PCRA)
   retrograde
   rotational
   rotational coronary
   transcutaneous extraction catheter
atherectomy catheter
atherectomy device
   directional
   extraction
   percutaneous
   PET balloon Simpson
   rotational
atherectomy technique
   double-wire
   kissing
athero-occlusive disease
AtheroCath, Simpson
atheroembolism
atherogenesis
atheroma (pl. atheromata)
   carotid bifurcation
   coral reef
   protruding
atheroma formation, exuberant
atheroma molding

atheromatous cholesterol crystal
  embolization
atheromatous debris
atheromatous degeneration
atheromatous embolism
atheromatous material
atheromatous plaque breakup by
  balloon catheter
atheromatous stenosis
atherosclerosis
  accelerated
  atherosclerotic
  carotid
  coronary
  extracranial carotid artery
  fatty streak
  fibrous plaque
  intimal
  intracranial carotid artery
  juxtarenal aortic
  native
  pararenal aortic
  virulent
atherosclerosis obliterans (ASO)
atherosclerotic aortic ulcer
atherosclerotic cardiovascular disease
  (ASCVD)
atherosclerotic carotid artery disease
  (ACAD)
atherosclerotic debris
atherosclerotic fatty streaks
atherosclerotic gangrene
atherosclerotic narrowing
atherosclerotic occlusive syndrome
atherosclerotic plaque
atherosclerotic stenosis
atherostenosis
atherothrombotic brain infarction
athlete's pseudonephritis
athletic heart
Atkin epiphyseal fracture

ATL (anterior tricuspid leaflet)
  ATL Mark 600 real-time sector
    scanner
  ATL Neurosector real-time scanner
  ATL ultrasound system
atlantoaxial articulation
atlantoaxial fixation
atlantoaxial instability
atlantoaxial interval
atlantoaxial joint
atlantoaxial posterior membrane
atlantoaxial separation
atlantoaxial subluxation
atlantomastoid
atlanto-odontoid
atlanto-occipital fusion
atlanto-occipital junction
atlanto-occipital membrane
atlas (C1, first cervical vertebra)
  arch of
  burst fracture of
  compression fracture of
  transverse ligaments of
Atlas LP PTCA balloon dilatation
  catheter
atlas matching
Atlas ULP balloon dilatation catheter
ATM (asynchronous transfer mode)
atm. (atmospheres)
atonic bladder
atonic esophagus
atonic ureter
atony (atonia)
  gastric
  intestinal
  sphincter
atraumatic occlusion of vessels
atresia
  anal
  aortic
  aortic arch
  aortic valve

atresia *(cont.)*
  biliary
  choanal
  congenital biliary
  congenital laryngeal
  duodenal
  esophageal
  extrahepatic biliary (EBA)
  familial
  infundibular
  intestinal
  intrahepatic (IHA)
  laryngeal
  mitral
  mitral valve
  nasopharyneal
  prepyloric
  pulmonary
  pulmonary valve
  pulmonary vein
  pulmonic
  tricuspid
  valvular
  ventricular
atresic
atria (pl. of atrium)
atrial activation mapping, retrograde
atrial activation time
atrial appendage
atrial arrhythmia
atrial cuff
atrial disk
atrial ectopic automatic tachycardia
atrial ectopy
atrial-femoral bypass
atrial infarction
atrial kick
atrial myxoma
atrial pacing wire, temporary
atrial partition
atrial phasic volumetric function
atrial right-to-left shunting

atrial septal aneurysm
atrial septal defect (ASD)
atrial septal defect occlusion (buttoned
  device)
atrial septal defect with mitral stenosis
atrial septum
atrial single and double extrastimulation
atrial situs
atrial situs solitus
atrial standstill
atrial systole
atrial thrombosis
atrial transposition
atrialized ventricle
atriocaval junction
atriofascicular tract
atriography
  contrast left
  negative contrast left
atrio-His (atriohisian)
atrio-His bypass tract
atrio-His fiber
atrio-His pathway
atrioseptal defect
atrioventricular (AV)
atrioventricular annulus
atrioventricular canal
atrioventricular groove
atrioventricular nodal bypass tract
atrioventricular node mesothelioma
atrioventricular orifice
atrioventricular ostium
atrioventricular ring
atrioventricular septal defect
atrioventricular septum
atrioventricular sequential pacing
atrioventricular valves (mitral and
  tricuspid)
atrium (pl. atria)
  common
  giant left
  high right

atrium *(cont.)*
   left (LA)
   low septal right
   nontrabeculated
   oblique vein of left
   pulmonary
   respiratory
   right (RA)
   single
   thin-walled
   trabeculated
   ventricular
atrium cordis
atrium dextrum/sinistrum cordis
atrium pulmonale
atrium sinistrum
atrophic emphysema
atrophic fracture
atrophic gastritis
atrophic lesion
atrophic nonunion
atrophic thrombosis
atrophy
   alveolar
   brachial muscular
   brain
   cerebellar
   cerebral surface
   compensatory
   compression
   cortical
   degenerative
   denervation
   disuse
   divopontocerebellar
   dorsum sellae
   eccentric
   frontotemporal
   gastric
   hemisphere
   interstitial
   kidney

atrophy *(cont.)*
   lesser (of disuse)
   lobar
   lobular lung
   localized muscular
   multiple system (MSA)
   muscle
   neurogenic
   olivopontocerebellar
   parenchymatous
   peroneal muscular
   physiologic
   postneuritic
   primary optic
   progressive neuropathic muscle
   progressive post-polio muscle
     (PPPMA)
   quadriceps
   scapuloperoneal muscular
   spinal muscular (SMA)
   subacute denervation
   subcortical
   Sudeck osteoporotic
   sulcal
   temporal horn
   vascular
   villous
atropine flush
attachment
   capsular
   cerebellar
   commissural
   dural
   fibrous
   Hudson cerebellar
   intimate (of diseased vessel)
   ligamentous
   mesenteric
   Pearson
   peritoneal
   tendinous
   vascular

attenuate
attenuated image
attenuated lumen
attenuating
attenuation
   aortic
   breast
   decreased
   diaphragmatic
   expiratory
   gamma ray
   ground-glass
   hemidiaphragm
   increased
   linear
   photon
   Picker SPECT attenuation
     correction
   tendon
   theophylline
   valve
attenuation artifact
attenuation coefficient on MRI scan
attenuation correction
attenuation effect
attenuation threshold
attenuation scan
attenuation value on MRI scan
attic adhesion
attrition rupture of tendon
ATV (anterior terminal vein)
atypical angina
atypical aortic valve stenosis
atypical chest pain
atypical interstitial pneumonia
atypical subisthmic coarctation
atypical verrucous endocarditis
198Au (gold) brachytherapy
Auenbrugger sign
Auerbach mesenteric plexus
Auger electron emitter
augmentation, abnormal

augmented filling of right ventricle
augmented stroke volume
auricle
   left
   right
auricular fissure
Aurora MR (magnetic resonance)
   breast imaging system
Aussies-Isseis unstable scoliosis
autoecholalia
autofusion
autogenous antigen
autologous patch graft
autologous pericardium
autologous vein graft
automated airway tree segmentation
   method
automated angle encoder system
automated border detection by
   echocardiography
automated cardiac flow measurement
   (ACM) ultrasound technology
automated cerebral blood flow analyzer
automated computerized axial
   tomography (ACAT)
automated quantification
automated synthesis
automatic extraction
automatic lumen edge segmentation
automatic motion correction
autonomic denervation
autonomic dysfunction
autonomic hyperventilation
autonomic insufficiency
autonomic nervous system
autonomous nodule
autoprescanning
autoradiograph
autoradiographic localization
autoradiography, calcium-45
autoregulation of cerebral blood flow
autosomal recessive polycystic kidney
   disease

AutoSPECT
autostereoscopic
autotopagnosia
AV (arteriovenous)
AV (atrioventricular)
AVA (aortic valve area)
avascular necrosis (AVN)
avascularity
AVCO aortic balloon
AVD (aortic valvular disease)
$AVDO_2$ (cerebral arteriovenous
   oxygen content difference)
Avellis syndrome
average pixel projection (APP)
averaging
   partial volume
   spike
   volume
AVF (arteriovenous fistula)
AVG (aortic valve gradient)
aviator's astragalus
AVM (arteriovenous malformation)
AVM radiotherapy
AVN (avascular necrosis)
AV-Paceport thermodilution catheter
AVR (aortic valve replacement)
AVSD (acquired ventricular septal
   defect)
avulse
avulsed fracture fragment
avulsion
   arterial
   bony
   coracoid tip
   epiphysis
   iatrogenic
   ligament
   nail plate
   spinal nerve root
   traumatic
   venous
avulsion chip fracture

avulsion fracture
avulsion fragment
AVVM (angiographically visualized
   vascular malformation)
axial compression forces
axial compression fracture
axial compression injury
axial dimension
axial gradient echo image
axial hiatal hernia
axial images, multi-echo
axial manual traction test
axial musculature
axial neuritis
axial plane
axial scan
axial section
axial skeleton
axial slice
axial spin density
axial spinal system
axial transabdominal image
axilla (pl. axillae)
axillary-axillary bypass graft
axillary-brachial bypass graft
axillary-femoral bypass graft
axillary-femorofemoral bypass graft
axillary node
axillary tail of Spence
axillary vein traumatic thrombosis
axillobifemoral bypass graft
axillofemoral approach
axillofemoral bypass graft
Axiom DG balloon angioplasty
   catheter
axis (C2, second cervical vertebra)
axis (pl. axes)
   anatomic
   ankle mortise
   basibregmatic
   basicranial
   bimalleolar foot

axis *(cont.)*
   bowel
   celiac
   coordinate
   cortical hinge
   craniospinal
   distal reference (DRA)
   eccentric axis of ankle rotation
   enteroinsular
   femoral shaft
   flexion-extension
   hypothalamic-pituitary
   hypothalamic-pituitary-adrenal
   hypothalamoneurohypophyseal
     (HNA)
   leg
   long
   longitudinal
   mechanical
   metatarsal

axis *(cont.)*
   proximal reference (PRA)
   rotation
   single (on knee prosthesis)
   spinal
   subtalar
   transcondylar (TCA)
   vertical
   weightbearing
   Z-
axis of heart
axoid
axonopathic neurogenic thoracic outlet
   syndrome
axoplasmic flow and papilledema
Ayerza-Arrillaga disease
azotemic osteodystrophy
azygos blood flow
azygos lobe of lung
azygos vein distension

B, b

baby formula with ferrous sulfate
   contrast
Baccelli sign of pleural effusion
Bachmann, anterior internodal tract of
bacillary angiomatosis
bacillary embolism
back, arching of
back-angle anomaly
back-bleeding
back crease
backfire fracture
backflow from arterial line
backflow of blood into atria
backflux
background subtraction technique
back manipulation
backrush of blood into left ventricle
backscatter characteristics of blood
backscatter electrons
backscattering
back stroke volume
backup of blood
backward flow
backward heart failure
bacterial meningitis
bacterial pneumonia or pneumonitis
Baffe anastomosis

baffle
   atrial
   construction of intra-atrial
   hemi-Mustard pericardial
   interatrial
   intra-atrial
   intracardiac
   Mustard
   pericardial
   Senning type of intra-atrial
baffled tunnel
baffle leak
bag (see also *pouch*)
   bile
   ostomy
   stomal
bagassosis
bagpipe sign
Baillinger, inner stripe of (in brain)
bailout catheter
Baim pacing catheter
baked brain phenomenon
baker's leg (genu valgum)
balance, mass
balanced ischemia
bald gastric fundus
Balint syndrome

Balkan fracture frame
Balke protocol for cardiac exercise
  stress testing
Balke-Ware treadmill exercise (stress
  testing) protocol
ball and seat valve
ball-and-socket joint
ball-bearing, Steinmann pin with
ball-occluder valve
ball of foot
ballism
ballismus
ballistic injury
ballistocardiography
balloon
  ACS SULP II
  AVCO aortic
  Ballobes gastric
  banana-shaped
  barium enema retention
  bifoil
  Blue Max
  esophageal
  Extractor three-lumen retrieval
  Fogarty
  Garren-Edwards
  gastric
  Gau gastric
  Grüntzig (Gruentzig)
  Hartzler angioplasty
  hydrostatic
  intra-aortic (IAB)
  intragastric
  kissing
  Kontron intra-aortic
  LPS
  Mansfield
  mercury-containing
  nondistensible
  Percival gastric
  Percor DL-II (dual-lumen)
    intra-aortic

balloon (cont.)
  Percor-Stat intra-aortic
  PET (positron emission
    tomography)
  pulsation
  rectal
  Riepe-Bard gastric
  Sci-Med Express Monorail
  scintigraphic
  self-positioning
  slave
  Soto USCI
  Spiegelberg epidural
  Stack autoperfusion balloon
  Taylor gastric
  trefoil
  Tru-Trac high-pressure PTA
  waist in the
  Vas-Cath PTA
  Wilson-Cook gastric
balloon and coil embolization
balloon angioplasty
balloon aortoplasty
balloon catheter fenestration
balloon counterpulsation
balloon decompression
ballooned floor of ventricle
balloon embolization (therapeutic)
balloon-expandable flexible coil stent
balloon-expandable intravascular stent
balloon-expandable metallic stent
balloon-flotation pacing catheter
balloon inflation
  sequential
  simultaneous
ballooning mitral valve prolapse
  syndrome
balloon occlusion
balloon occlusion arteriography
balloon occlusion pulmonary
  angiography
Balloon-on-a-Wire catheter

balloon pump
balloon sizing
balloon tamponade
balloon test occlusion
balloon-tipped catheter
ball-valve obstruction
ball valve thrombus
ball-valve tumor
ball-wedge catheter
Baló sclerosis
Bamberger-Marie disease
Bamberger sign
banana sign
band
   alpha
   alpha frequency
   amniotic
   anogenital
   anterior (of colon)
   AO tension
   aponeurotic
   atrioventricular
   Broca diagonal
   calf
   Clado
   constriction
   coronary
   external
   fascial
   fibroelastic
   fibromuscular
   fibrous
   free band of colon
   Gennari
   H
   Harris
   His
   Hunter-Schreger
   iliotibial (IT)
   intercaval
   internal
   Ladd

band *(cont.)*
   Lane
   lateral
   longitudinal
   lucent
   Maissiat
   Marlex
   Meckel
   mesocolic
   metaphyseal
   moderator
   omental
   parenchymal
   Parham
   Parham-Martin
   parietal
   peritoneal
   pretendinous band of hand
   Reil
   RF saturation
   scar
   septal
   septomarginal
   septum
   silicone elastomer
   Simonart
   tendinous
   transverse
banding appearance
bandlike adhesion
bandlike shadow
band of Broca
band of colon
   anterior
   free
band of density
band of Gennari
bands of deossification
band tenodesis
bandwidth limitations
Bannister angioedema disease
Banti disease

bar
   Bill
   bony
   cartilaginous
   congenital
   fibrous
   hyoid
   median
   Passavant
   unsegmented vertebral
bar defect
barber pole sign
barber's chair sign
Barclay niche
Bard CPS system
Bardeen disk
Bard guiding catheter
Bardic cutdown catheter
Bardinet ligament
Baricon contrast medium
barium
   double tracking of
   residual
   retained
barium artifact
barium column, head of
barium enema (BE)
   air contrast
   double contrast
   full-column
   therapeutic
barium enema retention balloon
barium enema through colostomy
barium enema with air contrast
barium esophagram
barium GI series, motor meal
barium-impregnated poppet
barium injection (through colostomy)
barium meal
barium sulfate contrast medium
barium suspension
barium swallow

Barkow ligament
bar-like ventral defect on
   myelography
Barlow hip instability test
Barlow sign
Baro-CAT contrast medium
Baroflave contrast medium
Barosperse contrast medium
barotrauma, pulmonary
Barré-Lieou syndrome
barrel chest
Barrett disease
Barrett esophagus
barrier
   blood-brain (BBB)
   blood-spinal cord
   blood-tumor
Barth hernia
Barton fracture
Bartter syndrome
basal, basally
basal chordae
basal cistern
basal ganglia calcifications
basal ganglia of cerebellum
basal joint of thumb
basal layer
basal movements
basal neck fracture
basal short-axis slice
basal skull fracture
basal tuberculosis
basal vein of Rosenthal
basal zone
base
   cranial
   dorsal spinal cord horn
   Dycal
   lung
   posterior spinal cord horn
   skull
baseball elbow

baseball finger
baseball shoulder
base deficit
baseline
    Reid
    reproducible
    return to
baseline artifact
baseline mammogram
baseline of bulb
baseline standing blood pressure
baseline standing pulse rate
baseline tenting (BLT)
base of brain
base of heart
base of lung
base of metacarpal
base of phalanx
base of skull (BOS)
base of thumb
base of toe
basibregmatic axis
basic blood pressure (BP)
basic cycle length (BCL)
basic drive cycle length (BDCL)
basic rate
basicranial axis
basilar artery insufficiency
basilar artery syndrome
basilar atelectasis
basilar cistern
basilar ectasia
basilar fracture
basilar infiltration
basilar insufficiency
basilar intracerebral hemorrhage
basilar invagination
basilar neck fracture
basilar occlusion
basilar pneumonitis
basilar pneumothorax
basilar region

basilar skull fracture
basilar sulcus
basilar suture
basilar syndrome
basilar-vertebral artery disease
basilar zone infiltration
basilic vein
basioccipital bone
basiocciput tumor
basion
basket, pericardial
basketlike calcification
basocervical fracture
batch-reading of x-rays
Batson plexus
Batson vertebral brain system
Batten disease
bat wing appearance
bat wing distribution
bat wing formation
bat wing shadow
Baudelocque diameter
Bauman angle
bauxite fibrosis of lung
bauxite pneumoconiosis
Baxter catheter
bayesian image estimation (BIE)
Bayes theorem in exercise stress
    testing
Bayliss effect
Bayne classification of radial agenesis
bayonet dislocation
bayonet leg
bayonet position of fracture
Bazin disease
BB (metallic foreign body) shot
BBB (blood-brain barrier)
BBC (biceps, brachialis, coraco-
    brachialis) muscles
B bile
BCA (bell clapper anomaly)
BDA (bile duct adenoma)

BDCL (basic drive cycle length)
BE (barium enema)
beach chair position
beaded appearance of fibromuscular
    dysplasia
beaded hepatic duct
beaded thickening
beading of artery
beads
    methyl methacrylate
    targeting
beaked cervicomedullary junction
beaking of head of talus
beaking, talonavicular
beaklike osteophyte formation
beak sign of a cortical cyst
beam
    blended
    cobalt-60
    fan
    intensity-modulated photon
    lateral opposed
    lucite
    multifield
    open
    pencil
    radiation
    sound
    wedge-pair
    wedged
beam diffraction
beam dosimetry
    adjacent field x-ray
    four-field x-ray
    large-field x-ray
    single x-ray
beam energy
beam's eye view dosimetry
beam filtration, supplemental
beam hardening artifact
beam intensity
beam linear accelerator, high-energy
    bent

BEAM (brain electrical activity map)
    (or mapping)
bear claw ulcer
bear's paw hand
beat knee syndrome
beaten silver appearance of skull
Beath view
beats per minute (BPM or bpm)
Beatson combined ankle angle
beat-to-beat variability
Beau disease
Beau line
Beauvais disease
beavertail appearance of balloon
    profile
Beckenbaugh technique
Beck triad
Beclard hernia
becquerel (Bq)
bed
    bladder
    capillary
    gallbladder
    hepatic
    liver
    monitor
    nail
    portal vascular
    primary tumor
    pulmonary
    pulmonary vascular
    skeletal
    stomach
    tumor
    ulcer
    vascular
beep-o-gram
Beer-Bouguer theory
Beevor sign
Behçet disease
Behr syndrome
Bekhterev arthritis

Bekhterev layer
bell clapper anomaly (BCA)
Bell-Dally cervical dislocation
Bell phenomenon
belly of muscle
bend, hand-shaped
bending fracture
Benedict-Talbot body surface area
    method
benediction posture (of hand)
benign asbestos related pleural disease
benignity
Benink tarsal index
Bennett basic hand dislocation
Bennett basic hand fracture
Bennett lesion
Bennett fracture
benzamide imaging agent
benzene scintillator
benzodiazepine (BN) receptor
benzodiazepine (GABA) receptor
Berman angiographic catheter
Bernard-Horner syndrome
Berndt-Hardy classification of
    transchondral fracture
Berndt-Hardy talar lesion staging
Bernstein catheter
berry aneurysm
Bertel position
Bertillon cephalometer
beStent balloon-expandable arterial
    stent
beta decay
beta particle
beta-ray applicators
beta-spectra shapefactor coefficient
Bethea sign
Bethesda bone
Beuren syndrome
Bevatron accelerator
beveled anastomosis
beveled edge sign

beveled electron beam cone
beveling
bezoar
Biad camera
Biad SPECT imaging system
Bianchi nodules
biatrial myxoma
BIB (biliointestinal bypass)
bibasally
bibasilar atelectasis
bibasilar discoid atelectasis
bibeveled
bicaval cannulation
biceps
    long head of (LHB)
    short head of
biceps femoris muscle
bicerebral infarction
Bichat canal
Bichat fat pad
Bichat membrane
bicipital aponeurosis
bicipital groove
bicipital rib
bicipital tuberosity
bicommissural aortic valve
biconcave
biconcavity
bicondylar fracture
biconvex
bicornuate uterus
bicoronal synostosis
bicortical screw
bicuspid aortic valve
bicuspid atrioventricular valve
bicuspid valvular aortic stenosis
bicycle exercise radionuclide
    ventriculography
bidirectional cavopulmonary
    anastomosis
BIE (bayesian image estimation)
Bielschowsky-Jansky disease

bifascicular heart block
bifid precordial impulse
bifida, spina
bifocal manipulation with distraction
bifoil balloon
bifurcate
bifurcation
   aortic
   basilar artery
   carotid
   common bile duct
   common carotid artery
   hepatic duct
   iliac
   middle cerebral artery
   patent
   pulmonary artery
   pulmonary trunk
   tracheal
   ureteral bud
bifurcation graft
bifurcation lesion
bigeminal rhythm
   atrial
   atrioventricular nodal
   bisferious pulse
   escape-capture
   nodal
   reciprocal
   ventricular
bihemispheral insult
bi-ischial diameter
bilateral carotid stenosis
bilateral consolidation
bilaterality of ureteral duplication
bilaterally
Bilbao-Dotter catheter
bile concretion
bile duct
   common (CBD)
   infundibulum of
   interlobular

bile duct *(cont.)*
   preampullary portion of
   sphincter of
bile duct proliferation
bile duct scan
bile flow
bile lake
bile plug
bile stasis
bilharziasis
   cardiopulmonary
   protopulmonary
biliary atresia
biliary duct
biliary-duodenal pressure gradient
biliary dyskinesia
biliary mud
biliary obstruction
biliary passages
biliary radicle
biliary saturation index
biliary sludge
biliary stent
biliary stone
biliary structures
biliary-to-bowel transit
biliary tract
biliary tract imaging
biliary tree
Biligrafin contrast medium
biliointestinal bypass (BIB)
biliopancreatic bypass (BPB)
bilirubin pigment stones (gallstones)
Biliscopin contrast medium
Bilivist contrast medium
Bill bar (bone)
billowing mitral valve prolapse
Billroth I type anastomosis
Billroth II type anastomosis
bilobed mass
bilobed polypoid lesion
bilocular stomach

biloma
Bilopaque contrast medium
Biloptin contrast medium
bimalleolar ankle fracture
binarize
binary image
binding, receptor
Bing-Horton syndrome
binning, projection
binocular acuity change
biocompatibility
biodegradable magnetic microclusters
biodegradable stent
bioeffects algorithms
biologic age
biological half-life
biological osteosynthesis
biological tissue valve
biomagnetometer, Magnes
biomechanical analysis
biomechanical imbalance
biomechanics of limb length
 discrepancy
biometry, longitudinal ultrasonic
biomodulator
bioprosthesis
biopsy (pl. biopsies)
 CT (computed tomography)-guided
 point-in-space stereotactic
 ultrasound-guided
Biosound AU (Advanced
 Ultrasonography) system
Biospec imaging system
biparietal bossing
biparietal diameter (BPD)
biparietotemporal hypometabolism
bipartite patella
bipartite sesamoid
bipartition, facial
bipenniform muscles of hand
biphasic contrast-enhanced helical CT
biphasic CT

biphasic curve
biplanar aortography
biplanar MR imaging guidance
biplane area-length method
 (echocardiography)
biplane fluoroscopy
biplane left ventricular angiogram
biplane orthogonal views
biplane pelvic arteriography
biplane pelvic oblique study
biplane sector probe
biplane transesophageal
 echocardiography (TEE)
bipolar gradient
bipolar hip replacement
bipolar sensing, integrated
bipolar temporary pacemaker catheter
bird-beak configuration or narrowing
bird-beak taper at esophagogastric
 junction
bird breeder's lung
birdcage coils
birdcage splint
bird fancier's lung
bird handler's lung
bird's-eye views
bird's nest filter (or bird nest filter)
birth fracture
Bis-Gd-mesoporphyrine (Bis-Gd-MP)
 imaging agent
bisection, AP malleolar
bishop's nod
Bismuth classification of benign bile
 duct stricture
bispinous diameter
bit-rate allocation
bituberous diameter
bivalve
biventricular assist device (BVAD)
biventricular global systolic
 dysfunction
biventricular hypertrophy

biventricular transposed aorta
biventricularly
BKA (below-knee amputation)
black blood magnetic resonance
    angiography (MRA)
black blood T2-weighted inversion-
    recovery MR imaging
black boundary artifact
black comets artifact
black dot heel
black echo writing
Blackfan-Diamond syndrome
black lung disease
bladder
    apex of
    atonic
    automatic
    base of
    centrally uninhibited
    dome of urinary
    exstrophy of
    hypertrophic
    hypotonic
    motor paralytic
    neck of
    neurogenic
    papilloma of
    refluxing spastic neurogenic
    sensory paralytic
    spastic
    thickened
    trigone of
    uninhibited
    urinary
    uvula of
bladder contractility study
bladder diverticula
bladder emptying
    complete
    incomplete
bladder floor
BladderManager ultrasound device

bladder neck contracture
bladder perforation
bladder stasis
blade of grass appearance
blade plate
blanch
bland aortic aneurysm
bland embolism
blast chest
bleb
    emphysematous
    myelin
    ruptured emphysematous
    subpleural
Bleck classification of metatarsus
    adductus
bleed (noun)
    GI
    herald
bleeding ulcer
blended beam technique
blennorrhagic swelling
blennothorax
blind catheter
blind dimple in floor of left atrium
blind intestine
blind loop syndrome
blind pouch
blind tibial outflow tracts
blister (vesicle)
blister, fracture
blister of bone
blistering distal dactylitis (BDD)
Bloch equation
block
    acquired symptomatic AV
    air
    alveolar-capillary
    anodal
    anterior fascicular
    anterograde
    arborization

block *(cont.)*
  AV (atrioventricular)
  AV Wenckebach heart
  BBB (bundle branch)
  BBBB (bilateral bundle branch)
  bifascicular
  bifascicular bundle branch
  bifascicular heart
  bilateral bundle branch (BBBB)
  bone
  bundle branch (BBB)
  bundle branch heart
  cerrobend
  complete AV (CAVB)
  complete congenital heart
  complete heart (CHB)
  conduction
  congenital complete heart
  congenital heart
  congenital symptomatic AV
  custom
  deceleration-dependent
  divisional
  donor heart-lung
  entrance
  exit
  false bundle-branch
  familial heart
  fascicular
  filler
  first-degree AV
  first-degree heart
  fixed third-degree AV
  heart
  high-grade AV
  incomplete atrioventricular (IAVB)
  incomplete heart
  incomplete left bundle branch
    (ILBBB)
  incomplete right bundle branch
    (IRBBB)
  inflammatory heart

block *(cont.)*
  infra-His
  intermittent third-degree AV
  interventricular
  intra-atrial
  intra-His
  intra-Hisian or intrahisian
  intranodal
  intravenous (IV)
  intraventricular conduction
  intraventricular heart
  inverted Y
  ipsilateral bundle branch
  irregular
  left anterior fascicular (LAFB)
  left anterior hemiblock
  left bundle branch (LBBB)
  left posterior fascicular (LPFB)
  mantle
  Mobitz I or II second-degree AV
  multiple
  paroxysmal AV
  partial heart
  peri-infarction (PIB)
  posterior fascicular
  pseudo-AV
  retrograde
  right bundle branch (RBBB)
  second-degree AV
  second-degree heart
  simple
  sinoatrial (SAB)
  sinoatrial exit
  sinus
  sinus exit
  sinus node exit
  supra-Hisian or suprahisian
  third-degree AV
  third-degree heart
  transient AV
  transmission
  trifascicular

block *(cont.)*
  unidirectional
  unifascicular
  VA (ventriculoatrial)
  ventricular
  vesicular
  Wenckebach AV
  Wilson
Block right coronary guiding catheter
blockage
  bronchus
  pulmonary artery
blocked APC (atrial premature
  contraction)
blocked artery
blocked bronchus
blocked pleurisy
blocked vertex field
blocker's exostosis
blocking, alpha
Blom-Singer tracheoesophageal fistula
blood
  arterial
  deoxygenated
  egress of
  epidural
  extravasated
  heparinized
  intraparenchymal
  intraventricular
  occult
  parenchymal
  peripheral
  shunted
  sludged
  subdural
  upstream
  venous
blood-brain barrier (BBB)
  alteration in
  defects in
  intact

blood-brain barrier osmotic disruption
blood clearance half-time
blood clot
blood-clotting mechanism
blood flow
  altered
  antegrade
  azygos
  capillary
  cerebral
  Doppler study of
  microcirculatory
  regional
  regional cerebral
  supratentorial cerebral
blood flow analyzer, automated
  cerebral
blood flow extraction fraction
blood flow in heart at rest
blood flow in heart during exercise
blood flow in microcirculation with
    high frequency Doppler ultrasound
blood flow on Doppler echocardiogram
blood flow reserve
blood flow response
blood flow study
blood flow to tissue beyond
  obstruction
blood flow velocity
blood inflow
blood leak
bloodless fluid
blood perfusion
blood perfusion monitor (BPM)
blood plate thrombus
blood pool
  vascular
  white-appearing
blood-pool activity
blood-pool imaging
blood-pool phase image

blood-pool radionuclide angiography

blood-pool radionuclide echocardiography

blood-pool radionuclide scan

blood pressure response

blood speckle

blood-spinal cord barrier

blood stream or bloodstream

blood substitute, oxygenated
 perfluorocarbon

blood supply
 accessory
 dual
 longitudinal

blood-tumor barrier

blood vessel thermography

blood vessel tumor

blood volume
 central
 circulating
 fractional moving

blood volume per minute (vol./min.)

blooming, signal

Blount disease

blow-in fracture

blow-out, aortic stump

blow-out fracture

blowing pneumothorax

BLT (baseline tenting)

Blue FlexTip catheter

Blue Max triple-lumen catheter

blue rubber-bleb nevus syndrome

Blumenbach clivus

Blumensaat line

Blumer rectal shelf

blunt border of lung

blunt chest trauma

blunted costophrenic angle

blunting of posterior sulci

blunt injury

blunt trauma

blurring of aortic knob

blurring of costophrenic angle

blurring of disk margins

blush
 tumor (on cerebral angiography)
 vascular (of tumor on carotid
  angiography)

BM (bowel movement)

BMC (bone mineral content)

BMD (bone mineral density)

BMI (body mass indices)

BMIPP SPECT scan

BML (billowing mitral leaflet)

B-mode (B-scan)
 longitudinal
 pseudocolor

B-mode echocardiography

B-mode echography

BMP (bone marrow pressure)

B-19036 chelate

BN receptor

BO field variation

board
 Dome Imaging RX20
 Intel PC Link2

Bochdalek, foramen of

Bochdalek hernia

body (pl. bodies)
 alignment of vertebral
 carotid
 coccygeal
 esophageal
 foreign
 foreign (retained)
 geniculate
 height of vertebral
 intra-articular
 juxtarestiform
 Luys
 mamillary
 navicular
 ossified
 osteochondritic loose

body *(cont.)*
  pacchionian
  pineal
  restiform
  retained foreign
  rhinencephalic mamillary
  rice joint
  scapular
  trapezoid
body background activity
body box plethysmography
body coil
body contour orbit, body artifacts
  due to
body mass indices (BMI)
body of vertebra
body section radiography
body surface area (BSA)
body surface potential mapping
Boeck sarcoid
Boehler (Böhler) angle
boggy synovitis
boggy synovium
Bogros space
Böhler (see *Boehler*)
Bohr effect
BOLD effect
BOLD image
Boltzmann distribution factor
bolus
  air
  contrast
  dynamic
  electron
  intravenous
  simple
  special
  tracer
  water
bolus challenge test
bolus contrast enhancement
bolus intravenous injection

bolus tracking
bolus transit
bombardment, alpha particle
bonds, wedge
bone
  accessory
  accessory navicular
  acetabular
  acromial
  alar
  Albers-Schönberg (Schoenberg)
    marble
  Albrecht
  alveolar
  alveolar supporting
  ankle
  anvil
  arch of
  areolae of
  articular lamella of
  articular tubercle of temporal
  astragalar
  astragalus
  astragalocalcanean
  astragalocrural
  astragaloscaphoid
  astragalotibial
  atrophy of
  autogenous
  basal
  basilar
  basioccipital
  basisphenoid
  Bertin
  Bethesda
  bicortical iliac
  blade
  bleeding
  Bonfiglio
  breast
  bregmatic
  Breschet

bone *(cont.)*
  brittle
  bundle
  calcaneal
  calcaneus
  Calcitite
  calvarial
  cancellated
  cancellous
  cannon
  capitate
  carpal
  cartilage
  cavalry
  central
  chalky
  cheek
  chevron (V-shaped)
  coccygeal
  coccyx
  coffin
  collar
  compact
  continuity of
  convoluted
  coronary
  cortical
  cortical cancellous
  costal
  coxal
  cranial
  crest of iliac
  cribriform
  cubital
  cuboid
  cuneiform
  dead
  dense
  dense structure of
  depression of nasal
  dermal
  destruction of

bone *(cont.)*
  devitalized portion of
  diastasis of cranial
  displaced fragment of
  dorsal talonavicular
  eburnated
  elbow
  endochondral
  enetral
  epactal
  epihyal
  epihyoid
  epiphysis
  epipteric
  episternal
  erosion of epiphyseal
  ethmoid
  exercise
  exoccipital
  femoral
  fibular
  first cuneiform
  flank (ilium)
  flat
  Flower
  fourth turbinated
  fracture running length of
  fragile
  fragment of
  frontal
  Goethe
  greater multangular (trapezium)
  hamate
  haunch
  heel
  heterotopic
  highest turbinated
  hip
  hollow
  hooked
  humeral
  hyoid

bone *(cont.)*
   hyperplastic
   iliac
   iliac cancellous
   immature
   incarial
   incisive
   incomplete fracture of
   incus
   infected
   inferior turbinated
   inflammation of
   innominate
   intermaxillary
   intermediate cuneiform
   interparietal
   intracartilaginous
   intrachondral
   intramembranous
   irregular
   ischial
   ivory
   ivorylike
   jaw
   knuckle
   lacrimal
   lamellar
   lenticular (of hand)
   lentiform
   lesser multangular (trapezoid)
   lingual
   long
   long axis of
   lunate
   lunocapitate
   luxated
   malar
   malleolar
   malleolus
   marble
   mastoid

bone *(cont.)*
   mature
   maxillary
   maxilloturbinal
   medial cuneiform
   medullary
   membrane of
   metacarpal
   metatarsal
   metastasis to
   metatarsal
   middle cuneiform
   middle turbinate
   morcellized
   mortise of
   multangular
   nasal
   navicular
   necrotic
   neoplasm of
   newly woven
   Nicoll
   occipital
   odontoid
   orbicular
   orbitosphenoidal
   os calcis
   os trapezium
   os trapezoideum
   ossifying fibroma of long
   osteonal
   osteopenic
   osteoporosis of
   osteoporotic
   pagetoid
   palatine
   parietal
   pedal
   pelvic
   perichondral
   perilesional
   periosteal

bone *(cont.)*
  triangular wrist
  triquetral
  triquetrum
  tubular
  tuberculosis of
  tumor-bearing
  turbinate
  turbinated
  tympanic
  tympanohyal
  ulnar
  ulnar sesamoid
  unciform
  upper jaw
  vascular
  vesalian
  Vesalius
  vomer
  weightbearing
  wing of sphenoid
  wormian
  woven
  wrist triquetrum
  xiphoid
  yoke
  zygomatic
bone absorption
bone age according to Greulich
  and Pyle
bone age ratio
bone allograft
bone atrophy
bone block
bone cement, Surgical Simplex P
  radiopaque
bone chip
bone core
bone debris
bone demineralization
Bone Densitometer, QDR-1500 or
  QDR-2000

bone density, increased
bone density measurement
bone density study
bone deposits, endochondral
bone destruction, localized
bone destructive process
bone dysplasia
bone ends
bone erosion
bone formation
  new
    sparsity of
    subperiosteal new
bone-forming sarcoma
bone-forming tumor
bone fracture
bone fragment
bone graft
bone growth stimulator
bone imaging
bone implant
bone infarct
bone infection
bone island
bone length study
bonelet
bone marrow embolism
bone marrow scintigraphy
bone mass, loss of
bone maturation
bone metastases, occult
bone "mets" (slang for metastases)
bone mineral content (BMC) study
bone mineral density (BMD)
bone mineralization
bone or joint pathology
bone phase image
bone pinhole
bone plate
bone plug
bone powder
bone remodeling

brachiocephalic ischemia
brachiocephalic lymph nodes
brachiocephalic trunk of aorta
brachiocephalic vein
brachiocephalic vessel
brachiocubital
brachioradialis muscle
brachium (pl. brachia)
brachium of colliculus
brachycephalic head shape
brachycephaly
brachydactyly
brachymetatarsia
brachytherapy (radiotherapy)
    afterloading
    ^{198}Au (gold)
    endobronchial
    ^{125}I (iodine)
    ^{192}I (iodine)
    interstitial
    intracavitary
    intraluminal
    intraoperative high dose rate
      (IOHDR)
    ^{103}Pd (pallidium)
    permanent
    remote afterloading (RAB)
    Syed-Neblett
    volumetric interstitial
    ^{169}Yb (yterrbium)
brachytherapy boost
Bradbury-Eggleston syndrome
Bradbury-Eggleston triad
Braden flushing reservoir
bradykinin
bradyphemic
bradyphrenia
Bragard sign
Bragg angle
Bragg curve
Bragg ionization peak
Bragg law

Bragg peak photon beam therapy
Bragg peak radiosurgery
braided diagnostic catheter
brain
    architecture of
    atrophic lesion of the
    edematous
    inflammation of
    metastasis to
    split
    unicameral
    Virchow-Robin spaces of the
    water on the
    wet
brain abscess
brain activity
brain anoxia
brain contusion
brain cyst
brain-dead patient
brain death
brain disease, organic (OBD)
brain dysfunction
brain electrical activity map (or mapping) (BEAM)
brain function
brain ischemia
brain laceration
brain lesion, atrophic
brain mantle
brain map
brain mapping
brain mass
brain parenchyma, bleeding into
brain perfusion scintigraphy
brain perfusion SPECT
brain plasticity
brain scan (see *imaging*)
brain stem compression
brain stem demyelination
brain stem disease
brain stem displacement

brain stem glioma tumor
brain stem hemorrhage
brain stem infarct
brain stem infarction
brain stem ischemia
brain stem lesion
brain stem pyramidal tract
brain stem reticular formation
brain stem signs
brain surface matching technique
brain swelling
brain syndrome, organic (OBS)
brain-to-background ratio
brain tumor
brain window
branch (pl. branches) (see also *artery*)
   acute marginal
   anterior cutaneous
   arterial
   AV (atrioventricular) groove
   bifid aortic
   bifurcating
   bronchial
   caudal
   circumflex
   cutaneous lateral
   diagonal
   digital
   distal
   feeding
   first diagonal
   first major diagonal
   first septal perforator
   inferior cardiac
   inferior wall
   large obtuse marginal
   left bundle
   marginal
   midmarginal
   motor
   muscular
   nonlingular

branch *(cont.)*
   obtuse marginal (OMB)
   paired parietal
   paired visceral
   perforating
   phalangeal
   posterior descending
   posterior intercostal
   posterior ventricular
   proper digital nerve
   pudendal
   ramus
   ramus intermedius artery
   ramus medialis
   right bundle
   second diagonal
   segmental
   septal
   septal perforating
   side
   subcostal
   superior phrenic
   unpaired parietal
   unpaired visceral
   ventricular
branched calculus
branches of vein
branching line
branching linear structure
branching, mirror-image brachiocephalic
branching tubular structure
branch of artery
branch point
Branham sign (arteriovenous fistula)
Brasdor method
Braun tumor
bread-and-butter heart
bread-and-butter pericarditis
bread-crumbling movement
"bread-loaf" technique (for obtaining
   tomographic slices)
breakthrough vasodilatation

breakthrough visualization
breast
  accessory
  atrophic
  cystic
  cystic disease of
  fibroadenoma of
  fibrocystic
  shoemaker's
  tail of
breast artifact
breast attenuation
breast bone or breastbone
breast fibrocystic disease stages:
  adenosis
  cystic disease
  mazoplasia
breast localizer
breast mass lesion with poorly defined
  margins
breast microcalcifications
breast shadow
breaststroker's knee
breast thrombophlebitis
breast tissue, attenuation by
breast ultrasound
breath-hold cine MR
breath-hold contrast-enhanced three-
  dimensional MR angiography
breath-hold GRE sequences
breath-hold MR imaging
breath-hold T1-weighted MP-GRE
  MR imaging
breath-hold ungated imaging
breath-hold velocity-encoded cine MR
  imaging
breathing
  ataxic
  labored
breathing artifact
breathing feedback
breathless when wheezing

breath pentane measurement
breath, shortness of (SOB)
breech presentation
bregma
bregmatic bone
bremsstrahlung scan
Breschet sinus
Brett syndrome
Breuerton x-ray view of hand
bridegroom's palsy
bridge (bridging)
  arteriolovenular
  bone
  bony
  interthalamic
  meniseal
  mucosal
  osseous
  osteophytic
  skin
  ventral
  Wheatstone
bridge autograft
bridged loop-gap resonator
bridging osteophytes
bright contrast enhancement
bright highly mobile echoes
brightly increased renal parenchymal
  echogenicity
brightness-time curves
bright pixel values
bright red flush
brim sign
B ring of esophagus
Brinton disease
brisement therapy
Brissaud syndrome
Bristol-Myers system
brittle bone
brittle bones failure
broadband noise detection error
  artifact

broad band of pleural fluid
broadband transducer
broad-based
Broadbent inverted sign
broadening, dipolar
broad maxillary ridge
Broca convolution
Broca diagonal band
Broca motor speech area of the brain
Broca region
Brock middle lobe syndrome
Brockenbrough catheter, modified
    bipolar
Brockenbrough mapping catheter
Broden view
Brodie abscess
Brodie bursa
Brodie disease
Brodie knee
Brodie ligament
Brodmann cytoarchitectonic fields
Bromine-76 bromospirone
bromodeoxyuridine labeling index
bromophenol blue
bronchi (pl. of bronchus)
bronchial adenoma
bronchial annular cartilage
bronchial arteriography
bronchial artery embolization
bronchial asthma
bronchial branch
bronchial bud
bronchial calculus
bronchial caliber
bronchial cartilage, absent
bronchial collapse on forced
    expiration
bronchial collateral circulation
bronchial cyst
bronchial dehiscence
bronchial diameter

bronchial distortions
bronchial kinking
bronchial lumen
bronchial mucosa
bronchial mucosal edema
bronchial obstruction
bronchial provocation testing
bronchial reactivity
bronchial septum
bronchial smooth muscle spasm
bronchial spasm
bronchial stenosis
bronchial stricture
bronchial tree
bronchial type B disease
bronchial vessels
bronchiectasis
    acquired
    capillary
    congenital
    cylindrical
    cystic
    dry
    follicular
    fusiform
    Polynesian
    postinfectious
    recurrent
    saccular
    tuberculous
    varicose
bronchiectasis-bronchomalacia
        syndrome
bronchiectasis-ethmoid sinusitis
bronchiectatic pattern
bronchiolar carcinoma
bronchiolar edema
bronchiolar emphysema
bronchiolar narrowing
bronchiolar obstruction
bronchiolar passages, narrowing of

bronchiole (pl. bronchioli)
   alveolar
   conducting
   lobular
   respiratory
   terminal
bronchiolitis
   constrictive
   diffuse pan-
   exudative
   proliferative
   respiratory
   smoker's
   vesicular
bronchiolitis obliterans with
   organizing pneumonia (BOOP)
bronchioloalveolar carcinoma
bronchiolocentric abnormalities
bronchiolus (pl. bronchioli)
bronchiospasm
bronchiostenosis
bronchitic
bronchitis
bronchitis obliterans
bronchitis with bronchospasm
bronchoadenitis
bronchoalveolar cell carcinoma
bronchoarterial bundles
bronchocavernous
bronchocele
bronchocentric granulomatosis
bronchocentric inflammatory infiltrate
bronchoconstriction
   exercise-induced
   isocapnic hyperventilation-induced
bronchoconstrictor
bronchocutaneous fistula
bronchodilatation or bronchodilation
bronchogenic carcinoma
bronchogenic cyst
bronchogram
bronchographic

bronchography
   air
   bilateral
   fiberoptic
   fluid-filled
   tantalum
   unilateral
broncholith
broncholithiasis
bronchomalacia
bronchomediastinal lymph trunk
bronchoplegia
bronchopleural fistula with empyema
bronchopleuropneumonia
bronchopneumonia
   bibasilar
   hemorrhagic
   hypostatic
   inhalation
   postoperative
   subacute
   tuberculous
   virus
bronchopneumonitis
bronchopulmonary atelectasis
bronchopulmonary dysplasia (BPD)
bronchopulmonary lymph node
bronchopulmonary segment
bronchoradiography
bronchosinusitis
bronchospasm
   paradoxical
   uncontrolled
bronchospastic effects
bronchostaxis
bronchostenosis
bronchotracheal
bronchovascular bundles
bronchovascular markings
bronchus (pl. bronchi)
   anterior
   anterior basal

bronchus *(cont.)*
  apical
  apicoposterior
  beaded
  branch
  cardiac
  contracted
  dilated
  edematous
  eparterial
  extrapulmonary
  granulomatous inflammation of
  hyparterial
  inferior lobe
  inflamed
  inflammation of
  intermediate
  intrapulmonary
  lateral basal
  left main
  left main stem
  lingular
  lobar
  main stem
  major
  medial
  medial basal
  medium-sized
  middle lobe
  mucoid impaction of
  normal-appearing
  posterior basal
  primary (right and left)
  principal
  right lobe
  right main
  right main stem
  secondary
  secretion-filled
  segmental
  stem
  subapical

bronchus *(cont.)*
  subsegmental
  superior
  superior lobe
  tracheal
Brooker classification of heterotopic
  ossification
Brostrom-Gordon arthrography
Broviac atrial catheter
brown atrophy
Brown-Dodge method for angiography
brown induration of lung
brown lung
brown pulmonary induration
brown tumor (osteoclastoma)
brow presentation
Br-76 bromospiperone
Bruce protocol (exercise stress testing)
  modified
  standard
  treadmill exercise
brucellosis, cerebral
Bruck disease
Bruel-Kjaer ultrasound scanner
Bruker console
Bruker CSI MR system
Bruker NMR spectrometer
Bruker PC-10 relaxometer
Brunner gland adenoma
Brunner gland of duodenum
Brunnstrom-Fugl-Meyer (BFM) arm
  impairment assessment
Bryant sign
BSA (body surface area)
BSA ejection fraction
B-scan (B-mode) ultrasound
B-72.3 labeled with ^{111}In bubble
bubble
  gastric
  intragastric
bubble ventriculography

bubbly lung syndrome
bubbly opacity
Buchbinder Omniflex catheter
Buchbinder Thruflex catheter
bucket-handle fracture
bucket-handle tear
buckle fracture
buckle, wire-fixation
buckled innominate artery syndrome
buckling of mitral valve, midsystolic
Bucky view
bud
   bronchial
   capillary
   dorsal pancreatic
   end
   vascular
   ventral pancreatic
Budd-Chiari syndrome
Budge, ciliospinal center of
Budin-Chandler anteversion
   determination
Budlinger-Ludlof-Laewen disease
BUdR (bromodeoxyuridine or brox-
   uridine) radiosensitizer
Buerger-Gruetz disease
Buerger thromboangiitis obliterans
   disease
buffalo hump
bulb
   aortic
   arterial
   baroreceptor in the carotid
   baseline of
   carotid
   dental
   duodenal
   end
   heart
   high jugular (HJB)
   inferior jugular vein
   internal jugular

bulb *(cont.)*
   jugular
   olfactory
   superior jugular vein
bulbar abnormality
bulbar intracerebral hemorrhage
bulbar septum
bulb of occipital horn of lateral
   ventricle
bulb of posterior horn of lateral
   ventricle
bulbosity
bulbous stump
bulbous urethra
bulbus (noun), bulbous (adj.)
bulge
   bilateral anterior chest
   disk
   late systolic
   palpable presystolic
   parasternal
   precordial
   suprasternal
bulging disk
bulk laxative
bulk, muscle
bulk susceptibility artifact
bull neck appearance
bulla (pl. bullae)
bulla formation
bullet
   hollow-point
   stabilizing
   tri-point
bullous edema
bullous emphysema
bullous lung disease
bull's-eye deformity
bull's-eye images
bull's-eye map
bull's-eye mapping
bull's-eye polar map

bull's-eye sign
bump
   hip
   inion
   runner's
bumper fracture
bunamiodyl contrast medium
bundle
   aberrant
   artery-vein-nerve
   AV (atrioventricular)
   Bachmann
   bronchoarterial
   bronchovascular
   common
   fascicular
   Flechsig bundle in cerebellum
   Gierke respiratory
   Gowers bundle in cerebellum
   His
   intercostal
   intercostal neuromuscular
   James
   Keith sinoatrial
   Kent
   Kent-His
   maculoneural
   Mahaim
   main
   neurovascular
   Pick
   Schultze
   sinoatrial
   Thorel
   vascular
bundle bone
bundle branch block (BBB) (on EKG)
bundle branch reentry (BBR)
bundle function
bundle of His
bundle of Kent accessory bypass
   fibers

bundle of Stanley Kent
bundle of Vicq d'Azyr
bunk bed fracture
Burdach, column of
Burke syndrome
burned-out tabes
burning
   selective hole
   substernal
Burns space
bursa (pl. bursae)
   Achilles
   adventitious
   anserine
   bicipitoradial
   Brodie
   calcaneal
   Fleischmann
   flexor
   intermediate
   intermetatarsophalangeal
   ischiogluteal
   Luschka
   Monro
   olecranon
   omental
   plantar
   popliteal
   prepatellar
   radial
   retrocalcaneal
   subacromial
   subdeltoid
   suprapatellar
   trochanteric
   ulnar
bursal adhesion
   subacromial
   subdeltoid
bursal flap
bursal fluid
bursal sac

bursitis (pl. bursitides)
  anserine
  bicipital
  calcaneal
  chronic retrocalcaneal
  infracalcaneal
  intermetatarsophalangeal
  intertubercular
  ischiogluteal
  olecranon
  patellar
  pigmented villonodular (PVB)
  postcalcaneal (posterior calcaneal
      bursitis)
  posterior calcaneal
  prepatellar
  radiohumeral
  retrocalcaneal
  septic
  subacromial
  subdeltoid
  Tornwaldt
  trochanteric
bursography
bursolith
burst (compression) fracture of the
    atlas
burst fracture of spiral column
bursting fracture
Burton sign
Burwell-Charnley classification of
    fracture reduction
Busquet disease
butterfly flap
butterfly fracture fragment
butterfly pattern of infiltrates
butterfly shadow
butterfly-type glioma
buttock sign
button
  aortic
  duodenal

button (cont.)
  patellar
  subdural
button toe amputation
buttonhole fracture
buttonhole opening
buttonhole rupture
buttonhole stenosis
buttress plate
buttressing
BVAD (biventricular assist device)
BVR (basal vein of Rosenthal)
BVS (biventricular support system)
BV2 needle
bypass
  aorta-iliac-femoral
  aorta-renal
  aorta-subclavian-carotid
  aorta-subclavian-carotid-
      axillo-axillary
  aorta to first obtuse marginal
      branch
  aorta to LAD
  aorta to marginal branch
  aorta to posterior descending
  aortic-femoral
  aortic-superior mesenteric
  aortobifemoral
  aortocarotid
  aortoceliac
  aortocoronary
  aortocoronary-saphenous vein
  aortofemoral
  aortofemoral-thoracic
  aortoiliac
  aortoiliac-popliteal
  aortoiliofemoral
  aortopopliteal
  aortorenal
  apico-abdominal
  atrial-femoral artery
  axillary

bypass *(cont.)*
   axillary-brachial
   axillary-femoral
   axilloaxillary
   axillobifemoral
   axillofemoral
   axillopopliteal
   brachial
   cardiopulmonary (CPB)
   carotid-axillary
   carotid-carotid
   carotid-subclavian
   common hepatic-common
      iliac-renal
   coronary
   coronary artery (CAB)
   cross femoral-femoral
   crossover
   distal arterial
   dorsal pedal
   DTAF-F (descending thoracic
      aortofemoral-femoral)
   EC-IC (extracranial-intracranial)
   extended tibial in situ
   extra-anatomic
   extracranial-intracranial (EC-IC)
   fem-fem (femoral-femoral)
   femoral-above-knee popliteal
   femoral crossover
   femoral distal popliteal
   femoral-femoral
   femoral to tibial
   femoral vein-femoral artery
   femoral venoarterial
   femoral-popliteal
   femoral-tibial-peroneal
   femoroaxillary
   femorodistal
   femorofemoral
   femorofemoral crossover
   femorofemoropopliteal
   femoroperoneal

bypass *(cont.)*
   femoropopliteal
   femoropopliteal saphenous vein
   femorotibial
   "fem-pop" (femoral-popliteal)
   heart-lung
   hepatorenal saphenous vein
   hypothermic cardiopulmonary
   iliac-renal
   iliofemoral
   iliopopliteal
   ilioprofunda
   infracubital
   infrainguinal stenosis
   in situ
   intracranial arterial
   ipsilateral nonreversed greater
      saphenous vein
   left atrium to distal arterial aortic
   left heart
   lesser saphenous vein in situ
   Litwak left atrial-aortic
   mammary-coronary artery
   marginal circumflex
   microscope-aided pedal
   nonreversed translocated vein
   normothermic cardiopulmonary
   obtuse marginal
   partial
   partial cardiopulmonary
   percutaneous femoral-femoral
      cardiopulmonary
   popliteal
   popliteal in situ
   popliteal to distal in situ
   pulsatile cardiopulmonary
   renal artery-reverse saphenous vein
   reversed
   right heart
   saphenous vein
   sequential in situ
   subclavian-carotid

bypass *(cont.)*
   subclavian-subclavian
   superior mesenteric artery
   supraceliac aortofemoral
   temporary aortic shunt
   thoracic aorta-femoral artery
   tibial in situ
   total cardiopulmonary
   upper extremity in situ
bypass circuit

bypass graft
bypass tract
   atrio-Hisian or atriohisian
   AV (atrioventricular) nodal
   concealed
   fasiculoventricular bypass
   nodo-Hisian
   nodoventricular
   right ventricular
byte mode

C, c

C (carbon)
CA (coronary artery)
"cabbage" (CABG)
CABG (coronary artery bypass graft)
CABS (coronary artery bypass
    surgery)
Cacchione syndrome
cachexia, lymphatic
CAD (computer-aided [or assisted]
    design [or diagnostics])
CAD (coronary artery disease)
cadmium iodide detector
caecum (cecum)
CAEP (chronotropic assessment
    exercise protocol)
Caffey disease
CA15-3 antigen radioimmunoassay
    imaging agent
cage
    bony thoracic
    osseocartilaginous thoracic
CAH (congenital adrenal hyperplasia)
calamus scriptorius
calcaneal bone
calcaneal fracture
calcaneal spur

calcaneocavus (clubfoot)
    talipes calcaneus
    talipes cavus
calcaneoclavicular ligament
calcaneocuboid joint
calcaneocuboid ligament
calcaneofibular (CF) ligament
calcaneonavicular coalition
calcaneoplantar angle
calcaneotibial fusion
calcaneovalgocavus
calcaneovalgus flatfoot
calcaneovalgus, pes
calcaneus
    pes
    sulcus
    talipes
calcaneus altus
calcar avis
calcar femorale
calcar pedis
calcar, pivot of
calcareous deposits
calcarine cortex
calcarine fissure
calcarine sulcus
calcific aortic stenosis

calcific arteriosclerosis
calcific artery
calcification
   aneurysmal wall
   annular
   aortic
   aortic valve
   arterial
   artery
   basal ganglia
   basketlike
   cartilage
   cerebral
   choroid plexus
   coarse vascular
   conglomerate
   coronary artery
   costal cartilage
   curvilinear
   dentate nuclei
   dural
   dystrophic
   eggshell
   falx
   fine
   focal
   foci of
   free body
   glial tumor
   granulomatous
   gyriform
   idiopathic pleural
   intervertebral cartilage
   intervertebral disk
   intracardiac
   intracranial
   irregular
   laminated
   ligamentous
   linear
   lymph node
   medial collateral ligament

calcification *(cont.)*
   metastatic
   mitral annular
   mitral ring
   mitral valve
   Mönckeberg (Moenckeberg)
   mottled
   multiple
   myocardial
   node
   normal
   parietal pericardial
   Pellegrini-Stieda
   periarticular
   pericardial
   pericardium
   periductal
   periventricular
   pineal gland
   plaque
   plaquing
   popcorn
   premature
   renal mass
   secondary
   sella turcica
   soft tissue
   stippled
   subannular
   target
   thrombus
   thyroid adenoma
   tramline cortex
   valve
   valvular leaflet
   visceral pericardial
calcific matrix
calcific plaque
calcific round body
calcific spur
calcifying
calcinosis circumscripta

calcinosis, tumoral
calcis, os
calcium deposit
calcium deposition
calcium-45 imaging agent (autoradiography)
calcium hydroxyapatite
calcium, intracardiac
calcium layering
calculated clearance time
calculation
   bayesian
   Cerenkov
   gap
   Monte Carlo
   multiplane dosage
   radiation dosimetry
   spectrophotometric
   volume implant
calculus (pl. calculi)
   alvine
   articular
   biliary
   branched
   bronchial
   cat's eye (in common bile duct)
   decubitus
   echogenic
   encysted
   fibrin
   gallbladder
   gastric
   hemic
   hepatic
   impacted
   intestinal
   joint
   lacteal
   lucent
   lung
   mammary
   metabolic

calculus *(cont.)*
   mulberry
   nephritic
   nonopaque
   opaque
   pancreatic
   primary vesical
   pocketed
   prostatic
   radiopaque
   renal
   salivary
   spermatic
   staghorn
   stomach
   stonelike
   ureteral
   urinary tract
Caldani ligament
Caldwell occipitofrontal view
calf muscle pump (anatomical)
calf vein thrombus
caliber
   bronchus
   internal
   luminal
   medium
   modest
   narrow
   tracheal
   vessel
   wide
calibration, absolute-peak efficiency
calibration failure artifact
calibration method
calibrator
caliceal blunting
caliceal clubbing
caliceal dilatation
caliceal system
caliectasia (or caliectasis)
California disease (coccidioidomycosis)

calix (pl. calices) (also calyx, calyces)
   major
   minor
   renal
callosal dysgenesis
callosal formation
callosal gyrus
callosal lesion
callosal sulcus
callosomarginal artery
callosum, corpus
callous (adj.)
callus
   bony
   bridging
   central
   definitive
   ensheathing
   external
   florid
   fracture
   intermediate
   permanent
   provisional
callus distraction
callus formation (*not* callous)
callus weld
calvarial bone
calvarium (pl. calvaria)
Calvé-Perthes disease
calyx (see *calix*)
CAM 5.2 antibody
camelback sign
camera
   ADAC gamma
   Anger gamma
   Anger-type scintillation
   APEX 409
   APEX 415
   Biad
   CeraSPECT
   CID

camera (*cont.*)
   Cidtech
   Digirad gamma
   DSI
   dual-head gamma
   Elscint
   Elscint dual-detector cardiac
   four-head
   gamma
   GE gamma
   GE single-detector SPECT-
     capable
   GE Starcam
   GE Starcam single-crystal
     tomographic
   Haifa
   Helix
   Israel
   MEDX gamma
   multicrystal
   multicrystal gamma
   Picker
   Pixsys FlashPoint
   R&F
   rotating gamma
   scintillation
   Siemens gamma
   slip-ring
   SP6
   Starcam
   Technicare
   three-head
   Trionix
   Vertex
   Vision
cameral fistula
Camper chiasma
camptocormia
camptodactyly
Camurati-Engelmann disease
CAMV (congenital anomaly of mitral
   valve)

canal
- abdominal
- accessory
- adductor
- Alcock
- alimentary
- alveolar
- alveolodental
- ampulla of semicircular
- anal
- anterior condyloid
- anterior semicircular
- arachnoid
- Arantius
- archenteric
- Arnold
- arterial
- atrial
- atrioventricular (AV)
- auditory
- basipharyngeal
- Bernard
- Bichat
- biliary
- birth
- bony semicircular
- Böttcher
- Braune
- Breschet
- calciferous
- carotid
- caroticotympanic
- carotid
- carpal
- caudal
- central
- central spinal
- cerebrospinal
- cervical (of uterus)
- cervical axillary
- cervicoaxillary
- ciliary

canal *(cont.)*
- Civinini
- Cloquet
- cochlear
- common atrioventricular
- complex atrioventricular
- condylar
- condyloid
- connecting
- Corti
- Cotunnius
- craniopharyngeal
- crural
- Cuvier
- deferent
- dental
- dental root
- dentinal
- diploic
- Dorello
- Dupuytren
- endocervical
- endodermal
- ethmoid
- ethmoidal
- eustachian
- external auditory
- facial
- facial nerve
- fallopian
- femoral
- femoral medullary
- Ferrein
- flexor
- Fontana
- galactophorous
- ganglionic
- Gartner
- gastric
- genital
- greater palatine
- gubernacular

canal *(cont.)*
    Guyon
    gynecophoric
    Hannover
    haversian
    hemal
    Henle
    Hensen
    Hering
    hernial
    Hirschfeld
    His
    Huguier
    Hunter
    Huschke
    hyaloid
    hydrops
    hypoglossal
    iliac
    incisive
    incisor
    inferior dental
    infraorbital
    inguinal
    inioendineal
    interdental
    interfacial
    intersacral
    intestinal
    intramedullary
    Jacobson
    lacrimal
    lateral
    lateral semicircular
    Löwenberg (Loewenberg)
    lumbar
    mandibular
    marrow
    mastoid
    maxillary
    medullary
    mental

canal *(cont.)*
    Müller (Mueller)
    musculotubal
    narrowing of spinal
    nasal
    nasolacrimal
    nasopalatine
    neural
    neurenteric
    notochordal
    Nuck
    nutrient
    obstetric
    obturator
    olfactory
    optic
    orbital
    palatine
    palatomaxillary
    palatovaginal
    paraurethral
    parturient
    pelvic
    pericardioperitoneal
    perivascular
    persistent atrioventricular
    persistent common atrioventricular
    petrous carotid
    pharyngeal
    pleural
    pleuropericardial
    pleuroperitoneal
    portal
    posterior semicircular
    principal artery of pterygoid
    pterygoid
    pterygopalatine
    pudendal
    pulmoaortic
    pulp
    pyloric
    recurrent

canal *(cont.)*
    Reichert
    Richet tibio-astragalocalcaneal
    Rivinus
    root (of tooth)
    Rosenthal
    sacculocochlear
    sacculoutricular
    sacral
    Santorini
    Schlemm
    scleral
    semicircular
    sheathing
    small (of chorda tympani)
    Sondermann
    sphenopalatine
    sphenopharyngeal
    spinal
    spinal cord
    Stensen
    Stilling
    subsartorial
    Sucquet-Hoyer
    supraorbital
    tarsal
    temporal
    Theile
    tibial medullary
    tibio-astragalocalcaneal of Richet
    tight spinal
    Tourtual
    tubal
    tubotympanic
    tympanic
    umbilical
    uniting
    urogenital
    uterine
    uterocervical
    uterovaginal
    utriculosaccular

canal *(cont.)*
    vaginal
    Van Hoorne
    ventricular
    Verneuil
    vertebral
    vesicourethral
    vestibular
    vidian
    Volkmann
    vomerine
    vomerorostral
    vomerovaginal
    vulvouterine
    zygomaticofacial
    zygomaticotemporal
canal decompression
Canale-Kelly classification of talar
    neck fracture
canaliculus (pl. canaliculi)
    apical
    auricular
    bile
    bone
    cochlear
    haversian
    innominate
canalization
Canavan disease
Canavan-van Bogaert-Bertrand disease
cancellated bone
cancellous bone
cancellous tissue
cancellus
cancer (see *carcinoma, sarcoma,*
    tumor)
    aniline
    betel
    chimney-sweep's
    clay pipe
    contact
    cystic

cancer *(cont.)*
　　dendritic
　　dye worker's
　　hereditary
　　latent
　　melanotic
　　mule-spinner's
　　oat cell
　　occult
　　paraffin
　　pitch worker's
　　swamp
　　tar
　　tubular
cancer embolus
candle wax appearance of bone
C angle
Cannon-Boehm point
Cannon point
Cannon ring
Cannon segmentation
cannula (pl. cannulae, cannulas)
　　double-lumen
　　femoral artery
　　high-flow
　　inflow
　　infusion
　　inlet
　　internal jugular venous
　　intra-arterial
　　intraventricular
　　large-bore inflow
　　large-egress
　　LV (left ventricular) apex
　　metallic tip
　　needle
　　outlet
　　perfusion
　　peripheral
　　single-bore
　　small-egress
　　two-stage

cannula *(cont.)*
　　vena cava
　　venous
　　ventricular
　　washout
cannulation
　　aortic
　　arterial
　　atrial
　　bicaval
　　direct caval
　　left atrial
　　ostial
　　retrograde
　　selective
　　single-cannula atrial
　　two-stage venous
　　venoarterial
　　venous
　　venovenous
cannulation catheter
cannulization
　　selective
　　subselective
Canon scanner
Cantelli sign
cap
　　duodenal
　　fibrous
　　hilar
　　knee
　　phrygian
　　pleural
　　thin
capacious veins
capacitator, MOS
capacity
　　bladder
　　closing
　　cranial
　　functional bladder
　　lung

capacity *(cont.)*
 respiratory
 vasodilatory
capillary (pl. capillaries)
 arterial
 bile
 continuous
 lymph
 Meigs
 sinusoidal
 venous
capillary bed
capillary blood volume
capillary bud
capillary congestion
capillary density
capillary embolism
capillary filling, compensatory
capillary filling time
capillary fracture
capillary hydrostatic pressure
capillary hyperpermeability
capillary leak (or leakage)
capillary-lymphatic malformation
 (CLM)
capillary malformation (CM)
capillary permeability
capillary pneumonia
capillary pressure
capillary pulsation
capillary refill
capillary resistance test
capillary-venous malformation (CVM)
capillary walls
capillary wedge pressure, pulmonary
capital epiphysis (CE) angle
capital extension
capital flexor
capital fragment
capital mover
capitate bone
capitellum

capitolunate joint
capitular epiphysis
capitulum costae
capitulum fibulae
capitulum humeri
capitulum mandibulae
capitulum radii
capitulum ulnae
Caplan syndrome
capsular imbrication
capsular ligament rupture
capsular plane
capsular reefing
capsular thrombosis
capsule
 adrenal
 articular
 auditory
 Bowman
 cartilage
 cricoarytenoid articular
 cricothyroid articular
 dorsal
 external
 facet
 fatty renal
 fibrous
 fibrous renal
 Gerota
 Glisson
 hepatic
 internal
 joint
 limb of anterior
 metatarsophalangeal (MTP) joint
 liver
 organ
 plantar
 posterolateral
 redundant
 renal
 rim of

capsule *(cont.)*
    splenic
    suprasellar
    talonavicular
    thyroid
    tumor
    wrist
capsulocaudate infarction
capsulolabral complex
capsuloperiosteal envelope
capsuloputaminal infarction
capsuloputaminocaudate infarction
Captopril renal scan
capture, boron neutron
caput medusae
Carabello sign (rise in arterial blood
    pressure; do not confuse with
    Carabelli dental sign)
carbogen radiosensitizer imaging agent
carbon (C)
    ^{11}C acetate
    ^{11}C butanol
    ^{11}C carbon monoxide
    ^{11}C carfentanil
    ^{11}C deoxyglucose
    ^{11}C FLU
    ^{11}C flumazenil
    ^{11}C imaging agent
    ^{11}C labeled cocaine
    ^{11}C labeled fatty acids
    ^{11}C L-159
    ^{11}C L-884
    ^{11}C L-methylmethionine
    ^{11}C lumazenil
    ^{11}C methionine
    ^{11}C methoxystauro-sporine
    ^{11}C N-methylspiperone
    ^{11}C N-methylspiroperidol (NMS)
    ^{11}C nomifensine
    ^{11}C palmitate
    ^{11}C palmitic acid radioactive

carbon *(cont.)*
    ^{11}C raclopride
    ^{11}C thymidine
carbon dioxide (see CO_2)
carbon dioxide laser
carbon-loaded thermoluminescent
    dosimeter
carcinoid syndrome
carcinoma (also *cancer, sarcoma,*
    tumor)
    acinous cell
    adenocystic
    adenosquamous
    adnexal
    adrenocortical
    aldosterone-producing
    aldosterone-secreting
    alveolar
    alveolar cell
    ameloblastic
    anaplastic (of thyroid gland)
    apocrine
    basal cell
        alveolar
        comedo
        cystic
        multicentric
        nodulo-ulcerative
        pigmented
        sclerosing
        superficial
    basaloid
    basosquamous cell
    bile duct
    bilharzial
    bladder
    breast
    bronchioalveolar
    bronchiolar
    bronchogenic
    cavitary squamous cell

carcinoma *(cont.)*
   cavitating
   cerebriform
   cervical
   cholangio-
   cholangiocellular
   chorionic
   choroid plexus
   clear cell
   colloid
   colon
   colorectal
   comedo
   corpus
   cortisol-producing
   cribriform
   cylindrical
   ductal
   duct cell
   eccrine
   embryonal
   embryonal cell
   endobronchial
   endometrial
   epidermal
   epidermoid
   esophageal
   exophytic
   extrahepatic bile duct
   fibrolamellar hepatocellular
   FIGO stage
   fibrolamellar
   follicular
   gallbladder
   gastric
   gelatinous
   genital
   giant cell (of thyroid gland)
   glandular
   glans
   granulosa cell
   hepatic

carcinoma *(cont.)*
   hepatocellular
   Hürthle cell
   hypernephroid
   infantile embryonal
   infiltrating ductal
   infiltrating lobular
   inflammatory
   intraductal
   intraepidermal
   intraepithelial
   invasive
   invasive lobular
   juvenile embryonal
   Kulchitzky cell
   large cell
   lenticular
   leptomeningeal
   lobular
   lung
   medullary
   melanotic
   meningeal
   Merkel cell
   metastatic
   metatypical
   microinvasive
   micropapillary
   moderately well-differentiated
   mucinous
   mucoepidermoid
   mucous
   nasopharyngeal
   neuroendocrine
   noninfiltrating lobular
   non-small cell
   oat cell
   osteoid
   ovarian
   Paget
   pancreatic
   papillary

carcinoma *(cont.)*
   perforated
   periampullary
   polypoid
   poorly differentiated
   preinvasive
   prickle cell
   primary
   primary intraosseous
   pulmonary
   rectal
   rectosigmoid
   renal
   renal pelvic urothelial
   residual
   retinoblastoma hereditary human
   scar
   schistosomal bladder
   schneiderian
   scirrhous
   sclerosing hepatic (SHC)
   sebaceous
   sessile nodular
   sigmoid
   signet-ring
   small cell
   small cell lung (SCLC)
   small round cell
   spindle cell
   squamous cell (SCC)
   string cell
   superficial depressed
   superficial
   terminal
   thyroid
   tonsillar
   transitional cell (TCC)
   tubular
   undifferentiated
   undifferentiated squamous cell
   uterine cervix
   uterine corpus

carcinoma *(cont.)*
   vaginal
   verrucous
   villous
   well-differentiated
carcinoma de novo
carcinoma en cuirasse
carcinoma ex pleomorphic adenoma
carcinoma in situ
   ductal (DCIS)
   lobular (LCIS)
carcinoma-specific monoclonal antibody
carcinomatosis
carcinomatous meningitis
carcinosis
card, Intel Plink Ethernet
Cardarelli sign
cardia
   crescent of
   gastric
   patulous
cardiac antrum
cardiac apex
cardiac atrial shunt
cardiac blood pool imaging, gated
   equilibrium
cardiac border
cardiac branch
cardiac catheter
cardiac catheterization
cardiac compensation
cardiac compression
cardiac contractility
cardiac contraction
cardiac creep
cardiac cycle
cardiac death, sudden
cardiac decompensation
cardiac decompression
cardiac denervation
cardiac dilatation

cardiac dynamics
cardiac effusion
cardiac enlargement
cardiac failure
cardiac fibroma
cardiac fibrosarcoma
cardiac filling pressure
cardiac fossa
cardiac ganglion, Wrisberg
cardiac gated MRA
cardiac gated PGSE sequence
cardiac gated respiration
cardiac gating
cardiac hamartoma
cardiac hemangioma
cardiac hypertrophy
cardiac impression on liver
cardiac index (CI)
cardiac infarct
cardiac insufficiency
cardiac irritability
cardiac laminography
cardiac lipoma
cardiac long axis view
cardiac lung
cardiac lymphangioma
cardiac MRI
cardiac mapping
cardiac margins
cardiac monitor
cardiac muscle fibers
cardiac myxoma
cardiac node
cardiac notch
cardiac output (CO)
cardiac output = stroke volume x
    heart rate (vol./min.)
cardiac overload (or overloading)
cardiac perforation
cardiac positron emission tomography
    (PET)
cardiac pumping ability

cardiac radiation syndrome
cardiac radiography
cardiac recovery
cardiac reserve
cardiac rhabdomyoma
cardiac rhabdomyosarcoma
cardiac rupture
cardiac sarcoma
cardiac scan
cardiac series
cardiac shadow
cardiac shape
cardiac short axis view
cardiac shunt
cardiac silhouette
cardiac sling
cardiac standstill
cardiac steady state
cardiac stomach
cardiac tamponade
cardiac teratoma
cardiac thrombosis
cardiac tumor embolization
cardiac valve
cardiac valve mucoid degeneration
cardiac vasculature
cardiac vein, great
cardiac waist
cardiac wall motion
cardinal sign
cardioangiography
CardioCamera imaging system
cardiochalasia
CardioCoil self-expanding coronary
    stent
cardiocutaneous syndrome
Cardio Data MK3 Holter scanner
cardiodilator
cardiodynia
cardioesophageal (CE) junction
cardiofacial syndrome
cardiogenesis

cardiogenic embolic stroke
cardiogenic embolism
cardiogenic pulmonary edema
cardiogenic shock
Cardiografin imaging agent
cardiogram
cardiography
   apex (ACG)
   esophageal
   precordial
   ultrasonic (UCG)
   vector
cardiohepatic
cardiohepatomegaly
cardiointegram (CIG)
cardiokymography (CKG)
Cardiolite (^{99m}Tc sestamibi) imaging
   agent
cardiology, invasive
cardiomegaly
   alcoholic
   borderline
   familial
   globular
   hypertensive
   iatrogenic
   idiopathic
   postoperative
cardiomotility
cardiomyopathy
   alcoholic dilated
   amyloidotic
   apical hypertrophic (AHC)
   arrhythmogenic right ventricular
   beer-drinker's
   beriberi
   concentric hypertrophic
   congenital dilated
   congestive
   constrictive
   diabetic
   diffuse symmetric hypertrophic

cardiomyopathy *(cont.)*
   dilated (DCM)
   end-stage
   familial hypertrophic (FHC)
   Friedreich ataxic
   hypertrophic (HCM)
   hypertrophic obstructive (HOC or
     HOCM)
   idiopathic
   idiopathic dilated (IDC)
   idiopathic restrictive
   infantile
   infectious
   infiltrative
   ischemic
   ischemic congestive
   left ventricular
   metabolic
   mucopolysaccharidosis
   myotonia atrophica
   noncoronary
   nonischemic congestive
   nonobstructive
   obliterative
   obscure
   obstructive
   obstructive hypertrophic
   peripartum
   peripartum dilated
   postmyocarditis dilated
   postpartum
   primary
   restrictive (RCM)
   right ventricular
   right-sided
   secondary
   tachycardia-induced
   thyrotoxicotic
   toxic
cardionecrosis
cardionephric
cardioneural

cardiopathy
  hypertensive
  infarctoid
  obscure
cardiophrenic angle
cardiophrenic junction
cardioplegic needle
cardiopneumatic
cardioptosis, Wenckebach
cardiopulmonary arrest
cardiopulmonary bilharziasis
cardiopulmonary bypass (CPB)
cardiopulmonary deterioration
cardiopulmonary insufficiency
cardiopulmonary obesity
cardiopulmonary support system (CPS)
cardiopuncture
cardiopyloric
cardiorenal disease
cardiorespiratory sign
cardiorrhexis
cardiosclerosis
cardioselective agent
cardiospasm
Cardio Tactilaze peripheral
  angioplasty laser catheter
CardioTec (^{99m}Tc teboroxime)
  imaging agent
cardiotherapy
cardiothoracic index
cardiothoracic ratio (CTR)
Cardio3DScope imaging system
cardiothyrotoxicosis
cardiotocograph
cardiotocography
cardiovalvular
cardiovascular accident (CVA)
cardiovascular anomalies
cardiovascular renal disease
cardiovascular shunt
carina of trachea
Carleton spots

C-arm digital fluoroscopy
C-arm fluoroscopy
C-arm portable x-ray unit
Carney syndrome
Caroli disease
caroticocavernous fistula
carotid angiography
carotid artery
  kinking of
  redundant
carotid artery aneurysm
carotid artery-cavernous sinus fistula
carotid atherosclerotic disease
carotid bifurcation
carotid blowout syndrome
carotid bulb baroreceptor
carotid-carotid venous bypass graft
carotid cavernous fistula occlusion
carotid distribution TIA (transient
  ischemic attack)
carotid duplex study
carotid ejection time
carotid occlusive disease
carotid phonoangiography
carotid plexus
carotid pulse peak
carotid pulse tracing
carotid pulse upstroke
carotid shudder
carotid sinus hypersensitivity (CSH)
carotid sinus massage
carotid sinus syncope
carotid sinus syndrome
carotid siphon
carotid stenosis
carotid string sign
carotid-subclavian bypass
carotid vein
carpal arch
carpal bone
carpal deviation

carpal-metacarpal (see *carpometa-carpal*)
carpal navicular
carpal row
carpal scaphoid bone fracture
carpal tunnel release (CTR)
carpal tunnel syndrome (CTS)
carpal tunnel view
Carpenter syndrome
carpometacarpal (CMC) joint
carpophalangeal joint
carporadial articulation
carpus
Carrel, triangulation of
carrier
   GABA uptake
   radionuclide
carrier-free separation
Carr-Purcell-Meiboom-Gill sequence
carrying angle
Carswell grapes
Carter equation
Carter-Rowe view
Cartesian reference coordinate voxel
  array
cartilage
  accessory
  accessory nasal
  alar
  arthrodial
  articular
  annular
  arytenoid
  auditory
  auricular
  basilar
  branchial
  calcified
  cariniform
  ciliary
  circumferential
  conchal

cartilage *(cont.)*
  connecting
  corniculate
  costal
  cricoid
  cuneiform
  elastic
  ensiform
  epiglottic
  epiphyseal
  falciform
  fibroelastic
  fibrous
  floating
  hyaline
  hyaline articular
  interarticular
  loss of elasticity of
  physeal
  pitted
  quadrangle
  roughened
  scored
  semilunar
  thinned
  thyroid
  tracheal
  triradial
  yellow
cartilage articulation
cartilage bone
cartilage joint
  primary
  secondary
  symphysis
cartilage joint space
cartilaginous ring
cartographic projection
cartwheel fracture
Carvallo sign in tricuspid regurgitation
CAS (coronary artery scan)

cascade (pl. cascades)
  abdominal
  diagnostic
cascade stomach
Castellani disease
Castellino sign
Castillo catheter
Castleman disease
CAT-CAM conversion
cat's eye calculi in common bile duct
cathartic colon
catheter
  Abramson
  Accu-Flo ventricular
  ACE
  Achiever balloon dilatation
  Ackrad balloon-bearing
  ACS (Advanced Catheter or
    Cardiac Systems) balloon
  ACS Endura coronary dilation
  ACSJL4
  ACS mini
  ACS RX coronary dilatation
  AL1 or AL-1
  Alzate
  Amplatz
  Angiocath PRN flexible
  angiographic balloon occlusion
  Angio-Kit
  Angiomedics
  angiopigtail
  angioplasty balloon
  angled balloon
  angulated
  Anthron heparinized
    antithrombogenic
  aortic flush pigtail
  aortic flush straight
  aortogram
  Arani double loop guiding
  Argyle Medicut R
  Arrow pulmonary artery

catheter *(cont.)*
  Arrow Twin Cath multilumen
    peripheral
  Arrow-Berman balloon
  ArrowGard Blue Line
  ArrowGard central venous
  Arrow-Howes multilumen
  arterial embolectomy
  AR-2 diagnostic guiding
  atherectomy
  AtheroCath
  Atlas LP PTCA balloon dilatation
  Atlas ULP balloon dilatation
  Atri-pace I bipolar-flared pacing
  Auth atherectomy
  AV-Paceport thermodilution
  Axiom DG balloon angioplasty
  bail-out
  Baim pacing
  Baim-Turi monitor/pacing
  balloon
  balloon biliary
  balloon dilatation
  balloon dilating
  balloon embolectomy
  balloon flotation
  balloon-flotation pacing
  balloon-tipped angiographic
  balloon-tipped end-hole
  ball-wedge
  Bard
  bat-wing
  Baxter
  Berman angiographic
  Bernstein
  bifoil balloon
  Bilbao-Dotter
  biliary
  bipolar pacing electrode
  bipolar temporary pacemaker
  blind
  Block right coronary guiding

catheter *(cont.)*
  Blue FlexTip
  Blue Max triple-lumen
  BPS spinal angiographic
  braided diagnostic
  Brockenbrough transseptal
  bronchial
  Bronchitrac L
  bronchospirometric
  Broviac
  Buchbinder Omniflex
  Buchbinder Thruflex
  Buerhenne steerable
  Camino ICP (intracranial pressure)
  cannulation
  Cardio Tactilaze peripheral
    angioplasty laser
  Cardiomarker
  Castillo
  Cath-Finder
  Cath-Track
  central venous (CVC)
  Chemo-Port
  cholangiographic
  cholangiography
  Cloverleaf
  coaxial
  coaxial Tracker
  Cobra and Cobra 2
  cobra-shaped
  coil-tipped
  Comfort Cath I and II
  conductance
  Cook arterial
  Cook pigtail
  Cope loop
  Cordis Brite Tip guiding
  Cordis Ducor I, II, and III coronary
  Cordis Ducor pigtail
  Cordis Son-II
  coronary sinus thermodilution
  corset balloon

catheter *(cont.)*
  coudé
  Councill
  Cournand cardiac
  CR Bard
  Critikon
  CVP (central venous pressure)
  Dacron
  Datascope DL-II percutaneous
    translucent balloon
  decapolar
  deflectable quadripolar
  diagnostic
  Diasonics
  dilatation balloon
  DLP cardioplegic
  Doppler coronary
  Dormia stone basket
  Dorros infusion/probing
  Dotter caged balloon
  Double J
  double-lumen
  Dow-Corning ileal pouch
  drainage
  Ducor balloon
  DVI Simpson atherocath
  EAC (expandable access catheter)
  EchoMark angiographic
  Edwards diagnostic
  eight-lumen esophageal manometry
  Elecath thermodilution
  electrode
  El Gamal coronary bypass
  Elite
  embolectomy
  end-hole
  Endosound endoscopic ultrasound
  Endotak C lead
  enhanced torque guiding
  epidural
  Eppendorf

catheter *(cont.)*
  ERCP (endoscopic retrograde
    cholangiopancreatography)
  Erythroflex hydromer-coated
    central venous
  expandable access (EAC)
  Express PTCA
  extraction
  extrusion balloon
  Faraday
  FAST (flow-assisted, short-term)
    balloon
  Finesse large-lumen guiding
  Flexguard Tip
  flotation
  flow-directed microcatheter
  flow-oximetry
  fluid-filled
  Fogarty balloon
  Fogarty balloon biliary
  Fogarty-Chin extrusion balloon
  Fogarty embolectomy
  Foley
  Foltz
  Force balloon dilatation
  French mushroom tip
  Ganz-Edwards coronary infusion
  Gensini coronary
  Gentle-Flo suction
  Goodale-Lubin cardiac
  Gorlin pacing
  Gould PentaCath 5-lumen
    thermodilution
  graft-seeking
  Grollman pigtail
  Groshong double-lumen
  Groshong tunneled
  Grüntzig (Gruentzig)
  Grüntzig balloon
  Grüntzig Dilaca
  guide
  guiding

catheter *(cont.)*
  Guidezilla guiding
  Halo
  Hanafee
  Hartzler ACX-II and RX-014
    balloon
  Hartzler LPS dilatation
  Hartzler Micro II and Micro XT
  headhunter
  helical-tip Halo
  helium-filled balloon
  HemoCath hemodialysis
  Heplock
  hexapolar
  Hickman indwelling
  Hickman tunneled
  Hidalgo
  Hieshima coaxial
  high-fidelity microtipped
  high-flow
  high-pressure
  high-speed rotation dynamic
    angioplasty
  HNB angiographic
  H-1-H (headhunter)
  hot-tip
  H/S (hysterosalpingography)
  HydraCross TLC PTCA
  Hydrolyser micro-
  hydrophilic-coated
  hydrostatic balloon
  hyperthermia
  IAB (intra-aortic balloon)
  ICP (intracranial pressure)
  Illumen-8 guiding
  ILUS (intraluminal ultrasound)
  indwelling
  Infiniti
  Infuse-a-port
  Inoue balloon
  internal-external drainage
  interstitial

catheter *(cont.)*
    intra-aortic balloon double-lumen
    intra-arterial
    intra-arterial chemotherapy
    Intracath
    intracoronary
    intrahepatic biliary drainage
    intratumoral
    intravascular ultrasound
    intravenous pacing
    intraventricular
    intrepid PTCA angioplasty
    ITC radiopaque balloon
    Jackman orthogonal
    Jackson-Pratt
    JB1
    JB3
    JCL 3.5 guiding
    Jelco intravenous
    JL4 (Judkins left 4 cm curve)
    JR5 (Judkins right 5 cm)
    Judkins USCI
    jugular
    KDF-2.3
    Kensey atherectomy
    Kifa
    King multipurpose coronary graft
    Kinsey atherectomy
    Kontron balloon
    large-bore
    large-caliber
    large-lumen
    laser
    left coronary
    left heart
    left ventricular sump
    Lehman ventriculography
    LeVeen
    Lo-Profile balloon and Lo-Profile
        II balloon
    Longdwel Teflon
    low-pressure

catheter *(cont.)*
    low-speed rotation angioplasty
    LPS
    Lumaguide
    Malecot
    Mallinckrodt angiographic
    Mani
    manometer-tipped cardiac
    manometric
    Mansfield Atri-Pace 1
    Mansfield orthogonal electrode
    Mansfield Scientific dilatation
        balloon
    Marathon guiding
    Match 35 PTA
    Max Force
    McGoon coronary perfusion
    McIntosh double-lumen
    Medicut
    Medi-Tech balloon
    medium-pressure
    Medtronic balloon
    Memory-Vu angiographic
    Micro-Guide
    micromanometer-tip
    Microvasive Rigiflex TTS balloon
    midstream aortogram
    Mikro-tip micromanometer-tipped
    Millar MPC-500
    Millenia balloon
    Mini-Profile dilatation
    Mirage over-the-wire balloon
    Mitsubishi angioscopic
    Molina needle
    Monorail balloon
    MPF
    MS Classique
    Mullins transseptal
    multi-electrode impedance
    Multi-Med triple-lumen infusion
    multifiber
    multilumen

catheter *(cont.)*
    multipolar impedance
    Multipurpose-SM
    mushroom
    MVP
    Mylar
    nasobiliary
    NBIH
    Neuhaus implantable port
    NIH (National Institutes of Health)
        left ventriculography
    nontraumatizing
    NoProfile balloon
    Nycore angiography
    octapolar
    Omniflex balloon
    one-hole angiographic
    Optiscope
    Oracle Focus PTCA
    Oracle Megasonics
    Oracle Micro Plus
    Orion balloon
    over-the-wire balloon
    oximetric
    Paceport
    Pacewedge dual-pressure bipolar
        pacing
    pacing
    Pathfinder
    PA Watch position-monitoring
    PE Plus II balloon dilatation
    Percor DL and DL-II balloon
    Percor-Stat-DL
    percutaneous
    percutaneous transhepatic biliary
        drainage (PTBD)
    percutaneous transhepatic pigtail
    perfusion
    peripheral atherectomy
    peripherally inserted central
        (PICC)
    peritoneal

catheter *(cont.)*
    peritoneal dialysis
    pervenous
    Pezzer
    Phantom V Plus
    PIBC (percutaneous intra-aortic
        balloon counterpulsation)
    pigtail
    pigtail angiographic
    polyethylene
    Polystan venous return
    portal
    Portnoy ventricular
    Positrol II
    preformed
    preshaped
    pressure
    probing
    Profile Plus dilatation
    Proflex 5 dilatation
    Pro-Flo
    Pruitt-Inahara balloon-tipped
        perfusion
    PTBD (percutaneous transhepatic
        biliary drainage)
    PTCA (percutaneous transluminal
        coronary angioplasty)
    Pudenz peritoneal
    pulmonary artery
    pulmonary flotation
    pusher
    quadripolar steerable electrode
    Quanticor
    Quinton Mahurkar dual-lumen
        peritoneal
    Raaf Cath vascular
    Raimondi spring
    Raimondi ventricular
    Ranfac LAP-013 cholangiographic
    Ranfac ORC-B cholangiographic
    Ranfac XL-11 cholangiographic
    Rashkind septostomy balloon

catheter *(cont.)*
    recessed balloon septostomy
    Reddick cystic duct cholangiogram
    RediFurl TaperSeal IAB
    red Robinson
    red rubber
    Rentrop infusion
    retroperfusion
    RF (radiofrequency-generated thermal) balloon
    right coronary
    right heart
    Rigiflex TTS balloon
    Ring-McLean
    Robinson
    Rodriguez-Alvarez
    Rosch
    rotatable pigtail
    Royal Flush angiographic flush
    Rsch-Uchida transjugular liver access needle-
    Rumel
    Sarns wire-reinforced
    Schneider-Shiley
    Schoonmaker multipurpose
    Schwarten balloon dilatation
    Sci-Med SSC "Skinny"
    Scott silicone ventricular
    Seldinger
    Seldinger cystic duct
    Seletz nonrigid ventricular
    sensing
    serrated
    shaver
    Shaw
    Sheldon
    Shiley-Ionescu
    SHJR4s (side-hole Judkins right, curve 4, short)
    short-arm Grollman
    side-hole
    sidewinder

catheter *(cont.)*
    Silastic
    silicone rubber Dacron-cuffed
    Silicore
    Simmons 1, 2, and 3
    Simplus PE/t dilatation
    Simpson peripheral AtheroCath
    Simpson Ultra Lo-Profile II balloon
    single-stage
    Skinny
    sliding rail
    Smec balloon
    snare
    Softip arteriography
    Softouch guiding
    Soft-Vu angiographic
    Soft-Vu Omni flush
    solid-state manometry
    SoloPass
    Sones Cardio-Marker
    Sones Hi-Flow
    Sones Positrol
    special steering
    Speedy balloon
    split sheath
    Squibb
    Stack perfusion coronary dilatation
    Stamey-Malecot
    standard Lehman
    steerable electrode
    steering
    Steerocath
    Stertzer guiding
    stimulating
    straight flush percutaneous
    subarachnoid
    subclavian
    subcutaneous ventricular reservoir
    subdural drainage
    SULP II
    sump

catheter *(cont.)*
Swan-Ganz Guidewire TD
Swan-Ganz Pacing TD
Swan-Ganz thermodilution
swan-neck
TAC atherectomy
Taut cystic duct
TEC (transluminal endarterectomy)
Teflon
temporary pacing
Tenckhoff peritoneal
Tennis Racquet angiographic
tetrapolar esophageal
thermistor
thermodilution
thrombectomy
thrombosuction
Thruflex PTCA balloon
toposcopic
Torcon NB selective angiographic
Total-Cross PTA
Tracker
transcutaneous extraction
transducer-tipped
transluminal endarterectomy (TEC)
transluminal extraction (TEC)
transseptal
transvenous pacemaker
trefoil balloon
Triguide
triple thermistor coronary sinus
triple-lumen
tripolar
TTS (through-the-scope)
tunneled
Tygon
ULP (ultra-low profile)
UltraLite flow-directed micro-
ultrasonographic
umbilical
UMI
Ureflex

catheter *(cont.)*
ureteral
UroLume flow-directed micro-
USCI Bard
USCI Mini-Profile balloon
dilatation
valvuloplasty balloon
Van Andel
Van Tassel pigtail
Variflex
Vas-Cath PTA balloon
venous
venting
Ventra PTA
ventricular
ventriculography
VIPER PTA
Vitalcor venous
Voda
Vygon Nutricath S
Wanderer micro-
Was-Cath
washing
water-infusion esophageal
manometry
Webster coronary sinus
Webster orthogonal electrode
Wexler
Williams L-R guiding
Wilton-Webster coronary sinus
Wishard
Witzel enterostomy
Z-Med balloon
Zucker
catheter advanced under fluoroscopic
guidance
catheter artifact
catheter-borne transducer
catheter damping
catheter deployment
catheter exchanged over guide wire
catheter impact artifact

catheter-induced coronary artery
  spasm
catheterization
  cardiac
  Mullins modification of transseptal
  retrograde
  right heart
  selective
  simultaneous right and left heart
  superselective
  transnasal
  transseptal
catheter kinking
catheter mapping
catheter migration
catheter sheath
catheter-skin interface
catheter tip hockey-stick appearance
catheter tip motion artifact
catheter-tipped manometer
catheter-tissue contact
catheter with preformed curves
catheter whip artifact
CathTrack catheter locator system
CAT scan (computerized [or com-
    puted] axial tomography)
  enhanced
  nonenhanced
CAT scan cradle
CAT scan gantry
cat scratch disease
Catterall classification
cauda equina compression syndrome
caudad
caudal branch
caudal collaterals
caudal-cranial angulation
caudal regression
caudal tilt
caudal view
caudate nucleus
caudothalamic groove

cauliflower appearance
cauliflower-shaped filling defect
cava, juxtarenal
caval-atrial (or cavoatrial) junction
caval-pulmonary artery anastomosis
caval snare
caval tourniquet
CAVB (complete atrioventricular
  block)
cavernous angioma
cavernous angiosarcoma
cavernous sinus meningioma
cavitary mass
cavitary squamous cell carcinoma
cavitary tuberculosis
cavitating carcinoma
cavitating pattern
cavitation
cavity
  abdominal
  abdominopelvic
  absorption
  air
  amniotic
  ancyroid (also ankyroid)
  axillary
  body
  buccal
  chest
  cleavage
  coexistent
  cotyloid
  cranial
  crown
  endometrial
  epamniotic
  epidural
  funnel-shaped
  glenoid
  lung
  joint
  marrow

cavity *(cont.)*
  Meckel
  medullary
  oral
  pericardial
  peritoneal
  pleural
  popliteal
  pulmonary
  retroperitoneal
  saclike
  septum pellucidum
  sigmoid
  subarachnoid
  subdural
  synovial
  syringomyelic
  syrinx
  thoracic
  trigeminal
  tubular
  uterine
cavoatrial (caval-atrial) junction
cavogram
cavography
cavovalgus
  pes
  talipes
cavovarus
  pes
  talipes
cavovarus deformity
cavus
  global
  local
  pes
  post-traumatic
  talipes
cavus deformity
Cayler syndrome
CBF (cerebral blood flow)
CBI (convergent beam irradiation)

CBI stereotactic ring
CBT (corticobulbar tract)
CBV (cerebral blood volume)
CBV/CBF ratio
cc (cubic centimeter)
C-C (convexo-concave) heart valve
CCA (common carotid artery)
CCD (central collodiaphyseal) angle
CCD photodetectors
CCF (carotid cavernous fistula)
CCTA (coronal computed tomographic
  arthrography)
CD (Crohn disease)
CDAI (Crohn disease activity index)
CDC (Crohn disease of colon)
CDCA (chenodeoxycholic acid)
CDE (common duct exploration)
CDH (congenital dislocation [or
  dysplasia] of hip)
CDI (color Doppler imaging)
CE (capital epiphysis) angle of
  Wiberg
CE (cardioesophageal) junction
C-E amplitude of mitral valve
CEA (carcinoembryonic antigen)
CEA scan for colorectal carcinoma
cecal appendage
cecal serosa
cecal sphincter
cecal volvulus
cecum (caecum)
  antimesocolic side of
  coned
  mobile
  subhepatic
Cedell fracture of talus
Cedell-Magnusson classification of
  arthritis on x-ray
Ceelen-Gellerstedt syndrome
Cegka sign
CeI scintillator
celiac and mesenteric arteriography

celiac angiography
celiac artery compression syndrome
celiac axis syndrome
celiac ganglia
celiac plexus
celiac trunk
celiectasia
celioma
CEM (central extensor mechanism)
Cemax/Icon scanner
Cemax PACS platform
cement
   acrylic bone
   hydroxyapatite (HA)
   Implast bone
   methyl methacrylate
   orthopedic
   polymerized
   radiopaque bone
   surface
cementation
cementifying fibroma
cement line
cement mantle
cemento-ossifying fibroma
Cencit surface scanner
center
   anechoic
   ciliospinal center of Budge
   cortical
   diaphyseal
   emetic
   growth center of bone
   ossification
Center of Metabolic and Experimental
   Imaging
centigray (cGy)
centimeter (cm)
central axis depth dose
central canal
central collodiaphyseal angle (CCD)
central intraluminal saturation stripe

central motor pathways disease
central nervous system (CNS)
central neurogenic hyperventilation
central point artifact
central rays
central splanchnic venous thrombosis
   (CSVT)
central tegmental tract
central venous pressure (CVP) line
centriciput
centrilobular emphysema
centrilobular region of liver
centrilobular shadow
centroparietal head region
centrum commune
centrum ovale
centrum semiovale
cephalad
cephalic angulation
cephalic index
cephalic presentation of fetus
cephalic vein
cephalization of blood flow
cephalocaudad length
cephalofacial proportionality
cephalohematocele
cephalohematoma, parietal
cephalometry
cephalopelvic disproportion (CPD)
cephalopelvimetry
CeraSPECT camera
cerebellar degeneration
cerebellar disease
cerebellar fiber
cerebellar hemisphere
cerebellar hemorrhage
cerebellar herniation
cerebellar infarction
cerebellar mass
cerebellar pathway
cerebellar peduncle
cerebellar syndrome

cerebellar tonsillar herniation
cerebellar tract
cerebellar vermis
cerebellopontile angle (CPA) tumor
   (also cerebellopontine)
cerebellum
   dentate nucleus of
   midline
   petrosal
cerebral abscess
cerebral aneurysm
cerebral angiography
cerebral aqueduct
cerebral arteries
cerebral arteriography
cerebral arteriovenous fistula
cerebral atrophy
cerebral blood flow (CBF)
cerebral blood volume (CBV)
cerebral blood volume/cerebral blood
   flow ratio
cerebral brain death
cerebral brain flow
cerebral commissure
cerebral contusion
cerebral cortex
cerebral CT venography
cerebral dominance
cerebral dysfunction
cerebral dysrhythmia
cerebral edema
cerebral embolism
cerebral gigantism
cerebral hemidecortication
cerebral hemisphere
cerebral herniation
cerebral hypotension
cerebral infarct (infarction)
cerebral infundibulum
cerebral ischemia
cerebral ischemic event
cerebral mantle

cerebral metabolic rate for glucose
   (CMRglu)
cerebral metabolic rate of oxygen
   ($CMRO_2$)
cerebral metabolism
cerebral nocardiosis
cerebral operculum
cerebral parenchyma
cerebral peduncle
cerebral perfusion SPECT scan
cerebral revascularization
cerebral sign
cerebral SPECT
cerebral steal syndrome
cerebral thrombophlebitis
cerebral Whipple disease
cerebral white matter
cerebri (pl. of cerebrum)
   commotio
   contusio
   falx
   gliomatosis
   pseudotumor
cerebriform
cerebrohepatorenal syndrome
cerebromacular degeneration (CMD)
cerebromeningeal intracerebral
   hemorrhage
cerebropontocerebellar pathway
cerebrospinal fluid (CSF)
cerebrospinal fluid-containing lesion
cerebrospinal fluid fistula
cerebrospinal fluid flow measurement
cerebrospinal fluid leak study
cerebrospinal fluid pathway
cerebrovascular accident (CVA)
cerebrovascular occlusive disease
cerebrum (pl. cerebri)
   central cavity of
   cortex of
   first ventricle of
   great vein of

cerebrum *(cont.)*
  lateral ventricle of
  second ventricle of
  third ventricle of
Cerenkov calculation
Cerenkov measurement
Cerenkov radiation
Cerenkov scintillation analysis
Ceretec imaging agent
cerium silicate imaging agent
cervical aorta syndrome
cervical aortic arch
cervical CT (computed tomography)
cervical disk disease
cervical dorsal outlet syndrome
cervical esophagus
cervical fracture
cervical intervertebral foraminal MR
  phlebography (CMRP)
cervical mover ligament
cervical musculature
cervical myelogram
cervical myelopathy
cervical nerve root
cervical outlet
cervical pleura
cervical rib
cervical spine (C1 to C7 vertebrae)
cervical spine dens view
cervical spondylosis of the spinal cord
cervical spondylosis, washboard effect
  on myelography in
cervical triangle
cervicocerebral
cervicography
cervicomedullary junction
cervico-occipital fusion
cervicothoracolumbar
cervicotrochanteric fracture
cervigram
cervix uteri

CES (cauda equina syndrome)
cesium chloride imaging agent
Céstan-Chenais syndrome
cestodic tuberculosis
CF or CX (circumflex) artery
CFR (coronary flow reserve)
CGI (common gateway interface)
CGR biplane angiographic system
cGy (centigray)
Chaddock sign
Chagas disease
chain, obturator nodal
chain of lakes sign
chalasia
chalk (or chalky) bones
challenge
  acetazolamide
  hypotensive
chamber
  cardiac
  false aneurysmal
  infundibular
  ionization
  irradiation
  left atrial
  left ventricular
  right atrial
  right ventricular
  rudimentary outlet
  well-type ionization
  Wilson cloud
chamber compression
chamber dilatation
chamber enlargement
chamber of heart
Chamberlain line
Chamberlain-Towne view
champagne-bottle legs in Charcot-
  Marie-Tooth disease
Chance spinal fracture
Chandra-Khetarpal syndrome

change (pl. changes)
   cystic
   degenerative
   dystrophic
   ECMO-induced
   fibrotic
   fMRI signal
   focal degenerative
   lytic
   osteoarthritic
   paroxysmal
   pre-slip
   radiation-induced
   residual-limb shape
   spondylitic
   vasomotor
change-coupled device
channel (pl. channels)
   blood
   central
   deep venous
   enlarged vascular
   gastric
   pancreaticobiliary common
   pyloric
Chaput tubercle
character cell terminal
characteristic, echo
charcoal trap
Charcot-Bouchard intracerebral
   microaneurysm
Charcot chondroma
Charcot cirrhosis
Charcot-Marie-Tooth disease
Charcot joint
Charcot triad
charge-coupled device digitizer
charged particles
chauffeur's fracture
Chauffard point
Chausse view
CHD (congenital heart disease)

check-valve sheath
Chédiak-Higashi syndrome
cheek bone
cheese handler's (or washer's) disease
cheiromegaly
cheirospasm
chemically induced dynamic nuclear
   polarization
chemical-selective fat saturation MR
chemical-shift artifact
chemical-shift phenomena artifact
chemical-shift ratio
chemiluminescence
chemodectoma
chemoembolization
   therapeutic
   transcatheter arterial
   transcatheter oily
Chemo-Port catheter
chemoradiation therapy
chemotherapy
   adjuvant
   CT-guided intra-arterial
   intra-arterial
   multiagent
   neoadjuvant
   superselective intra-arterial
Chen-Smith image coder
Cherry keyboard
CHESS method
chest
   alar (flat)
   barrel
   blast
   cobbler's
   cylindrical
   flail
   foveated
   funnel
   globular
   hollow
   keeled

cholecystectasia
cholecystitis
  acalculous
  acute
  calculous
  chronic
  emphysematous
  gaseous
  perforated
cholecystitis with cholelithiasis
cholecystocholangiogram
cholecystocholangiography
cholecystoduodenal ligament
cholecystogram, oral (OCG)
cholecystography
cholecystokinetic food
cholecystokinin (CCK)
cholecystokinin-pancreozymin
  (CCK-PZ)
cholecystolithiasis
cholecystopathy
cholecystoptosis
cholecystostomy
  percutaneous transhepatic
  ultrasound-guided percutaneous
choledochal cyst
choledochocele
choledocholithiasis
cholelith
cholelithiasis
cholelithoptysis
cholescintigram
cholescintigraphy, morphine augmented
cholestatic liver disease
cholesteatoma
cholesterol embolization
  diffuse
  disseminated
cholesterolosis of gallbladder
Cholografin meglumine imaging agent
chololith (cholelith)
chondral fragment
chondrification

chondroblastoma
chondrodiastasis
chondrodystrophia calcificans
chondrodystrophia fetalis
chondrofibroma
chondrogenic tumor
chondroid matrix
chondroitin sulfate iron colloid (CSIS)
  enhanced MRI
chondrolipoma
chondrolysis
chondroma
  Charcot
  juxtacortical
chondromalacia patellae
chondromatosis
  Henderson-Jones
  synovial
chondromatous hamartoma
chondromyofibroma
chondromyxoid fibroma (CMF)
chondromyxoma
chondromyxosarcoma
chondronecrosis
chondro-osteodystrophy
chondrophyte
chondroporosis
chondrosarcoma
chondrosarcomatosis
chondrosteoma
chondrosternal junction
Chopart ankle dislocation
Chopart joint
Choquet fuzzy integral
chorda (pl. chordae)
  basal
  cleft
  commissural
  first order
  second order
  strut
  third order

chorda magna
chorda tympani
chordae tendineae cordis
chordae Willisii
chordal rupture
chordocarcinoma
chordoepithelioma
chordosarcoma
choriocarcinoma
chorionic villus sampling
choroid glomera
choroid plexus papilloma (CPP)
choroidal fissure
choroidal pericallosal artery
Christmas tree appearance on MR
chromatographic separations
chromium (Cr)
    Cr-HIDA chelate
    Cr-HIDA imaging agent
    ^{51}Cr-labeled red blood cells
chromium-labeled red blood cells
chronologic age
Churg-Strauss syndrome
Ci (curie)
CI (continuous imaging), Aspire
CID camera
Cidtech camera
CIG (cardiointegram)
cigarette smoking, pack-years of
CIIP (chronic idiopathic intestinal
    pseudo-obstruction)
ciliary ganglion
ciliated border
ciliospinal center of Budge
cineangiocardiography
cineangiogram
cineangiography
    aortic root
    biplane
    coronary
    left anterior oblique (LAO)
    left posterior oblique (LPO)

cineangiography *(cont.)*
    left ventricular (LV)
    radionuclide
    right anterior oblique (RAO)
    right posterior oblique (RPO)
    selective coronary
    Sones technique for
    ventricular
cine-based viewing
cinecardioangiography
cine CT (computed tomography)
    scanner
cinedefecogram
cine-esophagogram
cinefluorography
cinefluoroscopy
cine gradient-echo MR imaging
cine (high frame-rate) mode
cine-loop
cine magnetic resonance tagging
Cine Memory with color flow
    Doppler imaging
cine PC imaging
cine projector, Tagarno 3SD (for
    angiography)
cineradiography
cine view in MUGA (multiple gated
    acquisition) scan
cineventriculogram
cineventriculography
cingulate gyrus
cingulate herniation
cingulate sulcus
cipher
    product
    transposition
circadian event recorder
circadian periodicity
circle
    arterial
    articular vascular
circle of Vieussens

circle of Weber
circle of Willis
Circon video camera
circuit
    anticoincidence
    application-specific integrated
      (ASIC)
    arrhythmia
    ASIC
    bypass
    coincidence
    doubly broadband triple resonance
      NMR probe
    macroreentrant
    magnetoresistive sensor
    microreentrant
    reentry
    shunting
circular muscles
circular plane
circular syncytium
circulation
    allantoic
    arrested
    assisted
    balanced
    cerebrospinal fluid
    codominant
    collateral
    compensatory
    cutaneous collateral
    derivative
    extracorporeal
    fetal
    greater
    intervillous
    peripheral
    placental
    spider-web
    systemic
    thebesian
circulation time

circulatory collapse
circulatory compromise
circulatory disturbance
circulatory embarrassment
circulatory failure
circulatory hyperkinetic syndrome
circulatory impairment
circulatory shock
circulatory stasis
circumference (of anatomical structure)
circumferential echodense layer
circumferential fracture
circumferentially
circumflex (circ., CF, CX)
circumflex artery
circumflex branches
circumflex coronary artery
circumflex groove artery
circumflex vessels
circumscribed edema
circumscribed infiltrate
circumscribed pleurisy
circumscript aneurysm
cirrhosis
    acholangic biliary
    acute juvenile
    alcoholic
    atrophic
    biliary
    Budd
    calculus
    cardiac
    Charcot
    cholangitic biliary
    congestive
    Cruveilhier-Baumgarten
    cryptogenic
    decompensated alcoholic
    diffuse septal
    end-stage
    fatty
    focal biliary

classification *(cont.)*
  Key-Conwell pelvic fracture
  Kiel non-Hodgkin lymphoma
  Kilfoyle condylar fracture
  King classification of thoracic
    scoliosis
  Kistler subarachnoid hemorrhage
  Klatskin tumor
  Kocher-Lorenz capitellum fracture
  Kostuik-Errico spinal stability
  Kyle fracture
  Lauge-Hansen ankle fracture
  Lukes-Butler non-Hodgkin
    lymphoma
  Mason radial fracture
  Mazur ankle evaluation
  McLain-Weinstein spinal tumor
  Merland perimedullary
    arteriovenous fistula
  Meyers-McKeever tibial fracture
  Milch elbow fracture
  Modic
  MSTS (Musculoskeletal Tumor
    Society) staging system
  Mueller humerus fracture
  multiaxial
  Neer shoulder fractures I, II,
    and III
  Neer-Horowitz humerus fracture
  Nevaiser frozen shoulder
  Newman radial fracture
  Nurick spondylosis
  NYHA (New York Heart Associa-
    tion) congestive heart failure
  O'Brien radial fracture
  Ogden epiphyseal fracture
  Olerud and Molander fracture
  Ovadia-Beals tibial plafond fracture
  osteoarthritis grading
  Pauwel femoral neck fracture
  Pipkin femoral fracture
  Poland epiphyseal fracture
  Rappaport lymphoma

classification *(cont.)*
  Ratliff avascular necrosis
  Riordan club hand
  Riseborough-Radin intercondylar
    fracture
  Rockwood acromioclavicular injury
  Rowe calcaneal fracture
  Rowe-Lowell fracture-dislocation
  Ruedi-Allgower tibial plafond
    fracture
  Russell-Rubinstein cerebrovascular
    malformation
  Rye Hodgkin disease
  Sage-Salvatore acromioclavicular
    joint injury
  Sakellarides calcaneal fracture
  Salter-Harris fracture
  Salter-Harris-Rang epiphyseal
    fracture
  Schatzker fracture
  Seinsheimer femoral fracture
  Shelton femur fracture
  Smith sesamoid position
  Sorbie calcaneal fracture
  Steinbrocker rheumatoid arthritis
  Steinert epiphyseal fracture
  Steward-Milford fracture
  talocalcaneal index
  Thompson-Epstein femoral fracture
  TNM (tumor size, nodal involve-
    ment, metastatic progress)
  Tronzo intertrochanteric fracture
  Trunkey fracture
  Vostal radial fracture
  Watanabe discoid meniscus
  Watson-Jones
  Wiberg patellar types
  Wilkins radial fracture
  Winquist-Hansen femoral fracture
  Wolfe breast carcinoma
  Zickel fracture
  Zlotsky-Ballard acromioclavicular
    injury

Claude syndrome
clavicle
clavicular head of sternocleidomastoid
clavicular notch
clavipectoral fascia
clawfoot deformity
  pes arcuatus
  pes cavus
claw hand (or clawhand)
clawtoe deformity
Claybrook sign
clay shoveler's fracture
CLC (Clerc-Levy-Cristeco) syndrome
clean shadow
clearance, aerosol
clearance curve
clearance half-time
clear zone
cleavage fracture
cleavage plane, subintimal
cleaving, plaque
Cleeman sign
cleft
  anal
  branchial
  first visceral
  gill
  interinnominoabdominal
  meniscal
  pudendal
  retrosomatic
  synaptic
  ventricular
cleft chordae
cleidocranial dysostosis
Cleland ligament in the hand
clenched fist view
Clerc-Levy-Cristeco (CLC) syndrome
clinical correlation
clinical sequelae
clinicopathological analysis
clinodactyly

clinoid ligament
clip
  aneurysm
  metallic
  surgical
clivus, Blumenbach
clivus meningioma tumor
CLO (congenital lobar overinflation)
cloacal anomaly
clockwise whirlpool sign
clonogen number
clonogenicity
C-loop of duodenum
closed-break fracture
closed dislocation
closed fracture
close-up view
closure
  growth center
  native aortic valve
  physeal
  threatened vessel
  tricuspid valve
  valve
clot
  agonal (or agony)
  blood
  chicken fat
  marantic
  passive
  preformed
  subarachnoid
  subdural
clot-filled lumen
clot lysis
clouding, alveolar
cloudy swelling of heart
Cloverleaf catheter
cloverleaf deformity
cloverleaf-shaped lumen
cloverleaf skull
clubfoot deformity

coil *(cont.)*
   modified birdcage
   opposed loop-pair quadrature
     NMR
   orthogonal RF
   platinum
   quadrature RF receiver
   radiofrequency (RF)
   receiver
   RF (radiofrequency)
   right ventricular
   saddle
   sensing
   shim
   solenoid surface
   surface
   three-axis gradient
   torso phased-array (TPAC)
coiled spring appearance of intus-
   suscepted bowel
coil embolization (therapeutic)
coil-tipped catheter
coil-to-vessel diameter
coincidence circuit
coincidence-summing correction
coin lesion
COLD (chronic obstructive lung
   disease)
cold nodule
cold spot myocardial imaging
colic impression on the liver
Colinet-Caplan syndrome
colitis
   chronic ulcerative (CUC)
   Crohn
   familial ulcerative
   focal
   fulminant
   fulminating ulcerative
   granulomatous transmural
   ischemic
   mucous

colitis *(cont.)*
   myxomembranous
   pseudomembranous (PMC)
   radiation
   radiation-induced
   regional
   single-stripe (SSC)
   transmural
   ulcerative (UC)
colitis polyposa
colitis ulcerosa gravis
collagen-filled interlocking detachable
   coils
collagen tissue proliferation
collagen vascular disease
collapse (of anatomical structure)
collar
   implant
   periosteal bone
collar bone
collar-button abscess
collar-button appearance in colon
collateral
   bridging
   porto-azygos
   retrograde
   septal
collateral blood flow
collateral blood supply
collateral branch
collateral channel
collateral circulation
collateral eminence
collateralization
collateral ligament
collateral sulcus
collateral system
collateral vessel
collecting system
collection of contrast material
Colles fracture
Colles ligament

colorectal (CR) mucosa
color flow Doppler
color flow Doppler real-time 2-D (two-dimensional) blood flow imaging
color flow duplex imaging
color flow mapping
colorimetric color reproduction
color power transcranial Doppler sonography
color reproduction, colorimetric
color space, C-Y
color space conversion
color space interpolator
color ultrasound
colosigmoid resection
colovaginal fistula
colovesical fistula
colpocele
colpoptosis
column
    anal
    anterior gray (of spinal cord)
    Bertin
    branchial efferent
    Clarke
    contrast medium
    Lissauer
    renal
    variceal
    vertebral
column extraction method
columning of dye
column mode sinogram images
column of Burdach
column of dye
column of Morgagni
CoLyte bowel prep
combination flow and pressure loads
combined flexion phenomenon
combined-modality radiation therapy
combined leukocyte-marrow imaging

combined multisection diffuse-weighted and hemodynamically weighted echo planar MR imaging
combined Myoscint/thallium imaging
combined thallium-Tc-HMPAO imaging
comma sign in truncus arteriosus
comminuted bursting fracture
comminuted fracture
commissural attachments
commissural chordae
commissural leaflet
commissural point
commissure
    anterior (AC)
    anteroseptal
    cerebral
    fused
    gray commissure of spinal cord
    posterior (PC)
    scalloped
    tectum
    valve
    vestigial
    white commissure of spinal cord
common bile duct (CBD)
common carotid artery (CCA)
common cavity phenomenon
common duct cholangiogram
common duct stone
common femoral artery
common gateway interface (CGI)
common iliac artery
communicating hydrocephalus
communicating vein
communication
    asyndetic
    interatrial
communis, extensor digitorum
Comolli sign
compact bone

comparison
  histopathologic
  yield
comparison view
compartment
  anterior
  anterior mediastinal
  deep posterior
  extensor
  extradural
  infracolic
  infratentorial
  lateral
  medial
  patellofemoral
  plantar
  posterior
  posterolateral
  posteromedial
  superficial posterior
  supracolic
compartment lesion, posterior
compartment syndrome
Compass stereotactic frame
compatible
compensated composite spin-lock
  pulse
compensated congestive heart failure
compensation
  cardiac
  cardiac gating
  respiratory
  scatter
  section-select flow
compensator
  scattering foil
  tissue deficit
compensatory emphysema
compensatory enlargement
compensatory hypertrophy
competent valve
competitive adsorption

complete atrioventricular block
complete atrioventricular dissociation
complete bladder emptying
complete dislocation
complete fracture
complete heart block
complex
  ankle joint (AJC)
  anterior communicating artery
  apical
  arcuate
  atrial
  auricular
  capsulolabral
  caudal pharyngeal
  diisocyanide-triisocyanide ^{99m}Tc
  discoligamentous
  Eisenmenger
  fabellofibular
  foot–ankle
  gadolinium
  gastrocnemius–soleus
  gastroduodenal artery
  Ghon
  hallux valgus–metatarsus primus
    varus
  hindfoot joint
  hippocampal-amygdaloid
  ligamentous
  MION-gene
  nipple-areola
  oxidized
  primary
  Ranke
  sesamoid
  sling ring
  subluxation
  superior olivary
  syndesmotic ligament
  tibiocalcaneal joint
  triangular fibrocartilage
  vertebrobasilar

complex blocking
complex dynamic pharyngeal and
   speech evaluation by cine recording
complex electron arc therapy
compound dislocation
compound fracture
compression
   aqueduct
   fingerprint image
   image
   interfragmental
   manual
   multiplanar
   nerve root
   plaque
   radicular
   root
   spot
   thermal
   wavelet
compression atelectasis
compression fracture (burst)
compression plate and screws
compression ratio
compression syndrome
compression ultrasonography
compromise
   circulatory
   respiratory
compromised flow
Compton scattering cross-section
Compton suppression spectrometer
Compuscan Hittman computerized
   electrocardioscanner
computed axial tomography (CAT)
   scan
computed ejection fraction
computed radiograph
computed sonography, Acuson
computed tomographic angiography
   (CTA)
computed tomography (see *CT*)

computed tomography angiographic
   portography (CTAP)
computed tomography dose index
   (CTDI)
computed tomography during arterial
   portography (CTAP)
computed tomography scan (see *CT*)
computed transmission tomography
computer-aided design (CAD)
computer-aided diagnosis scheme
computer, Aspect
computer-assisted intracranial navigation
computer-assisted stereotactic resection of deep-seated and superficial
   lesions
computer-assisted volumetric stereotactic resrection
computer-generated images
computerized (or computed)
   tomography (CT)
computerized axial tomography
   (CAT) with contrast
computerized axial tomography
   (CAT) without contrast
computerized cranial tomography
   (CCT)
computerized optical densitometry
   (COD)
computerized tomographic hepatic
   angiography (CTHA)
computerized tomography guidance
   for placement of radiation therapy
   fields
computerized tomography guidance
   for stereotactic localization
computerized tomography-guided
   needle biopsy
computerized transverse axial
   tomography (CTAT)
computer subtraction techniques
conal papillary muscle

conjugate, true
Conn syndrome
connection, ISDN (teleradiology)
connective tissue
    areolar
    dense
    peribronchial
    regular
    reticular
    subcutaneous
connective tissue proliferation
connective tissue septa
conoid ligament
conotruncal anomaly, congenital
conoventricular defect
Conrad-Bugg trapping of soft tissue in
    ankle fracture
Conradi-Hünermann syndrome
Conray imaging agent
Conray-60 imaging agent
Conray-280 imaging agent
consecutive dislocation
console
    Bruker
    SMIS
consolidated infiltrate
consolidation
    air-space
    alveolar
    bilateral
    confluent
    dense
    exudative
    ill-defined
    lobar
    lung parenchyma
    nonhomogeneous
    parenchymal
    patchy air-space
    peripheral
    pulmonary
    segmental
    unilateral

consolidative change
consolidative pneumonia
conspicuity
constant, Planck
constant tilt wave
constellation of findings; symptoms
constitutional symptoms
constriction
    airway
    hourglass
    occult pericardial
    postglomerular arteriolar
    tangential
construction artifact
constriction band syndrome
contact B-scan ultrasound
contents
    abdominal
    bone mineral (BMC)
    bowel
    brain water
    digestive tract
    gastric
    intestinal
contiguous images (in CT scan)
contiguous slices
continuity of bone
continuous imaging (CI), Aspire
continuous wave (CW)
continuous wave Doppler
    echocardiography
continuous wave Doppler
    ultrasonography
continuous wave laser system
continuous wave high frequency
    Doppler ultrasound system
contour
    irregular hazy luminal
    isodose
    S
    scalloping
    undulating

convolution *(cont.)*
  ascending parietal
  Broca
  cerebral
  Gratiolet
  Heschl
  occipitotemporal
  Zuckerkandl
convolution mask
Cook arterial catheter
Coopernail sign
coordinate axis (pl. axes)
coordinate, Cartesian
coordinates (X, Y, and Z) for target
  lesion
COPD (chronic obstructive pulmonary
  disease)
Cope point
coplanar contour points
copper (Cu)
  ^{62}Cu PTSM imaging agent
  ^{62}Cu pyruvaldehyde-bis-(4N-thio-
    semicarbazone) imaging agent
  Cu/Zn (copper-zinc)-SOD
copper filtration
co-precipitation
coprolith
coprostasis
cor (heart)
cor adiposum
cor arteriosum
cor biloculare
cor bovinum
cor dextrum
cor mobile
cor pendulum
cor pulmonale (c. pulmonale)
coracoacromial arch
coracoacromial ligament
coracoacromial process
coracohumeral ligament
coracoid notch

coracoid process
coracoid tuberosity
cord
  condyle
  fibrous
  hepatic
  Lissauer tracts of spinal
  medullary
  pretendinous
  rostral spinal
  sacral spinal
  spermatic
  spinal
  tethered
  vocal
  Weitbrecht
cordate pelvis
cord compression
cord embarrassment
Cordis Brite Tip guiding catheter
Cordis Ducor brachial I, II, and III
  coronary catheter
Cordis-Ducor-Judkins catheter
Cordis multipurpose access port
  (MPAP)
Cordis Son-II catheter
Cordis tantalum stent
cordlike mass
Cordonnier ureteroileal loop
corduroy arteries
corduroy artifact
corduroy cloth pattern on myelogram
core biopsy needle
core, bone
coregistration, morphological and
  physiological image
cork handler's lung disease
corkscrew appearance
corkscrew esophagus
Cornelia de Lange syndrome
Cornell protocol (exercise stress
  testing)

cornflake esophageal motility study
corn oil and ferric ammonium citrate
    contrast imaging agent
cornu (pl. cornua)
coronal computed tomographic
    arthrography (CCTA)
coronal image, multi-echo
coronal maximum-intensity projection
    (MIPcor)
coronal orientation
coronal plane
coronal projection
coronal section
coronal slab
coronal slice
coronal suture
coronal synostosis
coronal view
coronary angiography
   left (LCA)
   right (RCA)
coronary artery (see *artery*)
coronary artery disease (CAD)
coronary artery ostia
coronary (artery) perfusion pressure
    (CPP)
cardonary artery scan (CAS)
coronary artery steal syndrome
coronary artery tree
coronary atherosclerosis
coronary balloon angioplasty
coronary bypass graft patency
coronary-cameral fistula
coronary cineangiography
coronary cusp
coronary fistula
coronary flow reserve (CFR)
coronary groove
coronary heart disease (CHD)
coronary sinus (CS)
coronary sinus of Valsalva
coronary spasm

coronary steal phenomenon
coronary steal syndrome
coronary-subclavian steal syndrome
coronary sulcus
coronoid fossa
coronoid process
Coroskop C cardiac imaging
   system
corpora cavernosography
corpora fornicis
corpora restiformia
corpus callosum
corpus Luysii
corpus sterni
corpus striatum
corpus uteri
correction
   accidental
   automatic motion
   coincidence-summing
   fuzzy logic contrast
   inhomogeneity
   multi-illuminant color
   Picker SPECT attenuation
   summing
   surface variable attenuation
   trend
correlation
   clinical
   functional
   histologic
   histopathologic-CT
   imaging-anatomic
   imaging-pathologic
   in vivo
   mammographic-histopathologic
   morphological
   radiologic-anatomic
   radiologic-pathologic
correlation algorithms (CR)
Correra line
Corrigan sign

corrugated air column
corset balloon catheter
cortex (pl. cortices)
    adrenal
    articular
    auditory
    bilateral orbital frontal
    bone
    calcarine
    cerebellar
    cerebral
    entorhinal
    femoral
    frontal
    lymphatic
    mesial-frontal
    motor
    nonolfactory
    opercular
    orbitofrontal
    ovarian
    parastriate
    parietal
    perirolandic parietal
    peristriate
    perisylvian
    premotor
    primary auditory
    primary visual
    pyriform
    renal
    rolandic
    sensorimotor
    somatosensory
    striate
    visual
cortical activity
cortical adenoma
cortical atrophy
cortical bone
cortical branch
cortical defect

cortical deficit
cortical dysfunction
cortical gray matter
cortical hinge axis
cortical hyperintensity
cortical hyperostosis
cortical infarcts
cortical intracerebral hemorrhage
cortical ischemia
cortical motor area
cortical necrosis
cortical scintigraphy
cortical sign
cortical signet ring shadow
cortical sulci
cortical thumb
cortical tuber
cortical versus cancellous bone
cortical white matter
corticated border
corticocallosal dysgenesis
corticocancellous strut
corticocerebellar connection
corticogram
corticography
corticomedullary junction
corticomedullary phase (CP)
corticospinal motor pathway
Corti organ
corundum smelter's lung
Corvisart syndrome
cosine transform
costa fluctuans decima
costae spuriae
costae verae
costal angle
costal bone
costal cartilage
costal groove
costal interarticular cartilage
costal margin
costal margin syndrome

costal notch
costal pleura
costal pleural reflection
costal process
costal sulcus
costal surface
costal tubercle
costocervical artery
costocervical trunk
costochondral joint
costochondral junction
costochondritis
costoclavicular syndrome; test
costodiaphragmatic recess
costolateral
costomediastinal recess
costophrenic (CP) angle blunting
costophrenic recess
costophrenic septal lines
costophrenic sulcus
costosternal angle
costotransverse joint
costovertebral angle (CVA)
costovertebral articulation
costovertebral joint
costoxiphoid ligament
COSY H-1 MR spectroscopy
cottage loaf appearance
Cotton ankle fracture
Cotton-Berg syndrome
cotyloid cavity
cotyloid notch
couch view
cough fracture of rib
coulomb (C)
Councill catheter
count
    Cerenkov
    direct liquid scintillation
counter
    Geiger
    proportional

counter-current aortography
counter-occluder
counterpulsation
counting, double-label
coup
Cournand cardiac catheter
course (of anatomical structure)
coursing of gas
Courvoisier gallbladder
covered Gianturco stent
coxa adducta
coxa brevis
coxa flexa
coxa magna
coxa plana
coxa saltans
coxa senilis
coxa valga
coxa vara luxans
CP (costophrenic) angle
CPA (cerebellopontile or cerebello-
    pontine angle)
CPAD (chronic peripheral arterial
    disease)
CPB (cardiopulmonary bypass)
CPD (cephalopelvic disproportion)
CPI (conventional planar imaging)
CPMG sequence
c. pulmonale (cor pulmonale)
Cr (chromium)
CR (colorectal)
CR (computed radiology)
CR Bard catheter
CR-39 nuclear tract detector
crabmeat-like appearance
cranial and caudal angulations
cranial angled view
cranial nerves (12)
    I (olfactory)
    II (optic)
    III (oculomotor)
    IV (trochlear)

Cronkhite-Canada syndrome
cross-aortic
crossbridge cycle (cycling)
cross-collateralization
cross-correlation technique
crossed-coil design
crossed embolism
crossed-fused renal ectopia
crossed sciatica sign
crossed signs
cross-filling
cross ligament
cross-linked polystyrene (PET scan)
crossover of activity
cross-pelvic collateral vessel
cross-section, Compton scattering
cross-sectional image
cross-sectional zone
cross-table lateral film
cross-talk effect artifact
cross-union
Crouzon disease
crowding of bronchovascular mark-
    ings
Crowe pilot point
crown artifact
crown, halo
crown-rump length (CRL)
CRT (cathode ray tube)
cruciate ligament
crura of diaphragm (left and right)
crus (leg) (pl. crura)
    diaphragmatic
    lateral
    left
    medial
    right
crushing-type injury
Cruveilhier ulcer
crux cordis (crux of heart)
cryolesion
cryomagnet

cryosurgery, map-guided
crypt
    anal
    enamel
    epithelium
    ileal
    Lieberkühn
    Luschka
    Morgagni
crystallography
CS (coronary sinus)
CSA (cross-sectional area)
CSDH (chronic subdural hematoma)
CSF (cerebrospinal fluid)
CSF-suppressed T2-weighted 3D
    MP-RAGE MR imaging
CSI (coronary stenosis index)
    CSI-enhanced MRI
    CSI spectroscopy
C sign
C-60 teletherapy
CSL (central sacral line)
C-spine (cervical spine)
CSS (carotid sinus syndrome)
CST (contraction stress test)
CST (corticospinal tract)
CT (cardiothoracic) ratio
CT (computed tomography)
    biphasic
    cine
    collimation
    contrast-enhanced
    dual energy
    dual-isotope single-photon
    electron-beam\
    enhanced
    expiratory
    helical
    helical thin-section
    high resolution
    high spatial resolution cine
        (HSRCCT)

CT *(cont.)*
  high temporal resolution cine
    (HTRCCT)
  indirect
  lipiodol
  multiphasic
  nonenhanced
  peripheral quantitative (pQCT)
  quantitative spirometrically
    controlled CT angiography with
    volume rendering
  single-photon emission (SPECT)
  sliding-thin-slab maximum intensity
    projection
  slip-ring
  SPECT (single-photon emission)
  spiral
  superselective angio-
  thallium-201 single-photon emission
  thin-section
  thin-slice
  three-dimensional processed
    ultrafast
  transmission
  triphasic spiral
  two-phase helical
  ultrafast
  water-contrast
  Z-dependent
CT arterial portography (CTAP)
CT arteriography
CT arthrography
CT attenuation value
CT bone window photography
CT cisternogram, metrizamide
  (MCTC)
CT colography
CT densitometry
CT-directed hook wire localization
CT fluoroscopy, real-time
CT gantry
CT-guided aspiration

CT-guided intra-arterial chemotherapy
CT-guided needle biopsy
CT-guided percutaneous biopsy
CT-guided PEG (percutaneous endo-
  scopic gastrostomy)
CT-guided stereotactic surgery
CT-guided transsternal core biopsy
CT-guided ultrasound
CT holography (CTH)
CT imaging error
CT laser mammography (CTLM)
CT Max 640 scanner
CT myelography
CT PEG (CT-guided percutaneous
  endoscopic gastrostomy)
CT peritoneography
CT reconstruction image
C-TRAK hand-held gamma detector
CT scan directed needle biopsy
CT scan with contrast
CT scanner (see *scanner*)
CT sialography
CT/SPECT fusion
CT stereotaxic guide
CT with MR, single-photon emission
CT9000 scanner
CT9800 scanner
CTA (computed tomographic
  angiography)
CTA dosimetry
CTA-2 (second scan CT arterial
  portography)
CTAP (computed tomography during
  arterial portography)
CTAP-1 (first scan CT arterial
  portography)
CTAT (computerized transverse axial
  tomography)
CTDI (computed tomography dose
  index)
CTH (computerized tomographic
  holography)

CTHA (computerized tomographic
  hepatic angiography)
CTI 933/04 ECAT scanner
CTI PET scanner
CTLM (computerized tomographic
  laser mammography)
CTLV (cross-table lateral view)
CT/MRI-compatible stereotactic head-
  frame
CT/MRI-defined tumor slice image
CT/MRI-defined tumor volume image
CTR (cardiothoracic ratio)
CTS (carpal tunnel syndrome)
CTT (central tegmental tract)
Cu (copper)
cube vertices
cubic centimeter (cc)
cubic convolution interpolation
cubic packing
cubic voxels
cubital fossa
cubital tunnel syndrome
cubitocarpal
cubitoradial
cubitus valgus
cubitus varus
cuboid bone
cubonavicular joint
cue
  biopsy
  exclusionary
  inclusionary
  preclusionary
cue-based image analysis
cuff
  aortic
  atrial
  inflow
  musculotendinous
  rectal muscle
  right atrial
  rotator
  suprahepatic caval

cuffing, peribronchial
cuff rupture
cul-de-sac
  Douglas
  dural
Cullen sign
culprit lesion
culprit vessel
cumulative effect
cuneiform bone of carpus
cuneiform fracture-dislocation
cuneiform joint
cuneiform mortise
cuneus
cup
  acetabular
  hip replacement
  migration of acetabular
  prosthesis
  retroversion of acetabular
cup-and-spill stomach
CUP (cancer of unknown primary)
cupula
  diaphragmatic
  pleural
curie (Ci)
Curix Capacity Plus film processing
  system
Curling ulcer
Curracino-Silverman syndrome
Currarino triad
current
  gradient drive
  pulsing
  tube
curvature (see also *curve*)
  angular
  anterior
  backward
  cervical
  dorsal kyphotic
  flattening of normal lordotic

cyst *(cont.)*
    ovarian follicular
    pancreatic
    paratubal
    parovarian
    pericardial
    pineal
    pituitary
    primordial
    prostatic
    renal
    retention
    serous
    solitary bone
    tarsal
    testicular
    thin-walled
    thyroglossal duct
    unilocular
    wolffian
cystadenoma
cystic artery
cystic change
cystic duct cholangiogram
cystic duct remnant
cystic duct stump
cystic emphysema
cystic fibrosis
cystic hydroma
cystic hygroma
cystic lysis
cystic mazoplasia
cystic medionecrosis

cystic neoplasm
cystic osteofibromatosis
cystic pulmonary emphysema
cystic sac
cystic tumor
cystic wall
cysto-atrial shunt
cystocele, protrusion of
Cysto-Conray II contrast medium
Cystografin contrast medium
cystogram
cystography
    delayed
    double voiding
    excretory
    postdrainage
    postvoiding
    radionuclide
    retrograde
    stress
    triple voiding
    voiding
cystoscopic urography
cystourethrogram, voiding (VCUG)
cytoarchitectonic abnormality
cytoarchitectonic field, Brodmann
cytokine cascades
cytomegalic inclusion disease
cytomegalovirus pneumonitis
Cytomel suppression test
cytometry
    flow
    multicolor flow

D, d

D (diaphragmatic)
Dacron catheter
Dacron stent
dacryocystography
DAF (dynamic axial fixator)
Dagradi classification of esophageal
varices
DAI (diffuse axonal injury)
DALM (dysplasia with associated
lesion or mass)
D'Amato sign in pleural effusion
dammed-up CSF (cerebrospinal fluid)
dampened obstructive pulse
dampened pulsatile flow
dampened wave form
damping of catheter tip pressure
Dance sign
dancer's fracture
Dandy-Walker cyst
Dandy-Walker deformity
Dandy-Walker syndrome
Dane particle
Danis-Weber classification of ankle
fractures
D'Antonio classification of acetabular
abnormalities
DANTE sequence

DANTE-selective pulses
Dardik Biograft
dark pixel values
dark region
darkroom error
Darrach-Hughston-Milch fracture
DASA (distal articular set angle)
Daseler-Anson classification of
plantaris muscle anatomy
data
radiology outcomes
volumetric image
data acquisition time
data-clipping detection error artifact
data log, ICD
data sets
data spike detection error artifact
Datascope DL-II percutaneous
translucent balloon catheter
Datascope System 90 balloon pump
daughter product
Davies-Colley syndrome
Davies endomyocardial fibrosis
Dawbarn sign
DBM (demineralized bone matrix)
DBP (diastolic blood pressure)
DC (direct current) offset artifact

DC (dynamic compression) plate
DCA (directional color angiography)
DCA (directional coronary angioplasty)
DCA (directional coronary atherectomy)
DCBE (double contrast barium enema)
DCIS (ductal carcinoma in situ)
DCP (dynamic compression plate)
DCS (distal coronary sinus)
dD/dt (derived value on apex
cardiogram)
DDD (double-dose delay)
DDFP (dodecafluoropentane) imaging
agent
DDH (developmental dysplasia of hip)
dead space, anatomical
dead time
death
brain
cerebral
debilitation
debris
aspiration of
atheromatous
atherosclerotic
bone
calcium
cholesterol
extra-articular
foreign
gelatinous
grumous
intimal
intra-articular
joint
necrotic
particle
particulate
thallium
De Broglie wavelength
Debye-Scherrer photographic technique
decalcification

decalcified dorsum sellae
decannulated
decannulation
decapolar catheter
decay
beta
exponential
free induction
decay series
deceleration time
decelerative injury
dechondrification
decidua
decidual cyst
decidual reaction
decidual sac
deciduous
decimalized variance map
declamping
decoding
document image (DID)
Viterbi
decompensated congestive heart
failure
decompensation
cardiac
chronic respiratory
end-stage adult cardiac
end-stage fetal cardiac
hemodynamic
respiratory
ventricular
decompress
decompression
balloon
canal
cardiac
endoscopic
gastric
hydrostatic
intestinal
laser-assisted disk (LDD)

decompression *(cont.)*
  microvascular (MVD)
  percutaneous transhepatic (PTD)
  peripheral nerve
  portal
  surgical
  transduodenal endoscopic
  tube
  variceal
decompression tube
deconditioning
deconvolutional analysis
deconvolution, statistical
decortication
  cardiac
  chemical
  heart
  lung
decoupling
decreased attenuation
decryption algorithms
DecThreads software
decubitus film
decubitus position
  dorsal
  lateral
  ventral
decubitus ulcer
decubitus view
decussation
deep arch
deep artery
deep veins
deep cardiac plexus
deep Doppler velocity interrogation
deep hyperthermia treatment
deep lesion
deep respirations
deep-seated lesion
deep-seated tumor
deep-shelled acetabulum
deep vein thrombosis

deep venous aplasia
deep venous channel
deep venous incompetence
deep venous insufficiency (DVI)
deep venous thrombosis (DVT)
deep white matter track
defecation
defecogram
defography
defect (see also *deformity*)
  acquired ventricular septal (AVSD)
  anastomotic
  anteroapical
  aortic septal
  aorticopulmonary
  ASD (atrioseptal defect)
  atrial ostium primum
  atrioseptal (or atrial septal) (ASD)
  atrioventricular canal
  atrioventricular septal
  bar
  bar-like ventral (in myelography)
  birth
  bony
  bridging of
  cardiofacial
  cauliflower-shaped
  chain of lakes filling
  chiasmatic
  chondral
  cold
  concomitant
  congenital
  conoventricular
  contiguous ventricular septal
  cortical
  craniotomy
  crista supraventricularis septal
  curvilinear
  cushion
  developmental
  discoid filling

defect *(cont.)*
   supracristal ventricular
   supracristal ventriculoseptal
   Swiss cheese ventricular septal
   transient perfusion
   trochlear
   type I (supracristal) ventricular
      septal
   type II (infracristal) ventricular
      septal
   type III (canal type) ventricular
      septal
   type IV (muscular) ventricular
      septal
   V/Q (ventilation/perfusion)
   valvular
   ventilation
   ventilation/perfusion (V/Q)
   ventral hernia
   ventricular septal or
      ventriculoseptal (VSD)
   wedge-shaped
   wire-related
defective communication between
   cardiac chambers
defects in blood-brain barrier
deferential artery
deferens, ductus
defervesce
defervesced
deficit
deficiency
   Aitken femoral
   alpha-1-antitrypsin
   molybdenum cofactor
   pyruvate dehydrogenase complex
deficiency disease
deflectable quadripolar catheter
deflectable-tip catheter
deformans
   osteitis
   osteochondrodystrophia
   Paget osteitis

deformity (also see *defect*)
   Akerlund
   angular
   aortic valve
   Arnold-Chiari
   back-knee
   bell clapper
   biconcave
   bifid thumb
   bone
   bony
   boutonnière (of finger)
   bowing
   bull's-eye
   buttonhole
   calcaneus
   cavovarus
   cavus
   chain of lakes
   Charcot
   checkrein
   clawfoot
   clawhand
   clawtoe
   cloverleaf
   clubhand
   cock-up
   codfish
   compensatory
   congenital
   contracture
   cottage loaf
   coxa vara
   cranio-orbital
   cubitus valgus
   cubitus varus
   curly toe
   Dandy-Walker
   digital
   digitus flexus
   dinner-fork
   DISI (dorsal intercalary segment
      instability)

degeneration *(cont.)*
  liquefaction
  malignant
  Menzel olivopontocerebellar
  mitral valve
  Mönckeberg
  mucoid
  mucous
  mural
  muscular
  myocardial
  myocardial cellular
  myocardial fibers
  myxomatous
  olivopontocerebellar
  pancreas
  panceatic
  paraneoplastic cerebellar
  parenchymatous cerebellar
  paving stone
  primary progressive cerebellar
  progressive
  Regnauld-type great toe
  renal tubular
  retinal
  retrograde
  rim
  sclerotic
  secondary
  senile
  spinal
  spinocerebellar
  spongy
  spongy white matter
  subacute combined spinal cord
  testicular
  thyroid
  trabecular
  traumatic
  wear and tear
  Zenker

degenerative atrioventricular node
  disease
degenerative change
degenerative disease
degenerative disk disease
degenerative joint disease (DJD)
degenerative spurring
DeGimard syndrome
deglutition
deglutition mechanism
deglutition paralysis
deglutition syncope
Degos disease
degradation, image quality
degree, noncircularity
degree of correction
Dehio test
dehiscence
  bronchial
  perivalvular
  prosthesis
de la Camp sign
de Lange syndrome
Delarnette scanner
delay
  developmental
  regrowth
  temporal phase
  time (echo)
delayed excretion of contrast media
delayed films
delayed images
delayed phase
delayed gastric emptying
delayed transport of tracer
delayed traumatic intracerebral
  hematoma (DTICH)
delayed union
delayed visualization
delay time, echo
Delbet fracture classification
Delbet sign

deleterious effect
delicate crepitation
delivery, timed bolus
Delmege sign of tuberculosis
DELTAmanager MedImage system
deltoid branch of posterior tibial
   artery
deltoid ligament
deltopectoral groove
demagnetization field effect
demand (standby)
demarcate
demarcated
demarcation line
De Martini-Balestra syndrome
dementia
Demianoff sign
demifacets
demilune
demineralization, bone
demineralization from disuse
demineralized bone matrix (DBM)
demodulator
demographic data
Demons-Meigs syndrome
de Musset sign (aortic aneurysm)
de Mussey point or sign (pleurisy)
demyelinating disease
demyelination
   brain stem
   large-fiber
   posterior column
   postinfectious
   segmental
demyelinative disorder
denatured Tc-RBCs
dendritic lesion
denervated area
denervation atrophy
Denis classification of spinal injury
   (A to E)
de novo

dens (odontoid process of axis)
dens fracture
dens view of cervical spine
densitometer
   Achilles+
   bone
   CT
   DEXA (dual-energy x-ray
     absorptiometry)
   DPX-IQ
   dual-photon
   Expert-XL
   Hologic 2000
   Norland bone
   photon
   single-photon
densitometry
density (pl. densities)
   air
   bands of
   bone mineral (BMD)
   calcific
   calcified
   capillary
   diffuse reticular
   discrete perihilar
   double
   echo
   fluid
   ground glass
   hazy
   homogeneous soft tissue
   hydrogen
   ill-defined
   increased
   linear
   metallic
   mottled
   nodular
   patchy
   perihilar
   pleural

Dexter-Grossman classification of
   mitral regurgitation
dextrocardia
dextrocardiac
dextrogastria
dextrogastric
dextroposed
dextroposition
dextrorotatory
dextrorotoscoliosis
dextroscoliosis
dextrotransposition (D-transposition)
   of great arteries
dextrotropic
dextroversion of heart
DFA (hallux dorsiflexion angle)
DFP (diastolic filling pressure)
DGR (duodenogastric reflux)
diabetic gastroparesis
diacondylar fracture
diadochokinesia
diadochokinesis
diagnosis
   clinical
   differential
   empirical
   noninvasive
   pathologic
   postoperative
   preoperative
   presumptive
   radiologic
   remote
   roentgenographic
   sonographic
   tentative
   ultrasound
   working
diagnostic efficacy analysis
diagnostic procedure
diagnostic radiology
diagnostic radiopharmaceutical
diagnostic range ultrasound

diagonal branch of artery
diagonal conjugate diameter
diamagnetic shift
diamagnetic susceptibility
diametaphyseal
diametaphysis
diameter (or dimension)
   anteroposterior (AP)
   aortic (AD)
   aortic root
   artery
   Baudelocque
   bi-ischial
   biparietal (BPD)
   bronchial
   cardiac
   coccygeopubic
   coil-to-vessel
   conjugate
   Deventer
   diagonal conjugate
   gestational sac (GS)
   increased AP (anteroposterior)
   intercristal
   internal conjugate
   intertuberal
   left anterior internal (LAID)
   left ventricular internal (LVID)
   Lohlein
   luminal
   maximum AP (anteroposterior)
   midsagittal (MSD)
   minimal luminal
   narrow anteroposterior
   orthonormal
   pelvic
   right ventricular internal (RVID)
   sacropubic
   spinal cord
   stenosis
   transverse
   valve
   vessel

diffracting Doppler transducer device
diffraction
  beam
  high resolution
  high temperature
  x-ray
diffraction peak
diffuse axonal injury (DAI)
diffuse esophageal spasm (DES)
diffuse idiopathic sclerosis
  hyperostosis (DISH)
diffuse idiopathic skeletal hyperostosis
  (DISH)
diffuse uptake
diffusion
  anisotropic
  spectral
  thermal
diffusion and perfusion magnetic
  resonance imaging
diffusion coefficient
diffusion magnetic resonance imaging
diffusion pulse sequence
diffusion-weighted pulse sequence
DiGeorge syndrome
digestion
digestive system
digestive tract
Digirad gamma camera
digit (pl. digits)
  accessory
  arthrodesed
  flail
  replanted
  supernumerary
  syndactylization of
digital branches
digital equipment system
digital fluoroscopy, FluoroPlus
  Roadmapper
digital frequency analysis
digital imaging

Digital Imaging and Communications
  in Medicine (DICOM) protocol
digital imaging processing (DIP)
digitally fused CT and radiolabeled
  monoclonal antibody SPECT
  images
digital mammography
digital radiography
digital rotational angiography (DRA)
digital runoff
digital storage (in cineangiography)
digital subtraction angiography (DSA)
digital subtraction pulmonary
  angiogram
digital subtraction rotational
  angiography
digital-to-analog converter
digital unraveling
digital vascular imaging (DVI)
digital videoangiography
digitized slices
digitized spinography
digitizer (see *scanner*)
digitorum
Digitron digital subtraction imaging
  system
Digitron DVI/DSA computer
digiti manus (fingers)
digiti pedis (toes)
digitus annularis (ring finger)
digitus medius (middle finger)
digitus minimus (little finger)
digiti primus (thumb)
digitus secundus (index finger)
digitus valgus
digitus varus
dihydroxyphenylalanine (DOPA)
diisocyanide-triisocyanide ^{99m}Tc
  complexes
dilatation (dilation)
  alveolar
  anal

dilatation (dilation) *(cont.)*
   aneurysmal
   annular
   aortic root
   arterial
   artery by balloon catheter
   ascending aorta
   balloon
   bile duct
   biliary
   bowel
   bowel loop
   bronchial
   bronchiolar
   caliceal
   cardiac
   cavitary
   chamber
   colonic
   common duct
   diffuse aortic
   distal ureteral
   ductal
   Eder-Puestow
   endoscopic
   esophageal
   extrahepatic biliary cystic
   fusiform
   gastric
   hepatic web
   idiopathic pulmonary artery
   idiopathic right atrial
   intestinal
   intrahepatic biliary cystic
   intraluminal
   left ventricular
   megacolon
   multiple mural
   myocardial
   percutaneous balloon
   percutaneous transluminal balloon
     (PTBD)

dilatation (dilation) *(cont.)*
   periportal sinusoidal
   pneumatic bag esophageal
   pneumatic balloon catheter
   poststenotic
   probe
   prognathous (or prognathic)
   pulmonary artery
   pulmonary trunk idiopathic
   pulmonary valve stenosis
   rectal
   respiratory bronchiolar
   right ventricular
   sequential
   sulcus
   terminal bronchiolar
   tortuous vein
   transient left ventricular
   ureteral
   ureteric
   vein
   ventricular wall
dilatation and hypertrophy
dilate, dilated
dilation (see *dilatation*)
dilution curve
dilution, isotopic
DIMAQ integrated ultrasound workstation
dimension
   absolute artery
   aortic root
   arterial
   axial
   end-systolic
   intraluminal
   intrathoracic
   left atrial
   left ventricular end-diastolic
     (LVEDD)
   left ventricular end-systolic
     (LVESD)

dimension *(cont.)*
  left ventricular internal (LVID)
  left ventricular internal diastolic
    (LVIDD)
  left ventricular internal end-diastole
    (LVIDd)
  left ventricular internal end-systole
    (LVIDs)
  left ventricular systolic (LVs)
  luminal
  right ventricular (RVD)
diminished systemic perfusion
diminutive vessel
dimple of bone
dinner-fork deformity
diode detector
diode, infrared light-emitting
diode laser
Diodrast contrast medium
Dionosil contrast medium
DIP (desquamative interstitial
  pneumonia)
DIP (digital imaging processing)
  algorithms
DIP (distal interphalangeal) joint
diplegia spinalis brachialis traumatica
diploic
dipolar broadening
dipolar interaction
diprotrizoate contrast medium
dipyridamole echocardiography test
dipyridamole handgrip test
dipyridamole infusion test
dipyridamole thallium stress test
dipyridamole thallium-201
  scintigraphy
dipyridamole thallium
  ventriculography
dipyridamole tomographic thallium
  stress test
direct caval cannulation
direct current ablation (DCA)

direct current (DC) energy
direct fracture
direct hernia
direct liquid scintillation count
direct puncture phlebography
direct radioiodination
direct visualization
direction, aboral
directional color angiography (DCA)
directional coronary angioplasty
  (DCA)
directional coronary atherectomy
  (DCA)
directly coupled sample changer
  system
director, grooved
dirty shadowing
disarticulate
disarticulation
disc (see *disk*)
discernible findings
discogenic
discogram
discography
diskogram
diskography
discoid atelectasis
discoid lateral meniscus
discoid shadow
discoligamentous complex
discontinuity
discordant nodule
discrepancy, leg length
discreta, porokeratosis plantaris
discrete (separate) (not *discreet*)
discrete bleeding source
discrete lesion
discrete mass
discriminant analysis
discriminate
discrimination
discriminator

discus (disci)
disease (see radiology-related diseases
    listed alphabetically)
disease-free vessel wall
DISH (diffuse idiopathic sclerosing [or
    skeletal] hyperostosis)
dishpan fracture
DISI (dorsal intercalary segment
    instability)
DISIDA (diisopropyliminodiacetic
    acid) scan
disimpaction
disintegration of plaque by laser
    pulses
disjointing
disk (also disc)
    acromioclavicular joint
    anal
    articular
    atrial
    Bardeen primitive
    Bowman
    bulge (or bulging)
    cartilaginous (of epiphysis)
    cervical vertebral
    chorionic
    contained
    crescent-shaped fibrocartilaginous
    distal radioulnar joint
    embryonic
    epiphyseal
    extruded
    fibrocartilaginous
    fibrous ring of
    fixation
    frayed
    growth
    H
    hard
    Hensen
    herniated
    herniated cervical

disk *(cont.)*
    herniated intervertebral (HID)
    herniated lumbar
    herniated lumbosacral intervertebral
    herniated sacral
    herniated thoracic intervertebral
    I
    interarticular
    intervertebral
    intra-articular
    isotropic
    locking
    lumbar vertebral
    lumbosacral vertebral
    mandibular
    massive herniated
    Merkel tactile
    midline herniation of
    noncontained
    placental
    protruded (or protruding)
    ruptured
    sequestered
    slipped intervertebral
    soft
    sternoclavicular joint
    tactile
    temporomandibular joint
    thoracic vertebral
    thoracolumbar vertebral
    triangular
    vacuum
    vertebral
disk bulge
disk bulging
disk disease
disk extrusion
disk fragment
disk herniation
disk interspace
disk-like atelectasis
disk margin

disk maturation
diskogram
diskography (discography)
  intranuclear
  intervertebral
diskovertebral infection
disk plication
disk poppet
disk protrusion
disk space height
disk space narrowing
disk-to-magnetic field orientation
disk water signal
dislocate, dislocated
dislocation
  anterior
  anterior-inferior
  Bankart
  bayonet
  Bell-Dally
  Bennett
  boutonnière
  bursting
  central
  Chopart
  chronic recurrent
  closed
  complete
  complicated
  compound
  consecutive
  Desault
  divergent
  facet
  fracture
  frank
  gamekeeper's
  habitual
  Hill-Sachs
  incomplete
  irreducible
  isolated

dislocation (cont.)
  Jahss
  Kienböck (Kienboeck)
  Lisfranc
  lunate
  milkmaid's
  Monteggia
  Nélaton
  nonreducible
  nontraumatic
  open
  Otto
  partial
  pathologic
  perilunate
  posterior
  primitive
  recent
  recurrent
  simple
  Smith
  swivel
  traumatic
  volar
dislocation fracture
disobliteration, carotid
disorder
  esophageal motility
  evacuation
  functional
  gastric motor
  intrathoracic lymphoproliferative
  nonspecific esophageal motility
    (NEMD)
  right-left
disparate
disparity
disphenoid extraction
displaced fat pad sign
displacement, Ellis Jones peroneal
displacement field-fitting MR imaging

display
  multiparametric color composite
  pseudocolor B-mode
  real-time
  shaded surface
disproportion
  cephalopelvic (CPD)
  fiber-type
disrupted plaque
disruption, traumatic
dissecans
  osteochondritis (OD)
  osteochondrosis
dissect
dissecting aneurysm
dissecting hematoma
dissection
  aneurysmal
  aortic
  arterial
  descending aorta
  spontaneous
  Stanford type B aortic
disseminated atheromatous
  embolization
disseminated cholesterol embolization
disseminated disease
disseminated intravascular coagulation
  (DIC)
disseminated sclerosis
disseminated tuberculosis
distal articular set angle (DASA)
distal coronary sinus (CS)
distal interphalangeal (DIP) joint
distal splenorenal shunt (DSRS)
distally
distalward
distance
  interarch
  intercaudate
  interlaminar
  internuclear

distance *(cont.)*
  interopercular
  interorbital
  interpediculate
  interridge
  interslice
  interspinous
  source-skin (SSD)
  surface
distance-based block classification
distant metastases
distend
distended
distensible
distensibility
distention
  abdominal
  bladder
  colonic
  gaseous
  gastric
  intestinal
  neck vein
  pelvicaliceal
  postprandial
  rectal
  ureteral
  vesical
disto-occlusal
distortion
  geometric
  image
  pincushion
  radiographic pincushion
  S
  Y-shaped
distortion of limitations of image
  reconstruction algorithm artifact
distraction
  callus
  fracture fragment
  hyperflexion injury

divisionary line (in bipartite sesamoid)
divopontocerebellar atrophy
divot
Dixon method of fat suppression
Dixon method of phase unwrapping
DJD (degenerative joint disease)
DJJ (duodenojejunal junction)
DKS (Damus-Kaye-Stansel)
    anastomosis
D-loop, ventricular
D-loop ventricular situs
DMA (distal metatarsal angle)
D-malposition of aorta
DMI (Diagnostic Medical
    Instruments) analyzer
DMI (diaphragmatic myocardial
    infarction)
DMPE (99mTc-bis-dimethylphospho-
    noethane)
DMVA (direct mechanical ventricular
    actuation)
DNA ploidy pattern
DNA-MION
dobutamine echocardiography
dobutamine stress echocardiography
dobutamine thallium angiography
DOBV (double outlet both ventricles)
document image decoding (DID)
document-recognition algorithm
Dodd perforating vein group
dodecafluoropentane (DDFP) imaging
    agent
Dodge method for ejection fraction
dog artifact
dolichocephaly
dolichocolon
dolichoectasia
dolichoesophagus
dolichosigmoid
dolichostenomelia
DOLV (double outlet left ventricle)
domain, Fourier

dome
    anterior talar
    atrial
    diaphragmatic
    bladder
    liver
    shoulder
    talar
    weightbearing acetabular
dome and dart configuration on
    cardiac catheterization
Dome Imaging RX20 board
dome-shaped heart
dome-shaped roof of pleural cavity
dominance
    coronary artery
    hemispheric
    mixed
    right ventricular
    shared coronary artery
dominant
    anatomically
    autosomal
dominant hemisphere
dominant left coronary artery
dominant right coronary artery
doming, diastolic
doming of leaflets
doming of valve
D1 (diagonal branch #1)
donut sign (also doughnut)
dopamine D1 agonist
dopamine D2 receptor
dopamine transporter
Doplette monitor
Doppler
    color flow
    continuous wave
    contrast-enhanced color
    contrast-enhanced power
    duplex
    duplex B-mode

Doppler *(cont.)*
   gray-scale
   intraoperative
   pocket
   power
   pulsed wave
   range-gated pulsed
   real-time
   spectral
Doppler blood flow detector
Doppler blood flow monitor
Doppler blood flow velocity signal
Doppler blood pressure
Doppler color flow mapping
Doppler color spectral analysis
Doppler coronary catheter
Doppler-derived stroke distance
Doppler echocardiography
   continuous wave
   pulsed wave
Doppler flow probe study
Doppler flow signal
Doppler flow-imaging system, real-time two-dimensional
Doppler flowmetry
Doppler frequency shift
Doppler imaging
Doppler insonation
Doppler Intra-Dop intraoperative device
Doppler phenomenon
Doppler pulse
Doppler Resistive Index (DRI)
Doppler shift
Doppler shift principle
Doppler signal
Doppler signal enhancers
Doppler spectral analysis
Doppler spectral waveforms
Doppler tissue imaging (DTI)
Doppler ultrasonic blood flow detector
Doppler ultrasonic fetal heart monitor
Doppler ultrasonic velocity detector
Doppler ultrasonography
Doppler ultrasound, high frequency (HFD)
Doppler ultrasound segmental blood pressure testing
Doppler venous examination
Doppler waveform analysis
Dorendorf sign of aortic arch aneurysm
Dormia basket catheter
Dornier scanner
Dorros brachial internal mammary guiding catheter
dorsal branch
dorsal capsule
dorsal decubitus position
dorsal metacarpal ligament
dorsal pedal bypass
dorsal pedal pulse
dorsal position
dorsal ramus of spinal nerve
dorsal recumbent position
dorsal root entry zone (DREZ) lesion
dorsal root ganglia (DRG)
dorsal spine (D1 to D12)
dorsal spinocerebellar tracts
dorsal subaponeurotic space
dorsal subcutaneous space
dorsal wing fracture
dorsal wrist ligament
dorsalis pedis pulse
dorsalward
dorsiflexion
dorsiflexor
dorsoanterior
dorsocephalad
dorsolateral
dorsoplantar talonavicular angle
dorsoplantar view
dorsoposterior
dorsoradial

double spiral CT arterial portography
double strand, intracellular DNA
double systolic apical impulse
double tracking of barium
double-walled fibroserous sac
double wire atherectomy technique
doubly broadband triple resonance
　　NMR probe circuit
doughnut (also donut)
doughnut configuration on thallium
　　imaging
doughnut magnet
doughnut sign
Douglas bag method for determining
　　cardiac output
Douglas
　　cul-de-sac of
　　pouch of
Dow-Corning ileal pouch catheter
dowager's hump
dowel
Dow method for measuring cardiac
　　output
Down syndrome
downscatter
downstream sampling method
downward displacement of apical
　　impulse
downward sloping
dP/dt (upstroke pattern on apex car-
　　diogram), peak
DPA (double [or dual] photon absorp-
　　tiometry)
D point
DPTI (diastolic pressure-time index)
DPX-IQ densitometer
DRA (digital rotational angiography)
DRA (distal reference axis)
drainage
　　aberrent venous
　　percutaneous antegrade biliary
　　percutaneous transhepatic (PTD)
　　transvaginal ultrasound-guided

draining vein pressure (DVP)
draped aorta
DRC (dynamic range control) algo-
　　rithm used in digital radiography
Drennan metaphyseal-epiphyseal angle
Dressler post-myocardial infarction
　　syndrome
DREZ (dorsal root entry zone) lesion
DRG (dorsal root ganglia)
DRI (Doppler Resistive Index)
drifting wedge pressure
drip infusion cholangiography (DIC)
drooping lily appearance
drop finger
drop foot
dropsy (hydrops)
drop test for pneumoperitoneum
drowned lung
Drummond marginal artery
Drummond sign of aortic aneurysm
dry pleurisy
dry swallow on esophageal manometry
Drystar dry imager
DSA (digital subtraction angiography)
　　frameless stereotaxic
　　intra-arterial
　　intravenous
DSAS (discrete subvalvular aortic
　　stenosis)
DSC (dynamic susceptibility contrast)
　　MR imaging
D-shaped vessel lumen
DSI camera
D signal
DTAF-F (descending thoracic
　　aortofemoral-femoral) bypass
DTI (Doppler tissue imaging)
DTICH (delayed traumatic intracere-
　　bral hemorrhage [or hematoma])
D to E slope on echocardiography
DTPA (diethylenetriaminepentaacetic
　　acid)

DTPA renography
DTPA, technetium bound to
D-transposition (dextrotransposition)
  of great arteries
D2 dopamine receptors
dual atrioventricular node pathway
dual balloon method
dual blood supply
dual contrast study
dual echo DIET fast SE imaging
dual echo sequence
dual energy x-ray absorptiometry
  (DEXA)
dual GRE pulse sequences
dual head gamma camera system
dual head SPECT
dual isotope scanning
dual isotope single-photon emission
  CT
dual lookup table algorithm
dual phase scan
dual phase ^{99m}Tc-sestamibi imaging
dual photon absortiometry (DPA)
dual photon densitometry
dual x-ray absorptiometry (DXA)
Dubin-Johnson syndrome
Dubin-Sprinz disease
Ducor-Cordis pigtail catheter
Ducor HF (high-flow) catheter
duct
  aberrant
  aberrant bile
  accessory hepatic
  accessory pancreatic
  alveolar
  amniotic
  arterial
  Bartholin
  beaded hepatic
  bile
  biliary
  Botallo

duct *(cont.)*
  branchial
  bucconeural
  canalicular
  carotid
  choledochous
  cochlear
  common
  common bile (CBD)
  common gall
  common hepatic
  craniopharyngeal
  cystic
  cystic gall
  deferent
  distal bile
  efferent
  ejaculatory
  endolymphatic
  excretory
  extrahepatic bile
  frontonasal
  fusiform widening of
  galactophorous
  gall
  Gartner
  genital
  hepatic
  Hering
  His
  hypophyseal Rathke
  interlobular bile
  intrahepatic biliary
  involution of
  lacrimal
  lymph
  lymphatic
  main pancreatic (MPD)
  middle extrahepatic bile
  müllerian
  normal caliber
  obstruction of

duplex imaging, color-flow
duplex pulsed-Doppler sonography
duplex scan
   color-flow
   renal
duplex screening test
duplex ultrasound
duplicated renal collecting system
DuPont CRONEX x-ray film
DuPont Rare Earth Imaging System
DuPont scanner
Dupuytren contracture
Dupuytren fracture
dura
   attenuated
   bulging
dural arteriovenous malformation
dural attachment(s)
dural fold
dural impingement
dural sac
dural scar
dural sheath
dural sinus thrombosis (DST)
dural tear
dural trail sign
dural venous sinus thrombosis
dura mater of brain
dura mater of spinal cord
Duret lesion
Durham flatfoot
Duroziez mitral stenosis disease
DUS (dynamic ultrasound of
   shoulder)
Dusard syndrome
Duverney fracture
dV/dt (contractility)
DVI (deep venous insufficiency)
DVI (device-independent)
DVI (digital vascular imaging)
DVI Simpson atherocath
DVP (draining vein pressure)

DVT (deep venous thrombosis)
dwarfism
   achondroplastic
   deprivation
   Lorain-Lévi
   pituitary
   renal
   Russell-Silver
   Walt Disney
dwarf pelvis
DXA (dual x-ray absorptiometry)
^{166}Dy (dysprosium) ^{166}Ho
   holmium in vivo generator
Dy-DTPA-BMA imaging agent
dye (see *imaging agent*)
dye fluorescence index (DFI)
dye punch fracture
dynamic beat filtration
dynamic bolus
dynamic computerized tomography
   (CT)
dynamic conformal therapy
   (irradiation)
dynamic contrast-enhanced subtraction
   study
dynamic filtering
dynamic lineshape effects
dynamic multileaf collimation
dynamic pedobarography
dynamic radiotherapy
dynamic range control (DRC) algorithm used in digital radiography
dynamic snapshot
Dynamic Spatial Reconstructor (DSR)
   scanner
dynamic susceptibility contrast (DSC)
   magnetic resonance imaging
dynamic tagging magnetic resonance
   angiography
dynamic ultrasound of shoulder (DUS)
dynamic volume-rendered display
dynamic volumetric SPECT

dynamic wedge
Dynarad portable imaging system
dynode
dynograph
dyschezia
dyschondroplasia
dyscollagenosis
dyscrasic fracture
dysfunction
   positional
   swallowing
dysgenesis
   alar
   anorectal
   callosal
   corticocallosal
   epiphyseal
   gonadal
dyshormonogenesis
dyskinesia
   bile duct
   biliary
   regional
   tardive
   anterior wall
   anteroapical
   left ventricular
   segmental wall motion
   wall motion
dysmaturity, pulmonary
dysmotility, esophageal
dysosteogenesis
dysostosis
   cleidocranial
   craniofacial
   metaphyseal
dysostosis multiplex
dyspepsia
dyspeptic
dysphagia
   contractile ring
   esophageal

dysphagia *(cont.)*
   liquid food
   oropharyngeal
   postvagotomy
   pre-esophageal
   progressive
   sideropenic
   soft food
   solid food
   vallecular
dysphagia inflammatoria
dysphagia lusoria
dysphagia nervosa
dysphagia paralytica
dysphagia spastica
dysphagia valsalviana
dysplasia
   acropectorovertebral
   arteriohepatic
   bone
   bronchopulmonary
   cleidocranial
   congenital (of hip) (CDH)
   congenital polyvalvular
   cranioskeletal
   developmental
   diaphyseal
   endocardial
   epiarticular osteochondromatous
   familial arterial fibromuscular
   fibromuscular (FMD)
   fibrous
   foot
   mesomelic
   microscopic cortical
   mammary
   metaphyseal
   Mondini
   monostotic fibrous
   multiple epiphyseal
   Namaqualand hip
   oculoauriculovertebral (OAV)

dysplasia *(cont.)*
   odontoid
   osseous
   perimedial
   polyostotic fibrous
   polypoid
   progressive diaphyseal
   pulmonary valve (PVD)
   retroareolar
   right ventricular
   sheetlike
   Sponastrine
   spondyloepiphyseal
   Streeter
   tricuspid valve
   thymic
   ventricular
   ventriculo-radial
dysplasia with associated lesion or
   mass (DALM)
dyspnea on exertion

dysprosium analogue
dysprosium (^{166}Dy) ^{166}Ho holmium
   in vivo generator
dysprosium HP-DO3A imaging agent
dysraphism
   closed spinal
   occult spinal
   spinal
dyssynergia
   biliary
   detrusor-sphincter
   regional
   segmental
dyssynergy
dystocia
   fetal
   shoulder
dystopia
dystopic
dystrophy
dysuria

E, e

EAC (expandable access catheter)
E:A ratio on echocardiogram
early-phase termination
early venous filling
Eastman Kodak scanner
EBA (extrahepatic biliary atresia)
EBCT (electron beam computed
    tomography)
EBDA (effective balloon dilated area)
Eberth line
EBIORT (electron beam intraoperative
    radiotherapy)
EBRT (external beam radiation
    therapy)
Ebstein sign
eburnation, bony
ECA (external carotid artery)
E-CABG (endarterectomy and
    coronary artery bypass graft)
eccentrically placed lumen
eccentric atherosclerotic plaque
eccentric atrial activation
eccentric axis of rotation of the ankle
eccentric coronary artery
eccentric hypertrophy
eccentricity index
eccentric ledge

eccentric lesion
eccentric plaque disease
eccentric stenosis
eccentric vessel
ecchondroma
eccrine angiomatous hamartoma
ECG (electrocardiogram)
    ECG gating
    ECG-synchronized digital
        subtraction angiography
echo (slang for echocardiogram)
echo (pl. echoes)
    amphoric
    atrial
    bright
    dense
    highly mobile
    internal
    solid
    homogeneous
    inhomogeneous
    linear
    median level
    metallic
    navigator
    shower of
    sonographic

echo *(cont.)*
   specular
   spin
   swirling smokelike
   thick
   ultrasonographic
   ultrasound
   ventricular
echocardiogram
echocardiogram adenosine
echocardiographic automated border
echocardiography
   akinesis on
   ambulatory Holter
   A-mode
   anterior left ventricular wall
      motion
   apical
   apical five-chamber view
   apical left ventricular wall motion
      on
   apical two-chamber view
   B bump on anterior mitral valve
      leaflet
   B-mode
   biplane transesophageal
   blood pool radionuclide
   cardiac output
   color flow imaging Doppler
   continuous loop exercise
   continuous wave Doppler
   contrast
   contrast-enhanced
   cross-sectional two-dimensional
   CW (continuous wave) Doppler
   D-to-E slope on
   detection
   dipyridamole
   dobutamine stress
   Doppler
   dyskinesis on
   echo-free space on

echocardiography *(cont.)*
   echo intensity disappearance rate on
   epicardial Doppler
   E point on
   exercise
   Feigenbaum
   fetal (in utero)
   four-chamber
   hypokinesis on
   inferior left ventricular wall
      motion on
   intracardiac (ICE)
   intracoronary contrast
   intraoperative cardioplegic contrast
   late systolic posterior displacement
      on
   lateral left ventricular wall motion
      on
   left ventricular long-axis
   long-axis parasternal view
   loss of an "a" dip on
   MCE (myocardial contrast
      echocardiography)
   M-mode Doppler
   multiplanar transesophageal
   myocardial contrast (MCE)
   myocardial perfusion
   parasternal long-axis view
   parasternal short-axis view
   pharmacologic stress
   postcontrast
   posterior left ventricular wall
      motion on
   postexercise
   postinjection
   postmyocardial infarction
   precontrast
   preinjection
   premyocardial infarction
   pulsed Doppler
   pulsed-wave (PW) Doppler
   real-time

edema *(cont.)*
  plerocephalic
  postoperative pulmonary
  pulmonary
  reexpansion pulmonary
  renal
  solid (of lungs)
  stasis
  subglottic
  supraglottic
  terminal
  thalamic
  trace
  vasogenic
  venous
  vernal (of lung)
  visceral
edema fluid
edema neonatorum
edematous tissues
edentulous
edge
  boundary
  leading
  ligament reflecting
  ligament shelving
  liver
  Poupart ligament shelving
  sawtooth
  shelving
  sternal
  tentorial
  trailing
edge-boundary artifact
edge-detection angiography
edge effect
edge-enhanced error diffusion
  algorithm
edge misalignment artifact
edge profile acutance
edge-region pixel
edge ringing artifact

EDH (epidural hematoma)
EDL (extensor digitorum longus)
  muscle
Edmondson Grading System for
  hepatocellular carcinoma
EDQ (extensor digiti quinti) muscle
EDRT (endothelium-derived relaxant
  factor)
EDSRF spectrome
EDV (end-diastolic volume)
Edwards diagnostic catheter
EDXRF spectrometer
EF (ejection fraction)
EFF (electromagnetic focusing field)
  probe
efface, effacement
  cistern
  cisterna magna
  dural sac
  nerve root sheath
  sulcus
  ventricle
effect
  adverse
  anisotropic
  Anrep
  artifact
  attenuation
  Bayliss
  Bohr
  BOLD
  Bowditch
  bronchodilator
  bronchomotor
  cobra head
  collimator exchange
  Compton
  copper wire
  cumulative
  deleterious
  demagnetization field
  Dotter

electrocardiogram tracing
electrocardiographic gating
electrocardiographic variant
electrocardiography, electrocardiogram (ECG or EKG)
electrocardiography-gated echo-planar
 imaging
electrocardiophonogram
electrocardioscanner, Compuscan
 Hittman computerized
electrocorticographic evaluation
electrode monitoring
electrogastrogram
electrogastrography
electrolytes
electrolytic
electromagnet, structured coil
electromagnetic blood flow study
electromagnetic interference (EMI)
electromechanical dissociation (EMD)
 of heart
electrometer
electromyogram
electromyography
electron and x-ray diffraction patterns
electron arc therapy
electron beam boost
electron beam computed tomography
 (EBCT)
electron beam CT scanner
electron beam intraoperative
 radiotherapy (EBIORT)
electron bolus
electron dosimetry
electron equilibrium loss
electron linear accelerator
electron microscopy
electron photon field matching
electron production, secondary
electron spin resonance (ESR)
electronic portal imaging
electrons, backscatter

electrophilic radioiodination
electrophoresis
electrostatic potential
electrovectorcardiogram
electrovectorcardiography
element
 posterior
 neoplastic destruction of spinal
 subluxation of
elevated diaphragms
elevated hemidiaphragms
elimination kinetics
Elite double-loop catheter
Ellestad protocol for treadmill stress
 test
ellipsoid joint
elliptical
ellipticity index
Ellis-Garland line
Ellis line
Ellis sign
elongated heart
elongation and tortuosity
eloquent areas of brain
ELPIDA architecture
Elscint camera
Elscint dual-detector cardiac camera
Elscint Planar device
Elscint CT scanner
Elscint Twin CT scanner
Elsner syndrome
eluted
elution
elutriation
embarrassment
 circulatory
 cord
 midbrain function
 nerve root
 respiratory
embedding of stent coils
embolectomy, percutaneous balloon

embolization *(cont.)*
  coil (therapeutic)
  diffuse cholesterol
  disseminated atheromatous
  disseminated cholesterol
  endovascular
  flow-directed
  Gelfoam powder
  Ivalon
  massive
  microvascular
  percutaneous transvenous
  selective percutaneous transhepatic
  selective renal artery
  septic
  Silastic bead
  stent
  subsegmental transcatheter arterial (STAE)
  super selective
  therapeutic
  tract
  transarterial
  transcatheter oily chemo-embolization
  transcatheter variceal
  transhepatic (THE)
embolization transcatheter therapy
embolotherapy, catheter
embolus (pl. emboli) (see *embolism*)
embolus trap, Mobin-Uddin
embryonal cell carcinoma
embryonal tumor
embryonal vein
embryonic anastomosis
embryonic aortic arch
embryonic branchial arch
EMED scanner
emergent
emergently
emesis
EMF (endomyocardial fibrosis)

EMI CT scanner
eminence
  arcuate
  articular
  collateral
  cruciate
  cruciform
  deltoid
  facial
  frontal
  genital
  hypothenar
  iliopubic
  iliopectineal
  intercondylar
  intercondyloid
  medial
  median
  occipital
  pyramidal
  thenar
  thyroid
  tibial
emission and transmission data
emission probability
emitter
  alpha-particle
  Auger-electron
emphysema
  alveolar
  alveolar duct
  atrophic
  bronchiolar
  bullous
  centriacinar
  centrilobular
  chronic
  chronic hypertrophic
  chronic obstructive
  chronic tuberculous
  compensating
  compensatory

emphysema *(cont.)*
  congenital lobar
  cystic
  cystic pulmonary
  diffuse
  distal acinar
  distal lobular
  ectatic
  false
  focal-dust
  gangrenous
  generalized
  giant bullous
  glass blower's
  hypoplastic
  idiopathic unilobar
  infantile lobar
  interlobular
  interstitial
  intestinal
  liquefactive
  lobar
  localized obstructive
  lung
  mediastinal
  neck
  necrotizing
  neonatal cystic pulmonary
  obstructive
  oxygen-dependent
  panlobular
  paracicatricial
  paraseptal
  pericicatricial
  postoperative
  postsurgical
  pulmonary
  pulmonary interstitial (PIE)
  pulmonary subcutaneous
    encephalitis
  senile
  skeletal

emphysema *(cont.)*
  small-lunged
  subcutaneous
  substantial
  surgical
  traumatic
  unilateral
  unilateral pulmonary
  vesicular
emphysematous bleb
emphysematous bulla
emphysematous cholecystitis
emphysematous COPD (chronic
  obstructive pulmonary disease)
emphysematous gastritis
emphysematous lungs
emphysematous pyelonephritis
emphysematous type A disease
empirical therapy
emplaced (verb)
empty collapsed lung
emptying time
emptying, tortuous
empty sella syndrome
empyema
  chest
  gallbladder
  interlobar
  latent
  left-sided
  loculated
  metapneumonic
  pericardial
  pleural
  pulsating
  right-sided
  spinal
  subdural
  synpneumonic
  thoracic
  tuberculous
empyema with pachypleuritis

en bloc
encapsulated radioactive "seeds"
encephalitic
encephaloarteriography
encephalocele with cranium bifidum
encephaloclastic lesion
encephalocystocele
encephalodysplasia
encephaloid
encephalolith
encephaloma
encephalomalacia
encephalopathy
encerclage
enchondral ossification
enchondroma
enchondromatosis
encircle
encircled
encircling
encirclement
encoded-Fourier
encoded, wavelet-
encoding gradient
encroachment
   bony
   foraminal
   luminal
encryption algorithms
encryption, scheme
en cuirasse, cor
encysted pleurisy
endarterectomy and coronary artery
   bypass graft (E-CABG)
end diastole
end-diastolic flow
end-diastolic polar map
end-diastolic pressure
end-diastolic pressure-volume relation
end-diastolic velocity (EDV)
end-diastolic volume (EDV)
end-expiratory lung volume (FRC)

end-expiratory pressure
end-inspiratory pressure
endoanal coil
endoanal sonography
endobrachyesophagus
endobronchial brachytherapy
endobronchial carcinoma
endocardial activation mapping
endocardial catheter mapping
endocardial cushion defect
endocardial fibroelastosis
endocardial fibrosis, Davies
endocardial mapping
endocarditis
endocardium
   disc of
   wafer of
endocavitary applicator system
endochondral bone
endochondral ossification
EndoCoil biliary stent
endocranium
endocrine fracture
endodermal cyst
endoergic reaction
end of atrial systole
endogenous callus formation
endoluminal stent
endolymphatic duct
endolymphatic sac
endometrial echo
endometrial polyp
endometriosis
   colonic involvement of
   sciatic
   studding of
endomyocardial biopsy, ultrasonic
   guidance for
endomyocardial fibrosis, mural
end-on vessel
endophlebitis
Endo-P-Probe

endoprosthesis
  biliary
  double-lumen
  double-pigtail
  large-bore bile duct
  self-expanding metallic
endorectal coil
endorectal ileal pouch
endorectal ileal pull-through
endorectal ultrasonography
end-organ
endoscopic catheterization
endoscopic quadrature RF coil
endoscopic retrograde cholangiography
  (ERC)
endoscopic retrograde cholangiopan-
  creatography (ERCP)
endoscopic retrograde pancreatic duct
  cannulation
endoscopic retrograde parenchy-
  mography (ERP)
endoscopic sclerosing therapy
endoscopic ultrasound (EUS)
endoscopic washing pipe
endoscopic water pick
endoscopically
endoscopist
endoscopy, virtual
endoskeleton
EndoSonics IVUS/balloon dilatation
  catheter
endosonogram
endosonography
endosteal callus
endosteal revascularization
endosteal surface
endosteum
endosystolic volume (ESV)
endotenon
endothelialization of stent
endothelialized vascular grafts
endotheliomatous meningioma

endothelium
  arterial
  pulmonary capillary
  squamous
endothelium-derived contracting factor
endothelium-derived relaxant factor
  (EDRF)
Endotrac carpal tunnel release system
endotracheal (ET) tube intubation
endovaginal sonography
endovascular aortic graft
endovascular coil
endovascular embolization
endovascular flow wire study
endovascular stent-graft
endovascular therapy
endovascular ultrasonography
endplate
  hyaline-cartilage (of intervertebral
    disk)
  vertebral body
endpoint, measurable
end-pressure artifact
end-stage rejection
end-stage renal failure
end-systolic polar map
end-systolic pressure-volume relation
end-systolic reversal
end-systolic volume (ESV) indices
end-to-end anastomosis
end-to-side anastomosis
enema
  air
  air contrast barium
  analeptic
  barium (BE)
  blind
  contrast
  Cortenema retention
  double contrast barium (DCBE)
  flatus
  Fleet

enema *(cont.)*
   full column barium
   Gastrografin
   Harris flush
   hydrocortisone
   hydrogen peroxide
   Kayexalate
   lactulose
   mesalamine
   methylene blue
   nuclear
   phosphate
   phosphosoda
   prednisolone
   retention
   Rowasa
   saline cleansing
   single-contrast barium
   small bowel
   soapsuds (SSE)
   steroid foam
   sulfasalazine
   tap water
   theophylline olamine
   water soluble contrast
enemas administered until clear
energy
   beam
   kinetic
   low photon
   treatment
   variable
energy decays
energy transfer process
en face view
Engel-Recklinghausen disease
Engelmann disease
engorged collecting system
engorged tissues
engorged veins
engorgement
   vascular
   venous

Enhance deblurring method
enhanced imaging
enhancement
   contrast
   Doppler flow signal
   heterogeneous isodense
   isodense
   nodule
   nonhomogeneous
   PALA
   peak
   signal
   vascular MR contrast
enhancement morphology
enhancement pattern
enhancement rate, instantaneous
enhancing lesion
enlargement
   cardiac silhouette
   chamber
   compensatory
   hilar lymph node
   mediastinal lymph node
enophthalmic
en plaque, meningioma
ensiform appendix
ensiform process
ensued, ensuing
enteral alimentation
enteral nutrition (EN)
enterobiliary
enterocele sac
enterococcus
enterocutaneous fistula
enterocystoma
enteroenteral fistula
enteroinsular axis
enterolith
enteroperitoneal abscess
enteroptosis
enterourethral fistula
enterovesical fistula

erector spinae
ERF (external rotation in flexion)
ergonovine test
erosion
    articular
    bony
    bronchial
    duodenal
    gastric
    gastric antral
    graft-enteric
    linear
    osteoclastic
    pedicle
    plaque
    salt and pepper duodenal
    tumor
erosion of articular surface
erosive gastritis
ERP (effective refractory period)
ERP (endoscopic retrograde
    parenchymography)
    atrial
    ventricular
ERPF (effective renal plasma flow)
error
    darkroom
    Hausdorff
    isocenter placement
    magnification
    mean-square
    photoreceptor fractional velocity
    positioning
    raster spacing
    sensing
    size estimation
error diffusion method
error sum criterion
erythema of joint
erythematosus, systemic lupus
escape beat
escape interval

escape mechanism, ventricular
escape of air into lung connective
    tissue
escape-peak ratio
E sign on x-ray
ESIN (elastic stable intramedullary
    nailing)
ESOLAN program
EsophaCoil biliary stent
esophageal A ring
esophageal B ring
esophageal fold
esophageal hiatus
esophageal inlet
esophageal motility disorder,
    nonspecific (NEMD)
esophageal obturator airway
esophageal plexus
esophageal reflux
esophageal spasm
esophageal varices
esophageal web
esophageal window
esophagitis
esophagogastric fat pad
esophagogastric junction
esophagogram
esophagorespiratory fistula
esophagospasm
esophagram
    barium swallow
    contrast
esophagus
    achalasia of
    aperistaltic
    A ring of
    Barrett
    B ring of
    cervical
    columnar-lined
    corkscrew (diffuse esophageal
      spasm)

Evans syndrome
EVD (external ventricular drain)
even distribution of echoes in
    ultrasonography
event
    adverse
    atrial sensed (As)
    cardinal
    embolic
    inciting
    ischemic
    morbid
    precipitating
    untoward
    ventricular sensed
event counter
event marker
event recorder
eventration (peaking)
eventration of diaphragms
eversion sprain
evert, everted
evolution, stroke in
evolving stroke
Ewald test meal
Ewart sign
Ewing tumor
ex vacuo, hydrocephalus
ex vivo magnetic resonance imaging
exacerbate, exacerbated
exacerbation, acute
exam (examination)
exametazime imaging agent
exanthematous disease
excavatum, pectus
excellent prognosis
excessive joint play
exchange
    air
    catheter
    coupling
    guide wire
    narrowing

excimer (from "excited dimer") laser
excitation
    TCR rebound
    variable flip angle
    wave of
excitation function measurement
excitation profile
excitation-spoiled fat-suppressed T1-
    weighted SE images
exclusionary cue
exclusion-HPLC technique
exclusion, subtotal gastric
excrescence, bony
excrete
excretory intravenous pyelography
excretory phase
excretory urogram
excursion
exenteration, total pelvic
exercise echocardiography
exercise first-pass LVEF
exercise images
exercise-induced ischemia
exercise intolerance
exercise load (kpm/min)
exercise, modified stage
exercise oximetry
exercise strain gauge venous
    plethysmography
exercise stress-redistribution
    scintigraphy
exercise thallium-201 stress test
exercise thallium-201 tomography
exhalation
exit site of catheter
exit wound
Exner plexus
exocardia
exoccipital bone
exoergic reaction
exogenous obesity
exophytic adenocarcinoma

external iliac artery
external inguinal ring
external jugular vein
external oblique aponeurosis
external ring
external ventricular drain (EVD)
external wire fixation
extirpation of saphenous vein
extra-articular fracture
extra-adrenal chromaffin tissue
extra-adrenal sites
extra-articular resection
extra-axial fluid collection, crescent-
   shaped
extracapsular dissection
extracapsular fracture
extracardiac anomalies
extracardiac collateral circulation
extracardiac right-to-left shunt
extracavitary-infected graft
extracavitary prosthetic arterial graft
extracerebral intracranial glioneural
   hamartoma
extracorporeal membrane oxygenation
   (ECMO) therapy
extracorporeal photochemotherapy
extracorporeal shock wave lithotripsy
   (ESWL)
extracranial carotid artery atherosclerosis
extracranial carotid occlusive disease
extracranial cerebral circulation
extracranial-intracranial bypass (ECIC)
extracranial vessel
extraction
   automatic
   contour
   disphenoid
   first-pass
   fringe skeleton
   stone
   vascular segmentation and

extraction catheter
   transcutaneous
   transluminal
extraction catheter atherectomy
extraction column
extraction method
extradural artery
extradural compartment
extradural defect
extradural space
extradural tumor
extradural vertebral plexus of veins
extrahepatic bile ducts, dilated
extrahepatic biliary atresia (EBA)
extraintestinal
extraluminal air
extraluminal contrast medium
extraluminal endarterectomy
extramedullary hemangioma
extraneous material
extraovarian mass
extraparenchymal cyst
extrapericardial dissection
extraperitoneal rupture
extrapleural drainage
extrapleural hemorrhage
extrapleural space
extrapolate
extrapolation
extrapulmonary tuberculosis
extrapyramidal tract
extraskeletal osteosarcoma
extrathecal nerve roots
extrathoracic obstruction
extrauterine gestation
extrauterine pregnancy
extravasated blood
extravasated contrast
extravasation
   bile
   blood
   contrast

extravasation *(cont.)*
  dye
  fluid
  intravascular content
  joint fluid
  radiopaque fluid
  urinary
extravascular fluid
extravascular mass
extravascular pressure
extraventricular obstruction
extravesical opacification
extremity (pl. extremities)
  lower (LEs)
  upper (UEs)
extrinsic compression of trachea
extrinsic foot muscles
extrinsic lesion
extrinsic sick sinus syndrome
extrude

extruding
extrusion, disk
extubate, extubation
exuberant atheroma formation
exuberant granulation tissue
exudate
exudation
exudation of fibrin-rich fluid
exudative consolidation
exudative effusion
exudative pericardial fluid
exudative pleurisy
exudative tuberculosis
eye shield
  lead
  tungsten
eye view, beam's
eye-view 3D-CRT
eyelet, rod
E-Z-Paque barium suspension

F, f

F (fluorine)
FAB (French/American/British)
  classification
Fab (fragment antigen binding)
  fragment
fabella
fabellofibular complex
Fabry disease
face, en
facet (also facette)
  articular
  atlas
  capitate
  clavicular
  corneal
  costal
  flat
  hamate
  inferior
  inferior costal
  inferior medial
  Lenoir
  locked
  lunate
  scaphoid
  squatting
  superior

facet *(cont.)*
  superior articular
  superior costal
  transverse costal
facet capsule disruption
facet dislocation
facet joint
facet joint vacuum
facet surface of vertebra
facet syndrome
facet tropism
facetal imbrication
faceted gallstone
facial bipartition
facial fracture
facial nerve (seventh cranial nerve)
facial nerve canal
facies ossea
facile synthesis
facing of metacarpal heads
facioauriculovertebral (FAV)
    syndrome
faciostenosis
FACScan (fluorescence-activated cell
    sorter) flow cytometer
FACSVantage cell sorter
factitial

factor (pl. factors)
  Boltzmann
  EDRT
  endothelium-derived relaxant
    (EDRT)
  epidermal growth
  equilibrium
  geometry
  NOMOS correction
  overrelaxation
  prognostic
  recurrent human granulocyte colony
    stimulating (r-met HuG-CSF)
  technical
  wedge
Fahr-Volhard disease
FAI (functional aerobic impairment)
failed back surgery syndrome (FBSS)
failure
  adrenal
  cardiac
  congestive heart (CHF)
  hepatic
  liver
  heart
  multiple organ
  multisystem
  pituitary
  pulmonary
  renal
  respiratory
  vein graft
  ventricular
Fairbanks changes on x-ray
falciform ligament
falcine region
falcotentorial meningioma
falcula
falcular
fallopian tube
fallopian tube diverticula
fallopian tube occlusion

falloposcopy (with imaging)
Fallot, tetralogy of
fallout, signal
false aneurysm
false channel
false color scale
false diverticulum
false emphysema
false lumen
false sac
falx
  calcification of
  cerebral
falx cerebelli
falx cerebri
falx meningioma
familial adenomatous polyposis (FAP)
familial aortic dissection
familial avascular necrosis of
    phalangeal epiphysis
familial cardiomegaly
familial cavernous malformation
familial goiter
familial hypophosphatemic rickets
fan angle
fan beam
fan-beam collimator
fan-beam formula
fan-beam projection
fan-beam reconstruction
Fanconi-Hegglin syndrome
fan-shaped view
FAP (femoral artery pressure)
Faraday catheter
Farber disease
Farber syndrome
far field
farmer's lung
fascia
  anal
  antebrachial
  anterior rectus

fascia *(cont.)*
- axillary
- bicipital
- brachial
- broad
- buccopharyngeal
- Camper
- cervical
- clavipectoral
- Cloquet
- Colles
- cremasteric
- crural
- cribriform
- Cruveilhier
- deep
- deltoid
- dentate
- diaphragmatic
- endopelvic
- endothoracic
- extraperitoneal
- Gerota
- iliac
- infraspinous
- investing
- lateral oblique
- lateroconal
- lumbar
- medial geniculate
- obturator
- obturator internus
- palmar
- parietal pelvic
- pelvic
- perineal
- psoas
- quadratus femoris
- renal
- rim of
- Scarpa
- Sibson

fascia *(cont.)*
- subcutaneous
- superficial
- superficial temporalis
- superficial temporoparietal
- thoracolumbar
- visceral pelvic

fascia lata (but *tensor fasciae latae*)
fascial plane
fascial rent
fascial thickening
fascial tract
fasciculus (pl. fasciculi)
- arcuate
- lenticular
- longitudinal
- longitudinalis medialis
- medial longitudinal (MLF)

fasciogram
FAST (flow-assisted, short-term)
FAST balloon catheter
Fastcard
fast cardiac phase contrast cine imaging
fast dynamic volumetric x-ray CT
fast-FLAIR technique
fast-flow lesions
fast-flow malformation
fast-flow vascular anomaly
fast Fourier spectral analysis
fast Fourier transform (FFT)
fast fractionation
fast GE (Fastcard) sequences
fast low-angle shot (FLASH)
fast multiplanar spoiled gradient-recalled (FMPSPGR) imaging
fast-neutron therapy
fast PC cine MR sequence with echo-planar gradient
fast routine production
fast SE (FSE) imaging
fast SE and fast IR (FMPIR) imaging

fast SE train
fast short tau inversion recovery (fast STIR)
fast spin echo MR imaging
fast spin echo T2-weighted image
fast spoiled gradient-recalled MR imaging
fast STIR (short tau inversion recovery)
fat
   abdominal
   dietary
   digital process of
   extraperitoneal
   ischiorectal pad of
   pericolonic
   perihilar
   perinephric
   perirectal
   perirenal
   preperitoneal
   properitoneal
   protruding
   renal
   subcutaneous
fatal dose of radiation
fatal exsanguination
fatal herniation
fat embolism syndrome (FES)
fat embolus, cerebral
fatigability
fatigue damage
fatigue fracture
fatigue, progressively severe
fat line, subcutaneous
fat metabolism
fat pad
   abdominal
   antimesenteric
   foveal
   heel
   Hoffa

fat pad *(cont.)*
   intrapatellar
   ischiorectal
   pericardial
   scalene
fat pad sign
fat plane
fat selective presaturation
fat signal intensity
fat-suppressed three-dimensional spoiled gradient-echo FLASH MR imaging
fat suppression, double-echo three-point Dixon method
fat suppression pulse
fat suppression technique
fatty acid metabolism
fatty degeneration
fatty filum terminale
fatty infiltration of liver
fatty liver
fatty meal sonogram (FMS)
fatty streak atherosclerosis
fatty tumor
fat-water interface
fauces (pl. of faux)
   anterior pillar of
   arch of
fault, sagittal plane
faulty colloid preparation with excess aluminum
faulty RF (radiofrequency) shielding in MRI scanner room artifact
faux (see *fauces*)
faveolate
Favre disease
FB (foreign body)
FBP (filtered back-projection) method
FBS (failed back syndrome)
FBSS (failed back surgery syndrome)
FCR (flexor carpi radialis) muscle
FCR 9501HQ high-resolution storage phosphor imaging agent

FCS (full cervical spine) series of
  x-rays
FCU (flexor carpi ulnaris) muscle
FDC (flexor digitorum communis)
  muscle
FDG (fluorodeoxyglucose; fludeoxy-
  glucose F-18)
  FDG-blood flow mismatch
  FDG-labeled positron imaging
  FDG myocardial imaging
  FDG PET scan
  FDG SPECT
FDI (first digital interosseous) muscle
FDI (frequency domain imaging) in
  ultrasound
FDL (flexor digitorum longus) muscle
FDP (fibrin degradation products) on
  MRI
FDP (flexor digitorum profundus)
  muscle
FDQ (flexor digiti quinti) muscle
FDQB (flexor digiti quinti brevis)
  muscle
FDS (flexor digitorum sublimis)
  muscle
FDS (flexor digitorum superficialis)
  muscle
Fe-Ex orogastric tube magnet
feasible alternatives
feathery appearance
fecal impaction
fecal incontinence
fecal material, retained
fecal residue
fecalith
fecaloid
fecaloma
fecaluria
feces
  impacted
  inspissation of
feculence

feculent
Federici sign
feedback
  breathing
  real-time respiratory
feeder arteries
feeder veins
feeding artery to aneurysm
feeding branch of artery
feeding mean arterial pressure
  (FMAP)
feeding vessel
Feigenbaum echocardiogram
Feiss line
Feldaker syndrome
Feldkamp algorithm
felon
Felty syndrome
fem-pop (slang for femoral-popliteal)
  bypass
feminine aorta, small
feminizing tumor
femoral above-knee popliteal bypass
femoral anteversion
femoral aortic flush catheter
femoral approach for cardiac
  catheterization
femoral artery
femoral artery pressure
femoral bone
femoral capital epiphysis
femoral condyle
femoral-femoral bypass graft
femoral-femoral crossover
femoral head and neck
femoral head deformity
femoral head vascularity
femoral hernia
femoral neck
femoral-peroneal in situ vein bypass
  graft
femoral-popliteal bypass surgery

femoral-popliteal Gore-Tex graft
femoral pulse
femoral tuberosity
femoral vein
femoral vein percutaneous insertion
femoral venoarterial bypass
femoral venous approach
femoral view
femoroaxillary bypass
femorocrural graft
femorodistal bypass
femorodistal popliteal bypass graft
femorofemoral approach
femorofemoral bypass
femorofemoropopliteal
femoroperoneal bypass graft
femoropopliteal angioplasty
femoropopliteal artery
femoropopliteal atheromatous stenosis
femoropopliteal bypass
femoropopliteal thrombosis
femorotibial angle (FTA)
femorotibial bypass graft
femtoliter (fL)
femur (pl. femora)
   apex of
   body of
   greater trochanter of
   head and neck of
   head of
   lesser trochanter of
   neck of
   nutrient artery of
femur length (FL)
fender fracture
fenestra (pl. fenestrae)
fenestration
   aortopulmonary
   apical
   cusp
   interchordal space

fenestration of dissecting aneurysm
Fenwick disease
Feridex contrast medium
ferric ammonium citrate contrast
ferric ammonium citrate-cellulose
   paste
ferric chloride contrast
ferrioxamine methanesulfonate
   contrast
ferrocalcinosis, familial cerebral
ferromagnetic objects creating artifacts
    on imaging studies
   bra underwire
   button
   cigarette lighter
   clothing with metal object
   earring
   hair coloring
   hairpin
   make-up
   metal mesh in toupee or wig
   necklace
   paper clip
   pen
   political button
   probe
   ring
   shunt
   tooth filling
   watch
   zipper
ferromagnetic properties
ferromagnetic relaxation
ferruginous bodies
ferumoxides-enhanced MR imaging
ferumoxsil imaging agent
FES (fat embolism syndrome)
fetal biophysical profile
fetal bradycardia
fetal cardiac anomalies
fetal chromosome abnormality

fetal death
  early
  intermediate
  late
fetal echocardiography in utero
fetal gallbladder
fetal heart
fetal heart failure
fetal hydrops
fetal lobulation
fetal malformation
fetal midface
fetal motion or movement
fetal-pelvic disproportion
fetal-pelvic index
fetal placenta
fetal pole
fetal small parts
fetal sonography
fetal ultrasonography
fetal umbilical vein injection under
  sonographic guidance
fetometry
fetus (pl. fetuses)
  amorphous
  calcified
  growth-retarded
  impacted
  intrauterine
  maturity of
  nonviable
  paper-doll
  parasitic
  placenta of
  presentation of
  previable
  retained dead
  small parts of
  stunted
  tissue of
  umbilical artery in
  viable

fetus papyraceus
FFA (free fatty acid) scintigraphy,
  labeled
FFE sequences
F-4500 Fluorescence Spectrophotometer
FFP (fresh frozen plasma)
FFT (fast Fourier transform) image
FHB (flexor hallucis brevis) muscle
FHC (familial hypertrophic cardiomyopathy)
FHL (flexor hallucis longus) muscle
FI (full-scan with interpolation)
  method/projection
fiber (pl. fibers)
  cardiac muscle
  muscle
  myocardial
  skeletal muscle
  sling muscle
fiberoptic angioscopy
fiberoptic bronchography
fiberoptic light source
fiberoptic tapers
fiberoptic video glasses
fibrillate
fibrin clot
fibrin degradation products (FDP) on
  MRI
fibrin glue, percutaneous
fibrin mass
fibrinogen
  radiolabeled
  technetium ^{99m}Tc-labeled
fibrinogen degradation
fibrinolytic treatment
fibrinopurulent pleurisy
fibrin sleeve stripping
fibrin split products
fibroadenoma
fibroadipose tissue
fibroblast radiosensitivity

fibroblastic meningioma
fibroblastoma, perineural
fibrocalcific cusps
fibrocalcification
fibrocartilage
  circumferential
  intra-articular plates of
  triangular
fibrocartilaginous disk
fibrocartilaginous plate
fibrocollagenous connective tissue
fibrocystic breast syndrome
fibrocystic residual
fibrodysplasia ossificans progressiva
fibroelastoma of heart valve
fibroelastoma, papillary
fibroid
  calcified
  intramural
  pedunculated
  uterine
fibroid lung
fibroid myocarditis
fibroid uterus
fibrolamellar hepatocarcinoma
fibrolamellar hepatocellular carcinoma
fibrolipoma
fibroma
  aponeurotic
  cementifying
  cemento-ossifying
  chondromyxoid (CMF)
  desmoplastic
  heart
  juvenile ossifying
  meningeal
  nonossifying
  nonosteogenic
  ossifying
  osteogenic
  periosteal
  subcutaneous

fibroma-thecoma tumor of ovary
fibromatosis
fibromuscular dysplasia (FMD)
fibromuscular lesion
fibromuscular ridge
fibromyoma
fibromyxoma, odontogenic
fibronodular
fibro-osseous lesion
fibro-osseous tunnel
fibroretractive
fibrosarcoma
fibrosclerotic
fibrosed muscles
fibroserous pericardial sac
fibrosing inflammatory pseudotumor
fibrosis
  alcoholic
  arachnoid
  basilar
  confluent
  congenital hepatic (CHF)
  cystic
  diffuse interstitial pulmonary
    (DIPF)
  endocardial
  endomyocardial (EMF)
  idiopathic interstitial
  idiopathic pulmonary (IPF)
  interstitial
  interstitial pulmonary
  leptomeningeal
  mediastinal
  meningeal
  myocardial
  nodal
  nodular subepidermal
  noncirrhotic portal (NCPF)
  pericentral
  periductal
  perimuscular
  periportal

fill and spill of dye (in fallopian
  tubes)
filling
  atrial
  augmented
  capillary
  decreased left ventricular
  left atrial
  left ventricular
  passive
  peak
  rapid
  reduced
  retrograde
  ureteral
  venous
  ventricular
  vessel
filling defect
filling factor
filling phase, rapid
filling pressure
filling rate, peak
film (see also *position, projection,*
   view)
  Accu-Flo dura
  AP (anteroposterior)
  chest
  chiropractic
  comparison
  cross-table lateral
  decubitus
  digital subtraction
  DuPont Cronex x-ray
  expiratory
  flat plate
  GLP7
  high-contrast
  Knuttsen bending
  lateral
  lateral decubitus
  limited

film *(cont.)*
  low-contrast
  low-dose
  manual subtraction
  oblique
  outside
  overhead
  PA (posteroanterior)
  photo-plotter
  plain
  port
  portable
  postevacuation
  postvoid
  postvoiding
  preliminary
  prone
  radiochromic
  scout
  sequential
  serial
  skull
  spot
  stress
  suboptimal
  subtraction
  supine
  UP7
  upright
  working
film alternator
film-based viewing
film changer, Sanchez-Perez automatic
filmless imaging
film slippage
filter
  bird's nest percutaneous IVC
    (inferior vena cava)
  caval
  differencing
  Gianturco-Roehm bird's nest vena
    caval
  Greenfield vena caval

filter *(cont.)*
   inferior vena caval
   IVC (inferior vena cava)
   Kalman
   Kimray-Greenfield caval
   Mobin-Uddin umbrella
   Mobin-Uddin vena caval
   percutaneous inferior vena cava
      (IVC)
   prophylactic IVC
   Simon nitinol percutaneous IVC
   Simon nitinol vena cava filter
   translation-invariant
   umbrella
   Venatech percutaneous IVC
   wall
   Wiener
filtered-back projection
filtering, dynamic
filtration
   copper
   dynamic beat
   glomerular
   post beat
filum, fatty
filum terminale, fatty
fimbriated end of fallopian tube
finding (pl. findings)
   angiographic
   auscultatory
   cardinal
   characteristic
   concomitant
   equivocal
   focal
   lateralizing
   no discernible
   ominous
   pathognomonic
   salient physical
   scanty
   specious
   spurious

fine calcification
fine needle
fine-needle biopsy, ultrasound-guided
fine reticular pattern
fine-speckled appearance
Finesse large-lumen guiding catheter
finger
   angle
   baseball
   base of
   bolster
   clubbed
   drop
   fingers
   football
   index
   jammed
   jersey
   little
   long
   mallet
   middle
   pedicle
   pulley of
   pulp of
   replantation of
   replanted
   ring
   sausage
   spade
   speck
   spider
   stoved
   trigger
   webbedb
finger fracture
finger fracture dissection
fingerlike projection
finger of tumor
finger opposition
finger pad
fingerprint image compression

fingertip amputation
fingertip pad
firing of ectopic atrial focus
firing temperature
first-pass effect
first-pass extraction
first-pass imaging
first-pass MUGA
first-pass myocardial perfusion MR
first-pass radionuclide exercise
   angiocardiography
first-pass study
first-pass view
first portion of duodenum
first-trimester nuchal translucency
Fischer sign
fish-flesh appearance
fishmeal worker's lung
fishmouth configuration of mitral
   valve
fishmouth stenosis
fish-scale gallbladder
FISP (gradient echo sequence)
FISP sequence
Fissinger-Rendu syndrome
fission track analysis of urine
fissula
fissuration
fissure
   abdominal
   anal
   anterior median (of cord)
   antitragohelicine
   auricular
   brain
   calcarine
   callosomarginal
   central
   cerebellar
   cerebellopontine or cerebellopontile
   cerebral
   choroidal

fissure *(cont.)*
   chronic
   collateral
   cutaneous
   decidual
   dentate
   displacement of interhemispheric
   glaserian
   hippocampal
   horizontal
   interhemispheric
   lateral
   longitudinal
   lung
   main
   oblique
   occipital
   oral
   palpebral
   portal
   rolandic
   studded
   superior orbital
   supraorbital
   sylvian
   umbilical
fissure fracture
fissure in ano
fissure of Rolando
fissure of Sylvius
fissure sign
fistula
   abdominal
   anal
   anorectal
   aorta-left ventricular
   aorta-right ventricular
   aortic sinus
   aortic sinus to right ventricle
   aortocaval
   aortoduodenal
   aortoenteric

fistula *(cont.)*
    aortoesophageal
    aortopulmonary
    aortosigmoid
    AV (arteriovenous)
    biliary
    biliary-cutaneous
    biliary-duodenal
    biliary-enteric
    bilioenteric
    Blom-Singer tracheoesophageal
    branchial
    Brescia-Cimino AV
    bronchobiliary
    bronchocavitary
    bronchocutaneous
    bronchoesophageal
    bronchopleural
    cameral
    carotid artery-cavernous sinus
    carotid cavernous
    carotid-cavernous sinus
    cerebral arteriovenous
    cerebrospinal fluid
    cholecystenteric
    cholecystocholedochal
    cholecystocolonic
    cholecystoduodenal
    cholecystoduodenocolic
    choledochal-colonic
    choledochoduodenal
    chylous
    coil closure of coronary artery
    colocutaneous
    colonic
    colovaginal
    colovesical
    complex anorectal
    congenital
    congenital pulmonary arteriovenous
    coronary
    coronary arteriosystemic

fistula *(cont.)*
    coronary arteriovenous
    coronary artery cameral
    coronary artery-pulmonary artery
    coronary artery to right ventricular
    coronary-cameral
    coronary-pulmonary
    CSF (cerebrospinal fluid)
    cystic
    duodenocolic
    dural arteriovenous (AVF)
    durocutaneous
    Eck
    enterocutaneous
    enteroenteral
    enteroenteric
    enterourethral
    enterovaginal
    enterovesical
    esophagorespiratory
    external biliary
    extrasphincteric anal
    fecal
    gastric
    gastrocolic
    gastroduodenal
    gastrojejunal-colic
    gastrojejunocolic
    genitourinary
    graft-enteric
    hepatic
    hepatic arteriovenous
    hepatopleural
    horseshoe
    H-type
    iatrogenic
    ileosigmoid
    intersphincteric anal
    intradural arteriovenous
    intradural retromedullary
        arteriovenous
    intrahepatic AV

fistula *(cont.)*
   intrapulmonary arteriovenous
   jejunocolic
   Mann-Bollman
   mediastinal
   mesenteric
   microvenoarteriolar
   mucous
   orofacial
   pancreatic
   pancreatic cutaneous
   pancreaticopleural
   paraprosthetic-enteric
   parietal
   perineovaginal
   persistent bronchopleural
   pilonidal
   pleural
   pleurocutaneous
   premedullary arteriovenous
   pulmonary arteriovenous
   radial artery to cephalic vein
   radiation
   rectal
   rectovaginal
   rectovesical
   respiratory-esophageal
   retroperitoneal
   spinal dural arteriovenous
   splanchnic AV
   splenic AV
   suprasphincteric
   thoracic
   tracheobronchial
   tracheoesophageal (TE or TEF)
   transdural
   transsphincteric anal
   trigeminal cavernous
   ureteral
   ureterocutaneous
   ureterovaginal
   urethrovaginal

fistula *(cont.)*
   urinary
   vesical
   vesicovaginal
   vitelline
fistula in ano
fistula tract study
fistulogram
fistulography
fistulous formation
fistulous tract
5-chlorodeoxycytidine
511-keV high-energy imaging
5-iodoacetamidofluorescein imaging
   agent
5-iodo-2-deoxyuridine imaging agent
5 MHz sonography
5 MHz transducer (ultrasound)
5 mm collimation
five-view chest x-ray
fixed airway obstruction
fixed area of narrowing in large
   airway
fixed defect
fixed grid stereologic method
fixed intracavitary filling defect
fixed mass
fixed perfusion defect
fixed pulmonary valvular resistance
fixed segment of bowel
fixed shaped coplanar or nonplanar
   radiation beam bouquet
fL (femtoliter)
FL (femur length)
FL/AC ratio (femur length to
   abdominal circumference)
flabby heart
flaccid
Flack sinoatrial node
flail chest
flail digit
flail foot

flail joint
flail mitral valve
flail shoulder
FLAIR (fluid-attenuated inversion
    recovery) sequences
FLAIR-FLASH imaging (see *FLASH*)
flake fracture of the hamate
flaking of cartilage in osteoarthritis
flame appearance
flank bone (ilium)
flap
    bone
    entry
    intimal
    liver
    muscle
    necrotic
    osteoplastic
    pedicle
    pericardial
    pleural
    scimitar-shaped
    subclavian
flaplike valves
flap valve ventricular septal defect
flare
    condylar
    metaphyseal
    tibial
    trochanteric
flare phenomenon
FLASH (fast low-angle shot)
    FLASH images
    FLASH 3D sequence
flashlamp-pulsed dye laser
flask, vascular
Flatau-Schilder disease
flat bone
flatfoot deformity
flat-hand test
flat lined (verb)
flat-panel megavoltage imager

flat pelvis
flat plate of abdomen
flattened longitudinal arch of foot
flattening of normal lumbar curve
flat time-intensity profile
flaval ligament
flawed image
flax-dresser's disease
Flechsig tract
Fleet bowel prep
Fleischer disease
Fleischmann bursa
Fleischner sign
fleur de lis pattern
Flexguard tip catheter
flexibility
flexible cardiac valve
flexible suction cannula
flexible surface coil
flexible surface-coil-type resonator
    (FSCR)
flexion deformity
flexion-distraction injury of spine
flexion maneuver on cervical spine
    x-ray
flexion-rotation injury of spine
flexor carpi ulnaris (FCU) muscle
flexor digitorum profundus (FDP)
    muscle
flexor digitorum superficialis (FDS)
    muscle
flexor hallucis longus (FHL) muscle
flexor pollicis longus (FPL) muscle
flexor tendon
FlexStrand cable
flexure
    caudal
    cephalic
    cerebral
    cervical
    colonic
    cranial

fluid *(cont.)*
  spinal
  subgaleal cerebrospinal
  synovial
fluid accumulation in tissues
fluid-attenuated inversion recovery
  (FLAIR) imaging
fluid collection, loculated
fluid density
fluid enzymes
fluid expansion, rapid
fluid extravasation
fluid-filled bronchograms
fluid-filled mass in uterus
fluid flow between capillaries and
  interstitial tissue
fluid-fluid level
fluidification
fluid level
fluid mass
fluid overload
fluid resorption
fluid retention
fluid volume
fluid wave
fluke
  liver
  lung
fluorescein angiography
fluorescein uptake
fluorescence spectroscopy
fluorine (F)
  ^{18}F (fluorine-18, F-18)
  ^{18}FDG (fluorine-18 2-deoxy-D-
    glucose) PET scan
  ^{18}F estradiol (FES)
  ^{18}F fluoro-DOPA
  ^{18}F fluorodeoxyglucose
  ^{18}F fluorodeoxyglucose PET scan
  ^{18}F fluorotamoxifen
  ^{18}F labeled derivatives of
    m-tyrosine

fluorine *(cont.)*
  ^{18}F labeled HFA-134a
  ^{18}F labeled polyfluorinated ethyl
  ^{18}F N-methylspiperone
  ^{18}F spiperone
  ^{18}F 2-deoxyglucose (^{18}FDG)
    uptake on PET scan
  ^{18}F uptake
fluorocarbon-based ultrasound contrast
  agent
fluorodeoxyglucose (FDG) radioactive
  tracer
fluorography, spot-film
fluoroimmunoassay
fluorometer
fluorometry
  image intensification
  portable C-arm intensifier
  two-plane
FluoroPlus angiography
FluoroPlus Roadmapper digital
  fluoroscopy system
FluoroScan mini C-arm imaging
  system
fluoroscope (see *fluoroscopy*)
fluoroscopic assistance
fluoroscopic control, advanced under
fluoroscopic diskectomy
fluoroscopic guidance
fluoroscopic localization
fluoroscopic road-mapping technique
  in angioplastic vascular procedures
fluoroscopic view
fluoroscopy
  airway
  biplane
  C-arm
  C-arm digital
  chest
  digital
  electric joint
  FluoroPlus Roadmapper digital

fluoroscopy *(cont.)*
  mobile
  Orca C-arm
  real-time CT
  region-of-interest
FluoroPlus angiography
FluoroPlus Roadmapper digital
  fluoroscopy system
fluoroscopy-guided condylar lift-off
fluoroscopy-guided subarachnoid
  phenol block (SAPB)
Fluoro Tip cannula
flush aortogram
flush aortography
flushed
flushing of catheter
flutamide-associated liver toxicity
fluttering of valvular leaflet
fluximetry
fluxionary hyperemia
fly-through viewing, PVR
FMA cephalometric measurement
FMAP (feeding mean arterial pressure)
FMD (fibromuscular dysplasia)
FMH (first metatarsal head)
FMPIR (fast SE and fast IR) imaging
FMPSPGR (fast multiplanar spoiled
  gradient-recalled) imaging
FMPSPGR sequence
FMR (functional MR) imaging
fMRI or FMRI (functional magnetic
  resonance imaging)
fMRI signal change
FMS (fatty meal sonogram)
FNH (focal nodular hyperplasia)
FNTC (fine-needle transhepatic
  cholangiogram)
foam cell
foam embolus
foamy exudate in air spaces
focal abnormality
focal area of hemorrhage

focal area of hypometabolism
focal calcification
focal changes
focal damage
focal deficit
focal degenerative change
focal dilatations of air spaces
focal distortion
focal eccentric stenosis
focal edema
focal endocardial hemorrhage
focal hepatic hot spot
focal hyperinflation
focal inflammation in febrile
  granulocytopenia
focal interstitial infiltrate
focal intimal thickening
focal lesion
focal mass
focal nodular hyperplasia (FNH)
focal perivascular infiltrate
focal plaque-like defect
focal pooling of tracer
focal stenosis
focal uptake
focal wall motion abnormality
focal white matter signal abnormalities
foci of calcification
foci of tumor
focus (pl. foci)
  Assmann
  atrial
  ectopic
  epileptogenic
  hemorrhagic
  hypermetabolic activity
  junctional
  mesial frontal
  midline parasagittal
  multiple
  occipital
  radiolucent
  Simon

Fogarty adherent clot catheter
Fogarty arterial embolectomy catheter
Fogarty balloon biliary catheter
Fogarty-Chin extrusion balloon
  catheter
fog (or fogging) effect on CT
Foix-Alajouanine syndrome
fold
  adipose
  alar
  amniotic
  aryepiglottic
  caval
  cecal
  cholecystoduodenocolic
  circular
  circulator
  custocolic
  Douglas
  duodenojejunal
  duodenomesocolic
  epigastric
  esophageal
  falciform
  flattened duodenal
  gastric
  gastropancreatic
  genital
  giant gastric
  glossopalatine
  gluteal
  Guérin
  haustral
  Hensing
  hepatopancreatic
  ileocecal
  ileocolic
  Kerckring
  Kohlrausch
  mucosal
  Nélaton
  palatopharyngeal

fold *(cont.)*
  paraduodenal
  peritoneal
  prepyloric
  rectal
  rectouterine
  rugal
  sacrogenital
  semilunar
  sentinel
  sigmoid
  spiral
  superior duodenal
  superior transverse rectal
  thickened
  vestigial
folded fundus of gallbladder
folded step ramp
folding-potential analysis
Foley catheter
folinic acid, low-dose
follicle (pl. follicles)
  aggregated
  aggregated lymphatic
  anovular ovarian
  atretic ovarian
  gastric
  gastric lymphatic
  graafian
  intestinal
  malpighian
  nabothian
  ovarian
  primordial
  ruptured
  thyroid
  unruptured
follow-through, small-bowel
follow-up or followup (n., adj.)
  examination
follow up (v.)
Fonar Stand-Up MRI scanner

forefoot
  mid- and
  narrowing of
foreign body (FB)
  metallic
  retained
  tracheobronchial
foreign body aspiration
foreign body in respiratory passages
foreign body reaction
foreign body upper airway obstruction
foreign material artifact
Forestier disease
forking of sylvian aqueduct
form, wave
format
  cylindrical
  hemodynamic
  slice
  three-dimensional
  two-dimensional
formation
  bat-wing
  brain stem reticular
  bunion
  callosal
  callus
  Chiari
  eddy
  exuberant atheroma
  fistulous
  Gothic arch
  gray reticular
  hippocampal
  honeycomb
  lateral reticular
  marginal osteophyte
  mesencephalic reticular
  midbrain reticular (MRF)
  new bone
  osteophyte
  palisade

formation *(cont.)*
  paramedian pontine reticular
  periosteal bone
  pontine parareticular (PPRF)
  reticular
  rouleaux
  saccular
  spur
  thrombus
forme fruste (pl. formes frustes)
forme tardive
formication
formidable risk
formula
  Bayesian
  fan-beam
Forney syndrome
forniceal rupture
fornix (pl. fornices), flattening of
fornix cerebri
Forrester syndrome
forward failure
forward flow
forward flow of velocity
forward heart failure
forward subluxation
forward transport
forward triangle method
forward velocity (on Doppler)
fossa (pl. fossae)
  acetabular
  adipose
  amygdaloid
  anconeal (also anconal)
  antecubital
  anterior recess of ischiorectal
  articular
  axillary
  bony
  condylar
  coronoid
  cranial

fossa *(cont.)*
crural
cubital
digastric
digital
duodenal
duodenojejunal
epigastric
femoral
floccular
gallbladder
glenoid
Gruber
hyaloid
iliac
infraspinous
infrasternal
infratemporal
intercondylar
intercondyloid
interpeduncular
ischiorectal
Jobert
navicular
olecranon
ovarian
pararectal
paravesical
patellar
pituitary
popliteal
posterior
pterygopalatine
radial
retroappendiceal
rhomboid
Rosenmuller
sphenoidal
Sylvius
temporal
Treitz
valve of navicular
Waldeyer

fossa ovalis
fossa ovalis cordis
Foster-Kennedy syndrome
4-azido-2-([^{14}C]-methylamino)tri-
fluorobenzonitrile imaging agent
four-chamber apical view
four-chamber plane on echocardiography
four-dimensional (4D) image
four-head camera
Fourier analysis of electrocardiogram
Fourier coefficients
Fourier domain
Fourier-encoded
Fourier transform (or transformation)
imaging
Fourier transform infrared spectroscopy
Fourier transform Raman spectroscopy
Fourier transformation zeugmatography
Fourier two-dimensional (2D) imaging
Fourier two-dimensional (2D)
projection reconstruction
four-part fracture
fourth branchial cleft pouch
fourth compartment
fourth cranial nerve (trochlear nerve)
fourth intercostal space
fourth left interspace
fourth ventricle tumor
four-vessel cerebral angiography
four-view chest x-ray:
PA, lateral, both oblique
FOV (field of view) imaging
fovea
fovea centralis
fovea inferior
foveal fat pad
foveated chest
foveola, gastric

Fowler position
FP (frontopolar) artery
FPB (flexor pollicis brevis) muscle
FPL (flexor pollicis longus) muscle
F point of cardiac apex pulse
FR4 guiding catheter
fractal analysis
fractal-based method
fraction
   blood flow extraction
   ejection (EF)
   S-phase
   Teichholz ejection
   unattached
   ventricular ejection
fractional area
fractional moving blood volume
   estimation
fractional myocardial shortening
fractional shortening of left ventricle
fractionated radiation therapy
fractionated stereotaxic radiation therapy
fractionation
fraction dose
fracture
   abduction
   acute
   acute avulsion
   adduction
   agenetic
   Aitken classification of epiphyseal
   alveolar bone
   anatomic
   angulated
   ankle mortise
   annular
   AO classification of ankle
   apophyseal
   articular
   artificial
   Atkin epiphyseal

fracture *(cont.)*
   atrophic
   avulsion
   avulsion chip
   axial compression
   backfire
   Barton
   basal neck
   basal skull
   baseball finger
   basilar femoral neck
   basilar skull
   basocervical
   bending
   Bennett
   Berndt-Harty classification of
      transchondral
   bicondylar
   bimalleolar ankle
   bipartite
   birth
   blow-in
   blow-out
   boot-top
   Bosworth
   both-bone
   boxer's
   Boyd type II
   bucket-handle
   buckle
   bumper
   bunk bed
   burst (compression) (of atlas)
   bursting
   butterfly
   buttonhole
   Canale-Kelly talar neck
   capillary
   carpal navicular
   carpal scaphoid bone
   cartwheel
   Cedell (of talus)

fracture *(cont.)*
- cemental
- cementum
- cervical
- cervicotrochanteric
- Chance spinal
- chauffeur's
- chevron (V-shaped)
- chip
- chisel
- circumferential
- clay shoveler's
- cleavage
- closed
- closed break
- Colles
- collicular
- comminuted
- comminuted bursting
- comminuted intra-articular
- comminuted teardrop
- complete
- complex
- complicated
- composite
- compound
- compound skull
- compression (burst) (of atlas)
- condylar
- condylar compression
- condylar split
- congenital
- contrecoup
- cortical
- Cotton ankle
- cough (of a rib)
- crack
- craniofacial dysjunction
- crush
- cuboid
- cuneiform
- dancer's

fracture *(cont.)*
- Danis-Weber classification of ankle
- Darrach-Hughston-Milch
- dashboard
- decompression of
- Denis (A,B,C,D, or E) spinal
- dens
- dentate
- depressed
- depressed and compound skull
- depressed skull
- DeQuervain
- derby hat
- diacondylar
- diaphyseal
- diastatic
- direct
- dishpan
- dislocation
- displaced
- dogleg
- dome
- dorsal wing
- double
- Dupuytren
- Duverney
- dye punch
- dyscrasic
- endocrine
- epicondylar
- epiphyseal slip
- Essex-Lopresti calcaneal
- extra-articular
- extracapsular
- facial
- fatigue
- femoral neck
- fender
- fighter's
- finger
- fissure
- flake (of the hamate)

fracture *(cont.)*
    flexion-burst
    flexion-compression
    flexion distraction
    floating arch
    four-part
    Freiberg
    Frykman radial
    fulcrum
    Galeazzi (of radius)
    Garden femoral neck
    Gosselin
    greenstick
    grenade-thrower's
    gross
    growth plate
    Guérin
    gutter
    Hahn-Steinthal capitellum
    hairline
    hamate tail
    hangman's (C2)
    Hansen
    Hawkins talar neck
    healed
    heat
    hemicondylar
    Herbert scaphoid bone
    Hermodsson
    hockey-stick
    horizontal
    horizontal maxillary
    humeral head-splitting
    hyperextension teardrop
    hyperflexion
    hyperflexion teardrop
    idiopathic
    impacted
    impacted subcapital
    impacted valgus
    incomplete
    indented (of skull)

fracture *(cont.)*
    indirect
    inflammatory
    infraction
    insufficiency
    intercondylar
    internally fixed
    interperiosteal
    intertrochanteric
    intra-articular
    intracapsular
    intraperiosteal
    intrauterine (of fetus)
    irreducible
    ischioacetabular
    Jefferson burst
    joint
    joint depression
    Jones
    juvenile Tillaux
    juxta-articular
    Kocher
    Kocher-Lorenz classification of
        capitellum
    laryngeal
    lateral column calcaneal
    lateral wedge (of vertebral body)
    laterally displaced
    Lauge-Hansen classification of
        ankle
    Le Fort I, II, and III
    lead-pipe
    linear
    linear and depressed skull
    Lisfranc
    local compression
    local decompression
    long bone
    longitudinal
    loose
    lorry driver's
    low T humerus

fracture *(cont.)*
    lunate
    Maisonneuve fibular
    malar
    Malgaigne pelvic
    mallet
    malunited
    mandibular
    march
    maxillary
    medial column calcaneal
    medial epicondyle
    medial malleolar
    midfacial
    midshaft
    minimally displaced
    monomalleolar ankle
    Monteggia
    Monteggia fracture-dislocation
    Montercaux
    Moore
    Mueller classification of humerus
    multangular ridge
    multipartite
    multiple
    nasal
    navicular
    navicular body
    naviculocapitate
    neck
    Neer classification of shoulder
    neoplastic
    neurogenic
    neuropathic
    neurotrophic
    nightstick
    nonarticular radial head
    nondisplaced
    oblique
    occipital
    occult
    odontoid

fracture *(cont.)*
    Ogden classification of epiphyseal
    old
    olecranon
    olecranon tip
    one-part
    open
    open-break
    osteochondral
    Pais
    panfacial
    paratrooper
    parry
    patellar
    pathologic
    Pauwel
    pedicle
    pelvic rim
    pelvic ring
    perforating
    periarticular
    peripheral
    peritrochanteric
    phalangeal
    physeal plate
    Piedmont
    pillion
    pillow
    ping-pong
    plafond
    plaque
    plateau
    pond
    posterior element
    postmortem
    Pott ankle
    pressure
    puncture
    pyramidal
    Quervain (deQuervain)
    radial head
    radial styloid process

fracture *(cont.)*
    resecting
    retrodisplaced
    reverse Barton
    reverse Colles
    rib
    ring
    Rolando
    rotation burst
    Ruedi-Allgower tibial plafond
    sacral insufficiency
    Salter
    Salter-Harris (1 through 5)
    Salter-Harris-Rang classification of epiphyseal
    sandbagging (of long bones)
    scaphoid
    seat belt
    secondary
    segmental
    Segond
    senile subcapital
    SER-IV (supination, external rotation-type IV)
    shaft
    shear
    Shepherd
    sideswipe elbow
    silver-fork (Colles)
    simple
    simple skull
    skier's
    Skillern
    sleeve
    slice
    Smith
    Sneppen talar
    spiral
    splintered
    split compression
    spontaneous
    sprain

fracture *(cont.)*
    sprinter's
    stable
    stairstep
    Steinert classification of epiphyseal
    stellate
    stellate skull
    stellate undepressed
    step-off of
    Stieda
    straddle
    strain
    stress
    stress-type
    subcapital
    subcutaneous
    subperiosteal
    subtrochanteric
    supination (see *SER-IV*)
    supination-adduction
    supination-eversion
    supracondylar
    supracondylar femoral
    surgical neck
    T
    talar osteochondral
    T condylar
    T-shaped
    teardrop
    teardrop-shaped flexion-compression
    temporal bone
    thalamic (of calcaneal)
    three-part
    through-and-through
    tibial plafond
    tibial plateau
    tibiofibular
    Tillaux
    Tillaux-Kleiger
    tongue-type
    torsion

fracture *(cont.)*
   torus
   total condylar depression
   transcapitate
   transcervical femoral
   transchondral talar
   transcondylar
   transepiphyseal
   transhamate
   transscaphoid
   transtriquetral
   transverse
   trimalleolar ankle
   triplane
   triquetral
   trophic
   tuft
   two-part
   ulnar styloid
   undisplaced
   unilateral
   unstable
   ununited
   V-shaped (chevron)
   vertebra plana
   vertebral wedge compression
   vertical
   vertical shear
   wagon wheel
   Wagstaffe
   Watson-Jones navicular
   Watson-Jones spinal
   Weber C
   wedge
   wedge-compression
   wedged
   wedge flexion-compression
   willow
   Y
   Y-T
   Zickel
   zygomatic-malar complex (ZMC)

fracture classification
fracture deformity
fracture-dislocation, perilunate
   (PLFD)
fracture en rave
fracture fragment
fracture in close apposition
fracture line
fracture nonunion
fracture threshold
fracture zone
fragility, hereditary (of bone)
fragment
   alignment of fracture
   articular
   avulsed fracture
   avulsion
   bone
   bony
   butterfly fracture
   capital
   chondral
   cortical
   disk
   displaced
   displacement of fracture
   Fab (fragment antigen binding)
   fracture
   free
   free-floating cartilaginous
   loose
   major fracture
   osteochondral
   overriding of fracture
   retrolisthesed
   retropulsed bony
   smear
fragmentation myocarditis
fragmentation of apophysis
fragmentation therapy
frame
   robotics-controlled stereotactic
   stereotactic head

frameless stereotaxic DSA
frameless stereotaxic guidance tools
frank dislocation
frank hemorrhage
frank pulmonary edema
frank pus
Frank sign
Frank vectorcardiogram (VCG)
Frankel classification of spinal cord
    injury (Fraenkel)
Frankel white line
Frankfort horizontal plane
Frankfort mandibular incisor angle
fraught with error
fray
fraying of edges
fraying of meniscus
FRC (functional residual capacity)
free air
free air in body cavity
free air in diaphragm
free air passage
free air under diaphragm
free body in peritoneal cavity
free flap of cartilage
free-floating cartilaginous fragment
free fluid
free fragment
free hepatic venography
free induction decay (FID)
free induction delay curve
free induction signal
free intraperitoneal air
free intraperitoneal gas
free pericardial space
free pleural effusion
free radical
free-radical dosimeter
free wall, ventricular
free wall tract
freehand interventional sonography
freehand ultrasound

freely movable mass
Freiberg disease
Freiberg-Kohler disease
French 5 angiographic catheter
French MBIH catheter
French pigtail catheter
French scale for caliber of catheter
French shaft balloon
French T-tube
frequency analysis of Doppler signal
frequency domain imaging (FDI) in
    ultrasound
frequency
    halftone
    Larmor
    precisional
    raster
    vibration
frequency offset
frequency-related peak
friability
friable lesion
friable mass
friable mucosa
friable tumor
friable vegetation
friable wall
friction-reducing polymer
Friedel Pick syndrome
Friedreich foot
Frimodt-Moller syndrome
fringe field
fringe skeleton extraction
fringe, synovial
fringe thinning algorithms
frogleg view
frog-like appearance
Frohse ligamentous arcade
frond-like appearance
frontal bone
frontal defect

frontal foramina
frontal gyrus
frontal horn of lateral ventricle
frontal lobe
frontal lobe contusion
frontal lobe dysfunction
frontal lobe lesion
frontal lobe tumor
frontal plane
frontal plane loop
frontal pole
frontal sinus
frontal suture
frontal view
frontocentral convexity
frontocentral head region
frontoethmoidal encephalocele
fronto-orbital advancement
frontoparietal
frontoparietal suture
frontopolar region
frontosphenoid suture
frontosphenoidal encephalocele
frontotemporal (FT)
frontotemporal atrophy
frontotemporal muscle
frontotemporal region
frontozygomatic region
frothy colonic mucosa
Frykman classification of hand and
  wrist
FS (full scan) method/projection
FS-BURST MR imaging
FSCR, flexible surface-coil-type
FSE (fast SE) imaging
FSV (forward stroke volume)
FTA (femorotibial angle)
FTC (fibulotalocalacaneal) ligament
FTP (file transfer protocol)
F-1200 (and F-2000) Fluorescence
  Spectrophotometer

FUdR (5-fluorouracil deoxyribo-
  nucleoside)
Fuji AC2 storage phosphor computed
  radiology system
Fuji FCR9000 computed radiology
  system
Fukuyama congenital muscular
  dystrophy
fulcrum fracture
full-bladder ultrasound technique
full body echo planar system imager
full-blown cardiac tamponade
full-column barium enema
full energy peak efficiency
full-field digital mammography system
full-scan (FS) method/projection
full-scan with interpolation (FI)
  method/projection
full-thickness button of aortic wall
full-thickness Carrel button
full-thickness infarction of ventricular
  septum
full-volume loop spirometry
full width at half maximum (FWHM)
fulminant cerebral lymphoma (in
  AIDS)
fulminant course of disease
fulminant hepatic failure (FHF)
fulminant hydrocephalus
fulminant pulmonary edema
fulminant tuberculosis
fulminating ulcerative colitis
function
  atrial phasic volumetric
  commissural
  compromised ventricular
  depressed right ventricular
    contractile
  excitation
  exercise LV
  global ventricular

function *(cont.)*
  leaflet
  left atrial (LA)
  left ventricular (LV)
  left ventricular systolic/diastolic
  myocardial contractile
  point spread
  regional left ventricular
  regional ventricular
  reserve cardiac
  rest LV (left ventricular)
  rest RV (right ventricular)
  right and left atrial phasic
    volumetric
  right atrial (RA)
  right ventricular (RV)
  right ventricular systolic/diastolic
  sinusoid reference
  swallowing
  ventricular contractility (VCF)
  volumetric
functional abnormality
functional aerobic impairment (FAI)
functional bladder capacity
functional brain imaging
functional classification of congestive
  heart failure
functional correlation
functional cyst
functional disorder
functional disturbance
functional evaluation
functional impairment
functional magnetic resonance
  imaging (FMRI)
functional MRI (fMRI)
functional reentry
functional refractory period (FRP)
functional residual capacity (FRC)
functional ureteral obstruction
fundal

fundoplication
fundus
  aneurysmal
  bladder
  bald gastric
  eye
  gallbladder
  gastric
  stomach
  urinary bladder
  uterine
  vaginal
fundus of aneurysm
fundus uteri
fungal plaque
fungating
fungoides, mycosis
fungus ball
funic souffle
funicular souffle
funiculus (pl. funiculi)
funiculus cuneatus
funiculus dorsalis
funiculus gracilis
funiculus medullae spinalis
funiculus ventralis
funnel chest
funnel deformity
funnel pelvis
FUO (fever of undetermined origin)
Fürbringer sign (Fuerbringer)
furrier's lung
fused ankle
fused commissures
fused papillary muscle
fused physis
fusiform aneurysm
fusiform bronchiectasis
fusiform dilatation
fusiform narrowing of arteries
fusiform shadow

G, g

Ga (gallium)
GABA-BN complex
gadobenate dimeglumine imaging
    agent
gadodiamide imaging agent
gadolinium (Gd)
    Gd-BOPTA/Dimeg imaging agent
    Gd-DOTA contrast medium
    Gd-DOTA-enhanced subtraction
        dynamic study
    Gd-DTPA/Dimeg imaging agent
    Gd-DTPA-enhanced turbo FLASH
        MRI
    Gd-DTPA imaging agent
    Gd-DTPA-labeled albumin
    Gd-DTPA-labeled dextran
    Gd-DPTA PGTM imaging agent
    Gd-DTPA radioisotope
    Gd-DTPA with mannitol contrast
    Gd-enhanced imaging agent
    Gd-EOB-DTPA imaging agent
    Gd-FMPSPGR imaging
    Gd-HIDA chelate
    Gd-Hp-DO3A imaging agent
    Gd-labeled graft copolymer
    Gd-153 imaging agent
    Gd oxide contrast medium

gadolinium complex
gadolinium-enhanced MR imaging
gadopentetate dimeglumine imaging
    agent
gadoteridol contrast
Gaeltec catheter-tip pressure
    transducer
Gage sign
Gairdner disease
Gaisböck syndrome
galactography
galea aponeurotica
galeal extension of tumor
Galeazzi fracture-dislocation
Galeazzi fracture of radius
Galeazzi sign
Galen, great cerebral vein of
Galen Scan scanner
Galen teleradiology system
Gallannaugh bone plate
Gallavardin phenomenon
gallbladder
    bilobed
    body of
    chronically inflamed
    contracted
    Courvoisier

gallbladder *(cont.)*
  dilated
  distended
  double
  edematous
  fetal
  fish-scale
  floating
  folded fundus
  fundal portion of
  fundus of
  hourglass
  mobile
  multiseptate
  neck of
  nonvisualization of
  stasis
  thick-walled
  thin-walled
  wandering
gallbladder bed
gallbladder calculus
gallbladder ejection fraction
gallbladder hydrops
gallbladder lift
gallbladder polyp
gallbladder stasis
gallbladder study (oral cholecystogram)
gallbladder ultrasound
Gallie H-graft
gallium (Ga)
  ^{67}Ga bone scan
  ^{67}Ga citrate radioactive imaging
  ^{67}Ga exam
  ^{68}Ga GABA uptake carrier
  ^{67}Ga imaging agent
gallium scan (scanning)
gallium scintigraphy
gallstone (see also *stone*)
  asymptomatic
  dissolution of

gallstone *(cont.)*
  faceted
  floating
  innocent
  radiolucent
  retained
  silent
  symptomatic
gallstone migration
GALT (gut-associated lymphoid
  tissue)
gamekeeper's thumb
gamma camera (see *camera*)
gamma counter
gamma irradiation
gamma probe
gamma ray attenuation
gamma spectrometric analysis
gamma unit
gamma knife for radiosurgery
Gammex RMI DAP (dose area
  product) meter
Gammex RMI scanner
Gamna-Gandy nodule
Gandy-Nanta disease
ganglia (pl. of ganglion)
ganglioglioma
gangliolysis, radiofrequency
ganglion (pl. ganglia)
  aberrent
  acousticofacial
  aorticorenal
  Acrel
  auditory
  auricular
  basal
  calcification of basal
  cardiac
  carotid
  celiac
  cervical
  cervicothoracic

gassy
gas target
gastric air bubble
gastric antrum
gastric balloon (see *balloon*)
gastric bubble
gastric capacity
gastric catarrh
gastric channel
gastric contents
gastric distention
gastric fistula
gastric foveola
gastric fundus
gastric impression on liver
gastric mucosa imaging
gastric mucosal pattern
gastric outline
gastric partition
gastric pits
gastric pool
gastric pull-through segment
gastric reflux of bile
gastric remnant
gastric secretion
gastric ulcer
gastric window
gastrinoma, duodenal
gastritis
    acute
    antral
    atrophic
    chronic
    cirrhotic
    hemorrhagic
    hypertrophic
    necrotizing
    pseudomembranous radiation
gastroc (gastrocnemius muscle)
gastrocardiac syndrome
gastrocnemius muscle
gastrocnemius-soleus complex

gastrocnemius-soleus muscle group
gastrocolic ligament
gastrocolic omentum
gastroduodenal artery complex
gastroduodenitis
gastroduodenoscopy
gastroenteritis
gastroenterocolitis
gastroenteroptosis
gastroepiploic arcade
gastroepiploic artery
gastroepiploic vessel
gastroesophageal incompetence
gastroesophageal junction
gastroesophageal reflux (GER)
gastroesophageal reflux disease
    (GERD)
Gastrografin (meglumine diatrizoate)
    contrast medium
Gastrografin enema
gastrohepatic bare area
gastrohepatic omentum
gastrointestinal (GI)
    GI endoscopic ultrasound
    GI tract
gastrojejunocolic fistula
gastrolienal ligament
GastroMARK oral contrast medium
gastroparesis
Gastroport
gastroptosis
gastrosphincteric pressure gradient
Gastrovist contrast medium
gas ventilation study
gas volumes
gate arrays
gated blood (pool) cardiac wall
    motion study
gated blood pool ventriculogram
gated cardiac blood pool imaging
gated equilibrium blood pool scanning

gated exercise examination
gated imaging studies
gated inflow technique
gated magnetic resonance imaging
gated planar studies
gated radionuclide ventriculography
gated SPECT (GSPECT)
gated view (in MUGA, multiple gated
    acquisition scan)
gating (timing of images)
    cardiac
    diastolic
    ECG
    echocardiographic
    electrocardiogram
    heartbeat
    respiratory
    systolic
Gaucher disease
gauge
gauss
gaussian curve
gaussian dose-volume histogram
gaussian distribution
gaussian line saturation
gaussian mode profile laser beam
Gaynor-Hart position
GBM (glioblastoma multiforme)
GBP (gastric bypass)
GBS (Guillain-Barré syndrome)
GCSF, granulocyte colony stimulating
    factor
GCT (germ-cell tumor)
GCTSPS (germ-cell tumor with
    synchronous lesions in pineal and
    suprasellar regions)
GCVF (great cardiac vein flow)
Gd (gadolinium)
GE (gastroesophageal)
    GE junction
    GE reflux

GE (General Electric)
    GE CT Advantage scanner
    GE Advance PET scanner
    GE CT Hi-Speed Advantage
        system
    GE CT 8800 scanner
    GE CT Max scanner
    GE CT Pace scanner
    GE detector
    GE gamma camera
    GE GN300 7.05T/89 mm bore
        multinuclear spectrometer
    GE GN 500 MHz
    GE HiSpeed Advantage helical CT
        scanner
    GE HiSpeed CT scanner
    GE Medical Systems
    GE 9800 high-resolution CT
        scanner
    GE MR Max scanner
    GE MR Signa scanner
    GE MR Vectra scanner
    GE NMR spectrometer
    GE Omega 500 MHz
    GE QE 300 MHz GE PET scanner
    GE scanner
    GE Signa 5.4 Genesis MR imager
    GE Signa 5.5 Horizon EchoSpeed
        MR imager
    GE Signa MR system
    GE Signa 1.5 tesla scanner
    GE Signa 1.5 T magnet
    GE Signa 4.7 MRI scanner
    GE Signa 5.2 scanner
    GE Signa 5.2 scanner with SR-230
        3-axis EPI gradient upgrade
    GE single axis SR-230 echo-planar
        system
    GE single-detector SPECT-capable
        camera
    GE SPECT (single-photon emission
        computerized tomography)

GE (General Electric) *(cont.)*
  GE Spiral CT scanner
  GE Starcam single-crystal tomo-
    graphic scintillation camera
Gee-Herter disease
GEG (Garren-Edwards gastric) bubble
Geiger counter
gelatinous debris
gelatinous hematoma
Gelfoam powder embolization
gemellary pregnancy
gemellus (pl. gemelli) muscle
gene delivery imaging
general pattern matching
General Electric (see *GE*)
generalized
generator
  carbon dioxide
  ^{166}Dy (dysprosium)
  extraction
  ^{166}Ho (holmium in vivo)
  172Hf-172Lu
  molybdenum-99
  Van de Graaff
generator-produced ^{188}Re (rhenium)
genial tubercle of mandible
geniculate body
geniculate ganglion
geniculocalcarine region
geniculocalvarium
geniculum
genitourinary tuberculosis
Gennari
  band of
  line of
  stripe of (in brain)
Gensini catheter
Gentle-Flo suction catheter
genu valgum (knock-knee) deformity
genu varum (bowleg) deformity
geographic lesion
geometric distortion

geometry, coronary vessel
geometry factor
geophagia artifact
GER (gastroesophageal reflux)
GERD (gastroesophageal reflux
  disease)
Gerdy ligament
Gerdy tubercle in knee
Gerhardt sign
Gerhardt triangle
geriatric features on chest x-ray
germ-cell tumor (GCT), intracranial
germinal matrix
germinoma, primary central nervous
  system
Gertzbein classification of seat belt
  injury
gestation
  extrauterine
  intrauterine
gestational age
gestational sac diameter (GS)
gestational trophoblastic disease
gestational trophoblastic neoplasia
  (GTN)
GF cassette
GFR (glomerular filtration rate)
Ghon complex
Ghon primary lesion
Ghon-Sachs complex
Ghon tubercle
ghosting artifact
GI (gastrointestinal)
giant aneurysm
giant bullous emphysema
giant cell carcinoma
giant cell interstitial pneumonia (GIP)
giant gastric folds
Gianturco-Roehm bird's nest vena
  caval filter
Gianturco-Rösch Z-stent esophageal
  stent

Gianturco-Roubin flexible coil stent
Gianturco-Wallace venous stent
Gianturco wool-tufted wire coil stent
giardiasis
gibbous deformity
Gibbs artifact
Gibbs random field
gibbus (n.)
GIF (graphics interchange format)
gigantism, cerebral
GIP (giant cell interstitial pneumonia)
girdle
    limb
    pelvic
    shoulder
girth, abdominal
gland
    absorbent
    accessory
    admaxillary
    adrenal
    Albarran
    alveolar
    anteprostatic
    aortic
    apical
    aporic
    arterial
    arteriococcygeal
    axillary sweat
    Bartholin
    bulbocavernous
    bulbourethral
    calcification of pineal
    carotid
    coccygeal
    Cowper
    Duverney
    endocrine
    globate
    glomiform
    haversian

gland *(cont.)*
    hilar
    interscapular
    lacrimal
    lymph
    mammary
    ovaries
    pancreas
    parathyroid
    parotid
    pineal
    pituitary
    salivary
    Skene
    sublingual
    submandibular
    suprarenal
    testes
    urethral
    thymus
    thyroid
gland volume
glandular proliferation
glandular tissue
Glasgow sign
glass blower's emphysema
glass eye artifact
glass track detector
Gleason grade
Glénard disease
glenohumeral joint
glenohumeral ligament
glenoid cavity
glenoid fossa
glenoid process
GLF lymphography method
glial disease
glial nodule
glial scarring
glial tumor
Glidewire
    long taper/stiff shaft
    Radiofocus

glioblast
glioblastoma
glioblastoma multiforme (GBM)
glioma
   anaplastic cerebral
   brain stem
   butterfly-type
   cerebral
   high-grade
   intracranial
   low-grade
   malignant
   non-anaplastic
   optic nerve
   pontine
   rolandoparietal
   supratentorial
glioma tumor
gliomatosis cerebri
glioneural hamartoma
gliosarcoma
gliosis
   astrocytic
   progressive subcortical
   reactive
gliosis of sylvian aqueduct
Glisson capsule
global cardiac disease
global cerebral hypoperfusion
global cerebral ischemia
global cortical defect
global ejection fraction
global hypokinesis
global hypometabolism
global left ventricular dysfunction
global systolic left ventricular
   dysfunction
global tissue loss
global ventricular dysfunction
global wall motion abnormality
globally depressed ejection fraction
globe, optic

globe-orbit relationship
globoid heart
globular chest
globular sputum
globus hystericus
globus pallidus
glomeriform arteriovenous
   anastomosis
glomeriform arteriovenular
   anastomosis
glomerular basement membrane
glomerular filtration agent
glomerular filtration rate (GFR)
glomeruloid formation
glomerulonephritis
   acute
   membranous
   necrotizing
   proliferative
   segmental necrotizing
glomus (subungual) tumor
glomus-type arteriovenous
   malformation (AVM)
glossopharyngeal nerve (ninth cranial
   nerve)
glottic larynx
glottis
glove phenomenon (artifact)
gloves, radiation-attenuating surgical
glow curve
GLP7 film
glucagon
Glucarate ^{99m}Tc hot spot imaging
   agent
glucose metabolism within the
   myocardium
glue, percutaneous fibrin
glutamate spectroscopy
glutathione
gluteal bonnet
gluteal lines
gluteus maximus muscle

gluteus medius muscle
gluteus minimus muscle
gm (gram)
goiter
    Basedow
    colloid
    cystic
    diffuse
    diving
    exophthalmic
    familial
    fibrous
    intrathoracic
    iodide
    iodine deficiency
    lingual
    multinodular
    nodular
    parenchymous
    retrovascular
    simple
    substernal
    suffocative
    thyroid
    toxic
    toxic nodular
    vascular
    wandering
Golay coil
gold radioactive source
gold standard of diagnosis
gold-195m radionuclide
Goldblatt phenomenon
Goldenhar syndrome
golfer's elbow
GoLytely bowel prep
gonial angle (of mandible)
gonion-gnathion plane
Goodale-Lubin cardiac catheter
Goodpasture syndrome
gooseneck concept
gooseneck deformity of outflow tract

gooseneck shape of ventricular
    outflow
Gore-Tex catheter
gorge
gorging
Gorham disease
Gorlin catheter
Gorlin formula for aortic valve area
Gorlin hydraulic formula for mitral
    valve area
Gorlin method for cardiac output
Gorlin syndrome
Gosling pulsatility index
Gosselin fracture
Gosset, spiral band of
Gothic arch formation
Gottschalk staging
Gould PentaCath 5-lumen
    thermodilution catheter
Gould Statham pressure transducer
Gouley syndrome
gout, tophaceous
gouty tophus
Gowers bundle
Gowers column
Gowers fasciculus
Gowers syndrome
GP (gastroplasty)
graafian follicle
graafian vesicle
Grace method of ratio of metatarsal
    length
grade 1 tear
grade 2 tear
grade 3 tear
grade
    Gleason
    Hyams
    osteoarthritis
    placental
graded compression sonography
graded infusion

gradient
  aortic outflow
  aortic valve (AVG)
  aortic valve peak instantaneous
  arteriovenous pressure
  atrioventricular
  biliary-duodenal pressure
  brain-core
  conjugate
  coronary perfusion
  dephasing
  diastolic
  duodenobiliary pressure
  elevated
  encoding
  end-diastolic aortic–left ventricular
    pressure
  Ficoll
  gastrosphincteric pressure
  hepatic venous pressure
  holosystolic
  instantaneous
  left ventricular outflow pressure
  maximal estimated
  mean mitral valve
  mean systolic
  mitral valve
  negligible pressure
  outflow tract
  peak diastolic
  peak instantaneous
  peak pressure
  peak right ventricular–right atrial
    systolic
  peak systolic (PSG)
  peak-to-peak pressure
  perfusion
  pressure
  pressure-flow
  pulmonary artery diastolic and
    wedge pressure (PADP-PAWP)

gradient *(cont.)*
  pulmonary artery to right ventricle
    diastolic
  pulmonary outflow
  pulmonic valve
  rephasing
  residual
  right ventricular to main pulmonary
    artery pressure
  stenotic
  subvalvular
  systolic
  transaortic systolic
  translesional
  transmitral diastolic
  transpulmonic
  transstenotic pressure
  transtricuspid valve diastolic
  transvalvar
  transvalvular pressure
  tricuspid valve
  ventricular
gradient across valve
gradient amplifier
gradient coil
gradient drive current
gradient echo cine technique
gradient echo image
gradient echo imaging sequence
gradient echo MR with magnetization
  transfer
gradient echo pulse sequence
gradient echo sequence
gradient echo phase image
gradient echo pulse sequence
gradient echo sequence imaging
gradient magnetic field
gradient-recalled acquisition in a
  steady state (GRASS)
gradient-recalled echo (GRE)
gradient sheet coils
gradient waveforms

grading, histologic
graft
   coronary artery bypass (CABG)
   Dacron-covered stent
   endovascular aortic
graft copolymer
grafting
graft patency
graft-versus-host disease (GVHD)
Graham-Burford-Mayer syndrome
Graham-Cole cholecystography
grain-handler's lung
gram (gm)
Grancher sign
Grancher triad
grand mal seizure
Granger view
Grantham classification of femur
   fracture
granularity
granulated
granulation stenosis
granulation tissue
granulocyte colony stimulating factor
   (GCSF)
granulocytic leukemia
granuloma (pl. granulomata)
   amebic
   apical
   beryllium
   calcified
   cholesterol
   coccidioidal
   coli
   eosinophilic
   epithelioid
   extravascular
   fishtank
   foreign body
   frontoethmoidal giant cell
     reparative
   Hodgkin

granuloma *(cont.)*
   inguinal
   laryngeal
   lethal midline
   lipoid
   Majocchi
   malarial
   midline
   Mignon
   miliary
   noncaseating
   paracoccidioidal
   periapical
   pseudopyogenic
   reticulohistiocytic
   rheumatic
   silicotic
   stellate
   swimming pool
   thorium dioxide
   tricophytic
   tuberculous
   umbilical
   xanthomatous
granulomatosis
   allergic
   Wegener
granulomatous enterocolitis
granulomatous gastritis
granulomatous inflammation of
   bronchi
granulosa-theca cell tumor
granulovacuolar degeneration
graphics interchange format (GIF)
graphite fibrosis of lung
Graser diverticulum
GRASS (gradient-recalled acquisition
     in a steady state)
   GRASS MR imaging
   GRASS pulse sequence
Gratiolet convolutions
Graupner method

grave prognosis
Graves disease
gravid uterus
gravida
gravis, myasthenia
gravitational edema
gravity drainage
gray (Gy)
gray commissure (of spinal cord)
gray horns in spinal canal
gray matter
gray radiation absorbed dose (Gy rad)
gray-scale Doppler
gray-scale images (imaging)
gray-scale range
gray-scale ultrasound
gray to white matter activity ratio
gray to white matter utilization ratio
gray-white differentiation on CT scan
gray-white matter contrast ratio
gray-white matter junction
Grayson ligament in hand
GRE (gradient-recalled echo)
   GRE breath-hold hepatic imaging
   GRE-in images
   GRE-out images
   GRE magnetic resonance imaging
greater curvature of stomach
greater multangular bone
greater saphenous vein
greater sciatic notch
greater superficial petrosal nerve
greater trochanter
greater tuberosity
great vessels, transposition of
Greene sign
Greenfield IVC (inferior vena cava)
   filter
greenstick fracture
Greer EZ Access drainage pouch
grenade thrower's fracture
grenz ray

Greulich and Pyle, bone age
   according to
grey (see *gray*)
grid, megavoltage
grid therapy
Griesinger sign
Grollman pigtail catheter
groove
   alveolingual
   alveolobuccal
   alveololabial
   anal intersphincteric
   anterolateral
   anteromedian
   arterial
   atrioventricular (AV)
   auriculoventricular
   basilar
   bicipital
   bronchial
   buccal
   carotid
   carpal
   cavernous
   central
   coronary
   costal
   dental
   developmental
   digastric
   esophageal
   ethmoidal
   gastric
   genital
   gingivobuccal
   gingivolabial
   Harrison
   infraorbital
   interatrial
   intertubercular
   interventricular
   labial
   lacrimal

groove *(cont.)*
    Liebermeister
    neural
    paravertebral
    radial
    radial neck
    sagittal
    Sibson
    spindle colonic
    ulnar
    urethral
    venous
    Verga lacrimal
    vertebral
Groshong double-lumen catheter
Groshong tunneled catheter
Grossman scale for regurgitation
Grossman sign
ground-glass appearance of lungs
ground-glass attenuation
ground-glass density
ground-glass infiltrates in lungs
ground-glass opacity
ground plate
ground state
group viewing
growth arrest line
growth center of bone
growth plate arrest
growth plate fracture
growth plate injury
growth plate widening
Gruber fossa
Gruentzig (Grüntzig)
grumous debris
grumous tissue
Grüntzig (Gruentzig)
Grüntzig balloon catheter angioplasty
Grüntzig Dilaca catheter
Grüntzig technique for PTCA
GS (gestational sac)
GSA imaging agent for liver
    scintigraphy

Gsell-Erdheim syndrome
GSPECT (gated SPECT)
GSW (gunshot wound)
GSWH (gunshot wound to head)
GTN (gestational trophoblastic
    neoplasia)
guanylate cyclase (enzyme)
Guérin fracture
Guglielmi detachable coil (GDC)
guidance
    active biplanar MR imaging
    fluoroscopic
    radiologic
    under fluoroscopic
guide wire entrapment
Guidezilla guiding catheter
guiding catheter
guiding shots
guilt screen
Gull disease
gumma (pl. gummas or gummata)
gummas of rib
gun stock deformity
Gunn crossing sign
gunshot wound (GSW)
gunshot wound to head (GSWH)
Gustilo-Anderson classification of
    tibial plafond fracture
Gustilo classification of tibial fractures
gut (intestine)
    blind
    large
    mid-
    small
gutter
    lateral
    left
    paracolic
    parapelvic
    peritoneal
    right
    sacral

gutter fracture
Guyon canal
Gy (gray) radiation absorbed dose
gymnast's wrist
gynecoid pelvis
gyral crest
gyration
gyri cerebri
gyriform calcification
gyromagnetic ratio
Gyroscan, Philips
Gyroscan S15 scanner
gyrus (pl. gyri)
 angular (AG)
 annectant
 ascending parietal
 Broca
 callosal
 central
 cingulate
 contiguous supramarginal
 dentate
 fasciolar
 first temporal
 flattening of
 frontal
 fusiform
 Heschl transverse
 hippocampal
 inferior frontal
 inferior temporal
 infracalcarine
 insular
 lamination of
 lateral occipitotemporal
 lingual
 marginal

gyrus *(cont.)*
 medial occipitotemporal
 middle frontal
 middle temporal
 occipital
 occipitotemporal
 olfactory
 orbital
 paracentral
 parahippocampal
 paraterminal
 parietal
 postcentral
 posterior central
 precentral
 preinsular
 quadrate
 short insular
 subcallosal
 subcollateral
 superior frontal
 superior parietal lobule
 superior temporal
 supracallosal
 supramarginal
 temporal
 transverse temporal
 Turner marginal
 uncal
 uncinate
gyrus cerebelli
gyrus cingulatus
gyrus cinguli
gyrus fornicatus
gyrus hippocampi
gyrus isthmus fornicatus
gyrus rectus

H, h

H1 (halistatin-1) imaging agent
H1 spectroscopy
H_2 ^{15}O (water O-15) radioactive
diagnostic agent
H_2 ^{15}O PET (positron emission
tomography)
habenula
habitus
body
gracile
large
Haglund deformity
Hagner disease
Hahn-Steinthal classification of
capitellum fracture
Haifa camera
Haines-McDougall medial sesamoid
ligament
hairline crack in bone cortex
hairline fracture
Hale syndrome
half-Fourier acquisition single-shot
turbo spin-echo (HASTE)
half-Fourier imaging (HFI)
half-Fourier three-dimensional
technique
half-life
antibody
biological
effective
radioactive
short
half-moon artifact
half-moon shape
half-scan (HS) method/projection
half-scan with extrapolation (HE)
method/projection
half-scan with interpolation (HI)
method/projection
half-time, clearance
halftone banding
halftone frequency
half-wedged field technique
halistatin-1 (H1) imaging agent
Hallberg biliointestinal bypass
Hallermann-Streiff-François syndrome
hallucal pronation
hallux abductovalgus
hallux elevatus
hallux extensus
hallux flexus deformity
hallux interphalangeal joint

hallux interphalangeus angle
hallux limitus (HL)
hallux malleus deformity
hallux migration
hallux rigidus deformity
hallux valgus (HV)
    bilateral
    unilateral
hallux valgus angle (HVA)
hallux valgus deformity
hallux valgus interphalangeus angle
hallux valgus-metatarsus primus varus
    complex
hallux varus deformity
halo cast
halo effect
halo ring
halo sign
halogenated thymidine analogue
    (radiosensitizer)
HAMA (human anti-murine
    antibodies) response
hamartoma
    cardiac
    cartilaginous
    chondromatous
    duodenal wall
    glioneural
    pancreatic
    pulmonary
    subependymal
    vascular
    ventromedial hypothalamic
hamartomatous lesion
hamartomatous polyp
hamate bone
hamate tail fracture
Hamilton-Stewart formula for
    measuring cardiac output
Hamman pneumopericardium sign

Hamman-Rich syndrome (idiopathic
    pulmonary fibrosis)
hammer-marked skull secondary to
    thinning
hammer toe (or hammertoe)
    dynamic
    fixed
hammock mitral valve
hammock valve
hammocking of mitral valve leaflet
Hampton hump
Hampton line
hamstring muscle
Hanafee catheter
hand
    articulations of
    digital artery of
    phalanges of
hand grip exercise
hand-held probe
hand injection of contrast medium
Hand-Schüller-Christian disease
hangman's fracture
HAPE (high-altitude pulmonary
    edema)
Hara classification of gallbladder
    inflammation
Harbitz-Mueller syndrome
HARC-C wavelet compression
    technique
hard disk herniation
hard metal disease
hardening of arteries
hardware optimized trapezoid (HOT)
    pulse
Hardy-Clapham sesamoid classifica-
    tion
Harkavy syndrome
harmonic imaging
Harrison sulcus
Hartmann closure of rectum
Hartmann point

Hartmann pouch
Hartnup disease
Hartzler ACX-II or RX-014 balloon
    catheter
Hartzler angioplasty balloon
Hartzler LPS dilatation catheter
Hartzler Micro XT dilatation catheter
harvester lung
harvesting
    bone
    graft
    vein
Hashimoto thyroiditis
HASTE (half-Fourier acquisition
    single-shot turbo spin-echo) MR
    cholangiography
HAT-transformed images
Hatcher-Smith cervical fusion
hatchet-head deformity
Hatle method to calculate mitral valve
    area
Hausdorff error
Hausdorff metric measure
haustral blunting
haustral fold
haustral indentation
haustral markings
haustral pattern
haustral pouch
haustrations
haustrum (pl. haustra)
haversian canal
haversian gland
Hawkins breast localization needle
    with FlexStrand cable
Hawkins classification of talar neck
    fractures
Hawkins II talar neck fracture
Hawkins impingement sign
Hawkins line
Hayem-Widal syndrome

Haygarth node
hazy density
hazy infiltrate
HBCT (helical biphasic contrast CT)
H-benzapine imaging agent
HC (head circumference)
HC/AC ratio (head circumference to
    abdominal circumference)
HCTH (helical CT holography)
HDI (HDTV-interlaced)
HDI (high-definition imaging) 3000
    ultrasound system
HDIC (hepatodiaphragmatic
    interposition of the colon)
HDM bronchial provocation test
HDM challenge
HDR (high dose rate)
HE (half-scan with extrapolation)
    method/projection
head
    cartilaginous cap of phalangeal
    clavicular head of sternocleido-
        mastoid
    femoral
    first metatarsal (FMH)
    forward positioning of
    humeral
    long
    metatarsal
    pancreas
    radial
    short
    terminal
    transillumination of
    ulnar
head and neck, femoral
head circumference (HC)
headhunter catheter
head of barium column
healing infarct
health physics

heart
 abdominal
 air-driven artificial
 alcoholic
 ALVAD (intra-abdominal left
  ventricular assist device)
 artificial
 angiosarcoma of
 aortic opening of
 apex of
 armored
 artificial
 athlete's
 athletic
 axis of
 balloon-shaped
 Baylor total artificial
 beer
 beriberi
 boat-shaped
 bony
 booster
 boot-shaped
 bovine
 bread-and-butter
 bulb of
 cardiogenic shock
 cervical
 chaotic
 conical
 coronary artery of
 crisscross
 degeneration of
 diaphragmatic surface of
 dome-shaped
 donor
 drop
 dynamite
 enlargement of
 elongated
 empty
 encased

heart *(cont.)*
 enlarged
 failing
 fat
 fatty
 fibroid
 fibroma of
 flabby
 flask-shaped
 globoid
 hairy
 hanging (suspended)
 holiday
 horizontal
 hyperdynamic
 hyperkinetic
 hyperthyroid
 hypertrophied
 hypoplastic
 hypothermic
 inferior border of
 inflammation of
 intermediate
 irritable
 ischemic
 left (atrium and ventricle)
 left border of
 left ventricle of
 luxus
 lymphosarcoma of
 malposition of
 massively enlarged
 mildly enlarged
 movable
 myxedema of
 myxoma of
 one-ventricle
 ovoid
 ox
 paracorporeal
 parchment
 pear-shaped

heart *(cont.)*
- pectoral
- pendulous
- pulmonary
- Quain fatty
- resting
- rhabdomyoma of
- right (atrium and ventricle)
- right border of
- right ventricle of
- round
- sabot
- semihorizontal
- semivertical
- single-outlet
- snowman
- soldier's
- spastic
- sternocostal surface of
- stone
- superior border of
- superoinferior
- suspended
- systemic
- teardrop
- three-chambered
- thrush breast
- tiger
- tiger lily
- tobacco
- total artificial (TAH)
- transplanted
- transverse
- Traube
- triatrial
- trilocular
- univentricular
- University of Akron artificial
- upstairs-downstairs
- Utah artificial
- Utah TAH (total artificial heart)
- venous

heart *(cont.)*
- venting of
- vertical
- wandering
- water-bottle
- wooden shoe

heart and great vessels
heart and lung transplantation
heart apex
heart attack (myocardial infarction)
heart border
heart catheterization (also cardiac)
- femoral
- retrograde
- transseptal
- transvenous

heart in sinus rhythm
heart overload
heart decortication
heart disease, atherosclerotic
heart failure
- acute
- backward
- chronic
- compensated congestive
- congestive
- decompensated congestive
- diastolic
- fetal
- forward
- high-output
- left-sided
- low-output
- refractory
- right-sided
- systolic

heart-lung transplant (transplantation)
heart power failure
heart prosthesis
heart sac
heart tamponade
heart remnant

heart-to-background ratio
heart-to-lung ratio (HLR)
heat-damaged Tc-RBCs
heat-expandable stent
heat fracture
heat-generating source
Heath-Edwards classification of
    pulmonary vascular disease
heave and lift
heaving precordial motion
heavy-particle irradiation
Heberden disease
Heberden nodes
Heberden sign
Heckathorn disease
Hector, tendon of
heel bone
heel, Sorbol
heel tendon
Heerfordt syndrome
Hegglin syndrome
Heim-Kreysig sign
Helbing sign
helical biphasic contrast-enhanced CT
    (HBCT)
helical coil stent
helical computed tomography (CT)
helical CT holography (HCTH)
helical pattern
helical thin-section CT scan
helical-tip Halo catheter
Helios diagnostic imaging system
helium-filled balloon catheter
Helix camera
Helmholtz coil
Helmholtz configuration
heloma (pl. helomata)
heloma durum
heloma molle
hemal arch
hemangioblastoma tumor
hemangioendothelioma

hemangioma
    cavernous
    verrucous
hemangiomatosis
hemangiopericytoma
hematemesis
hematochezia
hematocystic spot (HCS)
hematogenous dissemination
hematogenous spread of metastases
hematologic parameters
hematoma
    aneurysmal
    balancing subdural
    carotid plaque
    chronic subdural (CSDH)
    corpus luteum
    dissecting aortic
    dural
    encapsulated subdural
    epidural (EDH)
    evolving
    extracerebral
    extradural
    gelatinous
    hemispheral
    intracerebral
    intracranial
    intramural
    intraparenchymal
    intrarenal
    intraventricular
    mural
    nasal septum
    organized
    perianal
    pericardial
    perirenal
    posterior fossa
    primary intracerebral
    rectus sheath
    retromembranous

Henry and Wrisberg, ligaments of
Hensing fold
heparin
heparinization
heparinized blood
hepatic angiography (angiogram)
hepatic angiomyolipoma
hepatic arterial phase (HAP)
hepatic arteriovenous fistula
hepatic artery thrombosis
hepatic bed
hepatic cirrhosis
hepatic congestion
hepatic cord
hepatic cyst
hepatic diverticulum
hepatic duct bifurcation
hepatic flexure of colon
hepatic insufficiency
hepatic necrosis
hepatic vein thrombosis
hepatic venography with hemodynamic
    evaluation
hepatic veno-occlusive disease
hepatic venous outflow
hepatic venous web disease
hepatic web dilation
hepatitis, fulminant
hepatization
hepatobiliary disease
hepatobiliary ductal system imaging
    with quantitative measurement of
    gallbladder function
hepatobiliary ductal system imaging
    with pharmacologic intervention
hepatobiliary imaging
hepatobiliary scintigraphy
hepatobiliary tree
hepatocarcinoma
hepatocellular carcinoma
hepatocellular dysfunction
hepatoclavicular view

hepatodiaphragmatic interposition of
    colon (HDIC)
hepatoduodenal-peritoneal reflection
hepatofugal flow
hepatojugular reflux
hepatolithiasis
hepatoma
hepatomalacia
hepatomegaly
hepatopetal flow
hepatopleural fistula
hepatoptosis
hepatorenal bypass graft
hepatorenal saphenous vein bypass
    graft
hepatorenal syndrome (HRS)
hepatosplenomegaly
hepatotoxicity
herald bleed
Herbert-Fisher fracture classification
    system
Hering canal
Hermodsson fracture
hernia (pl. hernias)
    abdominal wall
    axial hiatal
    Bochdalek
    cecal
    congenital
    diaphragmatic
    direct inguinal
    epigastric
    esophageal
    femoral
    funicular inguinal
    hiatal
    hiatus
    incarcerated
    incisional
    incomplete
    indirect inguinal
    inguinal

hernia *(cont.)*
  inguinofemoral
  interstitial
  intrapericardial diaphragmatic
  mediastinal
  obturator
  ovarian
  pantaloon
  paraesophageal hiatal
  paraileostomal
  parastomal
  peritoneal
  properitoneal
  rolling hiatal
  scrotal
  sliding hiatal
  sliding-type hiatal
  spigelian
  strangulated
  umbilical
  ventral
hernia defect
hernia pouch
hernia sac
herniated abdominal contents
herniated cerebellar tonsil
herniated cervical disk
herniated disk
herniated intervertebral disk (HID)
herniated nucleus pulposus (HNP)
herniated preperitoneal fat
herniation
  brain
  brain tissue
  central
  cerebellar
  cerebral
  cingulate
  concentric
  disk
  fatal
  foramen magnum

herniation *(cont.)*
  frank disk
  hard disk
  hippocampal
  impending
  internal disk
  intraspongy nuclear disk
  lumbosacral intervertebral disk
  phalangeal
  soft disk
  subfalcine (subfalcial)
  subligamentous disk
  supraligamentous disk
  temporal lobe
  tentorial notch
  thoracic intervertebral disk
  tonsillar
  transtentorial
  uncal
herniation of brain tissue
herniation of nucleus pulposus into
  adjacent vertebral body
HER-2 neu oncoprotein expression
Heschl convolution
Heschl transverse gyrus
Hesselbach ligament
Hesselbach triangle
heterocyclic free radicals
heterogeneous appearance
heterogeneous hyperattenuation
heterogeneous isodense enhancement
heterogeneous microdistribution
heterogeneous perfusion pattern
heterogeneous system disease
heterogeneous uptake
heterologous graft
heterotaxy
  abdominal
  visceral
heterotaxy syndrome
heterotopia
  gastric
  gray matter

heterotopic bone formation
heterotopic gray matter
heterotopic ossification
heterotopic pancreas
heterotopic pregnancy
Hetzel forward triangle method for
    cardiac output
Heubner, recurrent artery of
Hewlett-Packard color flow imager
Hewlett-Packard phased-array imaging
    system
Hewlett-Packard scanner
Hewlett-Packard ultrasound unit
Hexabrix contrast medium
hexadactyly
hexamethylpropyleneamine oxime
Hey amputation
HFD (high frequency Doppler) ultra-
    sound
HFLA duration
HI (half-scan with interpolation)
    method/projection
hiatal hernia
hiatus
    adductor
    diaphragmatic
    esophageal
    popliteal
hiatus hernia
Hibbs metatarsocalcaneal angle
hibernating myocardium
hibernation, myocardial
hibernoma
Hickman indwelling right atrial
    catheterf
Hickman tunneled catheter
hickory-stick fracture
HID (herniated intervertebral disk)
HIDA (hepatoiminodiacetic acid) scan
Hidalgo catheter
hierarchical information
hierarchical scanning pattern

Hieshima coaxial catheter
HIFU (high-intensity focused
    ultrasound)
high altitude pulmonary edema
    (HAPE)
high amplitude impulse
high attenuation
high contrast film
high defect in atrial septum
high definition imaging (HDI) 3000
    ultrasound system
high definition television (HDTV)
high density barium
high density linear array
high dose film dosimeter
high dose rate (HDR)
high dose rate remote afterloading
high energy imaging
high energy protons
high energy trauma
high field open MRI scanner
high field strength MR imaging
high field strength scanner
high field system
high filling pressure
high flow, low resistance pattern
high frequency Doppler ultrasound
high frequency miniature probe
high frequency therapeutic ultrasound
high frequency ultrasound imaging
high grade stenosis
high grade tumor
high impedance circulation
high interstitial pressure
high lateral wall myocardial infarction
high left main diagonal artery
high minute ventilation
Highmore, antrum cardiacum of
high order curve recognition
high osmolar media (HOM)
high output circulatory failure
high output heart failure

high-pitched signal
high pontine lesion
high power field
high power, thin section quantitative
   MT
high rate detect interval
high rate pacing
high rate ventricular response, atrial
   fibrillation with
high reflectivity
high resolution B-mode imaging
high resolution computed tomography
   (HRCT) scan
high resolution coronal cuts on CT
   scan
high resolution CT mammography
high resolution diffraction
high resolution EEG
high resolution infrared (HRI) imaging
high resolution, low-speed radiography
high resolution magnification
high resolution storage phosphor
   imaging
high-riding patella (patella alta)
high right atrium
high sensitivity measurement
high signal mass
high spatial frequency reconstruction
   algorithm
high spatial resolution cine CT (HSR-
   CCT)
high spatial resolution mode
   (volumetric imaging)
high speed rotation dynamic
   angioplasty catheter
high take-off of left coronary artery
high temperature diffraction
high temporal resolution cine CT
   (HTRCCT)
high temporal resolution mode
   (multi-time point imaging)
high torque (see *Hi-Torque*)

high velocity gunshot wound
high velocity jet
hilar area
hilar artery
hilar dance
hilar gland enlargement
hilar haze
hilar lymph node enlargement
hilar mass
hilar plate
hilar prominence
hilar reaction
hilar shadows
hilar structures
hilar vessels
Hilight Advantage System CT scanner
Hill sign
Hill-Sachs deformity
Hill-Sachs shoulder lesion
Hillock arch
Hilton law
hilum (formerly hilus) (pl. hila)
   hepatic
   kidney
   lips of
   lung
   renal
   splenic
hilus (pl. hili) tuberculosis
hindbrain deformity
hindfoot excursion
hindfoot instability
hindfoot joint complex
hindfoot valgus
hinged implant
hip
   congenital dislocation of (CDH)
   congenital dysplasia of (CDH)
   developmental dysplasia (DDH) of
   dislocated
   hanging
hip bone (os coxae)

hip bump
hip dislocation
Hippel-Lindau syndrome
hip prosthesis
hip replacement
hippocampal formation
hippocampal gyrus
hippocampal herniation
hippocampal infarction
hippocampal MR volumetry
hippocampal region
hippocampal sclerosis
hippocampal volume
hippocampus
Hippuran contrast medium
Hirschsprung-associated enterocolitis
   (HAEC)
His
   angle of
   atrioventricular node of
   atrioventricular opening of
   bundle of
His band
His bundle
His spindle
His-Haas muscle transfer
Hislop-Reid syndrome
Hispeed CT scanner
histamine
histiocytic origin
histiocytoma
   angiomatoid
   benign fibrous
   fibrous
   low-grade malignant
   malignant fibrous
Hi-Star midfield MRI system
histiocytosis, sinus
histiocytosis X
histogram
   dose-volume
   gaussian dose-volume
   multisectional dose-volume

histogram equalization algorithms
histologic grading
histology
histopathological subtype
histopathologic comparison
histopathologic-CT correlation
histoplasmoma
histoplasmosis
Hitachi CT scanner
Hitachi MR scanner
Hitachi Open MRI System
Hitachi ultrasound
Hi-Torque Floppy (HTF) guide wire
HIV-related metabolic abnormality
HIV-seronegative
HIV-seropositive
HJB (high jugular bulb)
HL (hallux limitus)
HLA (horizontal-long axial) images
HLHS (hypoplastic left heart
   syndrome)
HLR (heart-to-lung ratio)
H-mode echocardiography
HMPAO (hexamethyl propylene
   amine oxime) for SPECT scan
HNA (hypothalamoneurohypophyseal
   axis)
HNP (herniated nucleus pulposus)
Ho:YAG (holmium yttrium aluminum
   garnet) laser
Hobb view
HOC or HOCM (hypertrophic
   obstructive cardiomyopathy)
hockey-stick appearance of catheter tip
hockey-stick deformity of tricuspid
   valve
Hodgkin disease
Hodgkin lymphoma
Hodgkin tumor
Hodgson aneurysmal dilatation of the
   aorta
Hodgson disease

Hoffa disease
Hoffmann atrophy
Hofmeister anastomosis
Hohl tibia condylar fracture
   classification
Holdsworth classification of spinal
   injury
hole burning, selective
hole pattern
holiday heart syndrome
hollow chest syndrome
hollow foot
hollow-point bullet
Holmes cortical cerebellar
   degeneration
Holmes heart
Holmes syndrome
holmium (Ho)
holmium-166 imaging agent
holmium:YAG (yttrium aluminum
   garnet) laser for angioplasty
holocrania
Hologic QDR 1000W dual-energy
   x-ray absorptiometry scanner
Hologic 2000 scanner
hologram
holography
   MEVH
   multiple-exposure volumetric
     (MEVH)
   3-D
   volumetric multiplexed transmission
   Voxgram multiple exposure
holosystolic mitral valve prolapse
Holt-Oram syndrome
Holthouse hernia
Holzknecht space
Holzknecht stomach
HOM (high osmolar media)
homoartery
homogeneity
homogeneous appearance

homogeneous echo pattern
homogeneous opacity
homogeneous perfusion
homogeneous soft tissue density
homogeneous thallium distribution
homology mapping
homonuclear spin systems
homotransplantation
Honda sign appearance
H-1-H (headhunter) catheter
H-1 CSI scan
H-1 MR spectroscopic imaging
H1 spectroscopy
H_2 ^{15}O positron emission tomography
honeycomb formation
honeycomb lung
honeycomb pattern
honeycombing, fibrotic
hooklike osteophyte formation
hook-shaped ureter
hook wire localization, CT-directed
hoop-shaped loops of bowel
Hoover sign
Hope sign
horizontal fissure
horizontal fissure of lung
horizontal fracture
horizontal gaze
horizontal lie
horizontal long axis SPECT image
horizontal-long axial images (HLA)
horizontal plane
horizontal plane loop
horizontal striping
hormone, immunoreactive parathyroid
   (iPTH)
horn
   Ammon
   anterior
   central
   dorsal spinal cord
   enlarged frontal

horn *(cont.)*
    frontal
    lateral
    meniscal
    occipital
    posterior
    posterior gray (of spinal cord)
    projectile
    spinal cord
    spinal dorsal
    splaying of frontal
    temporal
    uterine
    ventral
    ventricular
Horner syndrome
horseshoe appearance
horseshoe configuration on thallium
    imaging
horseshoe kidney
horseshoe shape
Horsley anastomosis
Horton disease
hose-pipe appearance of terminal
    ileum
host, immunocompromised
hot area
"hot" contrast
hot-cross-bun skull
hot nodule
hot nose sign
hot spot artifact
hot spot imaging agent
hot spot on scan
hot-tip laser
Hough transform (HT)
Hounsfield calcium density
    measurement unit (on CT scan)
Hounsfield unit (HU) (on CT scan)
hourglass bladder
hourglass constriction of gallbladder

hourglass deformity on myelogram
hourglass-shaped lesion
hourglass stomach
House grading system
housemaid's knee
Howtek Scanmaster DX scanner
HPCD (hemostatic puncture closure
    device)
hpf (high-power field)
HPGe detector
HRA (high right atrium)
HRCT (high resolution computed
    tomography) image
HRI (high resolution infrared)
    imaging
HRS (hepatorenal syndrome)
HS (half-scan) method/projection
H/S or HSG (hysterosalpingography)
    catheter
HSS ligament rating scale
HSSG (hysterosalpingosonography)
HT (Hough transform)
HTML (hypertext markup language)
HTTP (also http) (hypertext transfer
    protocol)
HU (Hounsfield unit)
Huchard disease
Hughes-Stovin syndrome
Hughston Clinic classification of
    injury
Hughston view
human anti-murine antibodies
    (HAMA)
human serum-albumin imaging agent
human visual sensitivity weighting
humeral bone
humeral head-splitting fracture
humeroradial articulation
humeroulnar articulation
humerus
humidifier lung

hump
　buffalo
　hip
　dowager's
　Hampton
humpback
Hunter canal
Hunter syndrome
Hunter-Sessions inferior vena cava
　balloon occluder
hunterian ligation of aneurysm
Hunt-Hess aneurysm grading system
Hunt-Hess subarachnoid hemorrhage
　scale
Hunt-Kosnik classification of
　aneurysm
Huppert disease
Hurler syndrome
Huschke ligament
Hutchinson-type neuroblastoma
Hutinel-Pick syndrome
HV (hallux valgus)
HVA (hallux valgus angle)
Hx (history)
hyaline-cartilage endplate of the
　intervertebral disk
hyaline membrane disease
hyaloid fossa
hybrid MRI imaging agent
hybrid-RARE imaging
hydatid
　alveolar
　sessile
　Virchow
hydatid cyst
hydatidiform mole (molar pregnancy)
HydraCross TLC PTCA catheter
Hydradjust IV table
hydramnios
hydranencephaly
hydrocephalus
hydrated proteoglycan gel of annulus
　fibrosus

hydration
hydrencephalomeningocele
hydrencephaly
hydrocele
hydrocephalic
hydrocephalocele
hydrocephalus
　acquired
　acute
　asymptomatic
　bilateral
　chronic
　communicating
　congenital
　delayed
　idiopathic
　infantile
　noncommunicating
　normal-pressure (NPH)
　normotensive
　obstructive
　occult
　posthemorrhagic
　postinfectious
　post-traumatic
　primary
　progressive
　secondary
　symptomatic
　unilateral
　unshunted
hydrocephalus ex vacuo
hydrodynamic potential of disk
hydroencephalocele
hydroencephaly
hydrogen proton imaging
Hydrolyser microcatheter for
　thrombectomy systems
hydroma (see *hygroma*)
hydronephrosis
hydronephrotic kidney
hydropericardium

hydroperitoneum
hydrophilic-coated catheter
hydrophone, needle
hydropic changes
hydropic degeneration
hydropneumothorax
hydrops
   endolymphatic
   gallbladder
   labyrinthine
   semicircular canal
hydrosalpinx
hydrostatic pressure of blood
hydrosyringomyelia
hydrothorax
hydroureter
hydroureteronephrosis
hygroma
   cystic
   subdural
hyoid bone
hyoscine butylbromide imaging agent
Hypaque contrast medium
Hypaque-Cysto contrast medium
Hypaque-M contrast medium
Hypaque Meglumine contrast medium
Hypaque myelography
Hypaque-76 contrast media
Hypaque Sodium contrast medium
Hypaque swallow
hyparterial bronchi
hyperabduction maneuver
hyperacute renal transplant rejection
hyperacute stroke
hyperaeration
hyperaldosteronism
hyperattenuation, heterogeneous
hypercalcemia-supravalvular aortic
   stenosis
hyperconcentration of contrast medium
hyperdense middle cerebral artery
   sign

hyperdynamic abductor hallucis
hyperdynamic AV fistulae
hyperechoic area
hyperechoic region
hyperechoicity
hyperemia
   active
   arterial
   collateral
   diffuse
   fluxionary (active)
   mucous membrane
   passive
   reactive
   venous
hyperemic flow
hyperexpanded lobe
hyperexpansion, compensatory lobe
hyperextensibility of joints
hyperextension injury
hyperextension of neck
hyperextension teardrop fracture
hyperfixation
Hyperflex steerable wire
hyperflexion/hyperextension cervical
   injury
hyperflexion injury
hyperflexion teardrop fracture
hyperfractionated radiation therapy
hyperinflation
   dynamic pulmonary
   pulmonary
hyperintense marrow space
hyperintense mass
hyperintense ring sign
hyperintense signal
hyperintensity
   cortical
   white matter signal
hyperkinetic segmental wall motion
hyperlordosis, functional
hyperlucency

hyperlucent lung
hypermetabolic nodule
hypermetabolic region
hypermotility
hypermyelination
hypernephroma
hyperosmotic solution
hyperostosis
   ankylosing spinal
   Caffey
   diffuse idiopathic sclerosis (DISH)
   diffuse idiopathic skeletal (DISH)
   idiopathic cortical (ICH)
   infantile cortical
   senile ankylosing (of spine)
   skull
hyperostosis associated with venous
   malformation
hyperostosis frontalis interna
HyperPACS system
hyperperistalsis
hyperplasia
   adaptive
   adenomatous
   adrenal
   adrenocortical
   angiofollicular lymph node
   angiolymphoid
   benign prostatic
   compensatory
   congenital adrenal (CAH)
   cortical nodular
   ductal
   endometrial
   epiphyseal
   fibrous tissue
   focal nodular (FNH)
   follicular
   giant follicular
   hematopoietic bone marrow
   intravascular papillary endothelial
   lipoid adrenal

hyperplasia *(cont.)*
   lung lymphoid
   lymphoid
   mucosal
   myointimal
   neoplastic
   nodular adrenal
   nodular lymphoid
   nodular regenerative
   parathyroid
   pituitary
   prostatic
   pseudoangiomatous stromal
   reactive
   sinus
   smooth
   splenic
   Swiss-cheese
   thymus
   thyroid
hyperplastic adenomatous polyp
hyperplastic lesion
hyperpolarized He-3 imaging agent
hyperpolarized helium
hyperpolarized ^{129}Xe (xenon-129) gas
hyperprolactinemia
hyperrugosity
hypersplenism
hypertelorism
hypertension (HTN, Htn)
   benign intracranial (BIH)
   intracranial
   primary pulmonary (PPH)
   pulmonary artery
   renovascular
   striate hemorrhage in intracranial
hypertension injury
hypertensive cardiomegaly
hypertensive cardiopathy
hypertensive contrast concentration
hypertensive crisis
hypertensive diathesis

hypothermia
hypotonic duodenography
hypotonic patient
hypovolemia
hypovolemic shock
hypoxic brain damage
hypoxic cell sensitizer
hypoxic injury
hypoxic ischemic encephalopathy
hypoxic ischemic insults
hypoxic pulmonary hypertension

hypoxic pulmonary vasoconstriction
hypoxic vasoconstriction
hysterogram
hysterography
hysterosalpingogram
hysterosalpingography
hysterosalpingosonography (HSSG)
hysterosonography
hysterotubogram
Hz (hertz or cycles per second)

I, i

I (iodine)
IAB (intra-aortic balloon) catheter
IABP (intra-aortic balloon pump)
IADSA (intra-arterial digital subtraction angiography)
IAM (internal auditory meatus)
IAS (interatrial septum)
iatrogenic carotid-cavernous fistula
iatrogenic dural tear
iatrogenic injury
IBD (inflammatory bowel disease)
IBM field-cycling research relaxometer
IBM NMR spectrometer
IBM Speech Server clinical reporting system
I-B1 radiolabeled antibody
IBS (irritable bowel syndrome)
IBZP (chloro-hydroxy-iodophenyl-methyl-tetrahydro-H-benzapine) imaging agent
ICA (internal carotid artery)
ICAM-1 (intercellular adhesive molecule)
ICE (intracardiac echocardiography)
ICEDP (intracranial epidural pressure)

ICEUS (intracaval endovascular ultrasonography)
ice-pick view on M-mode echocardiogram
ICH (intracerebral hemorrhage)
ICP (intracranial pressure)
ICRU 50 radiotherapy
ICS (improved Chen-Smith) coder
ICS (intercostal space)
ictal hyperperfusion
ictal phase study
ictal SPECT
ictal technetium Tc-99m HMPAO brain SPECT
ictus site
ICU (intensive care unit)
ICUS (intracoronary ultrasound)
ICV (internal cerebral vein)
IDD (intraluminal duodenal diverticulum)
identification
    particle
    peak
    phase
    topographic
idiopathic calcium pyrophosphate dihydrate (iCPPD) deposition disease

idiopathic cardiomegaly
idiopathic disease
idiopathic fibrosis, pulmonary interstitial
idiopathic fracture
idiopathic hypertrophic subaortic stenosis (IHSS)
idiopathic inflammatory bowel disease (IBD)
idiopathic intestinal pseudo-obstruction
idiopathic megacolon
idiopathic mural endomyocardial disease
idiopathic pleural calcification
idiopathic pulmonary arteriosclerosis (IPA)
idiopathic pulmonary fibrosis
idiopathic scoliosis
idiopathic unilobar emphysema
idiopathic varicocele
IDIS (intraoperative digital subtraction) angiography system
IDK (internal derangement of knee)
IDSA (intraoperative digital subtraction angiography)
IDSI (Imaging Diagnostic Systems Inc.) scanner
IEA (inferior epigastric artery) graft
IgG autoantibodies
Ig2b kappa monoclonal antibody
IHSS (idiopathic hypertrophic subaortic stenosis)
IJV (internal jugular vein)
ileal conduit
ileal motility
ileal neo-bladder
ileal pouch-anal anastomosis
    H-shaped
    J-shaped
    S-shaped
    W-shaped

ileal reservoir
ileitis
    backwash
    Crohn
    distal
    granulomatous
    obstructive dysfunctional
    prestomal
    regional
    terminal
ileoanal endorectal pull-through
ileocecal fat pad
ileocecal junction
ileocecal region
ileocecal valve
    competent
    incompetent
ileococcygeus muscle
ileocolic disease
ileocolic fold
ileocolic vessel
ileocolitis
ileoconduit
ileogram
ileostogram (loopogram)
ileostomate
ileostomist
ileotransverse colon anastomosis
ileum, terminal
ileus
    adhesive
    adynamic
    adynamic/paralytic
    dynamic
    dynamic/spastic
    gallbladder
    gallstone
    mechanical
    meconium
    occlusive
    paralytic
    postoperative
    spastic

Ilfeld-Holder deformity
iliac artery angioplasty
iliac artery disease
iliac artery stent
iliac atherosclerotic occlusive disease
iliac bone
iliac crest
iliac dowel
iliac fossa
iliac lesion
iliac-renal bypass graft
iliac spine
iliac stenosis
iliac tuberosity
iliac vessel
iliac wing
iliocaval compression syndrome
iliocaval junction
iliocaval thrombolysis
iliocaval tree
iliofemoral bypass
iliofemoral vein thrombosis
iliofemoral venous stenosis
ilioinguinal ring
ilioinguinal syndrome
iliopectineal eminence
iliopectineal line
iliopopliteal bypass
ilioprofunda bypass graft
iliopsoas muscle
iliopsoas ring
iliotibial band friction syndrome
ilium
Ilizarov ring
ill-defined consolidation
ill-defined mass
Illumen-8 guiding catheter
ILP (interstitial laser photocoagulation)
IM (intermetatarsal) joint
IM (intramedullary) rod (rodding)
IMA (inferior mesenteric artery)

IMA (intermetatarsal angle)
IMA (internal mammary artery)
image (see *imaging*)
   artifact
   attenuated
   stereotactic CT scan
image acquisition gated examination
image acquisition time
image analysis system
image coder, Chen-Smith
image control
imaged (verb)
image edge profile acutance
image fusion
image-guided radiosurgery
image intensification
image intensifier
image matrix
image noise
Imagent GI imaging agent
image post-processing errors artifact
image quality degradation
imager (see *scanner*)
image reconstruction
image restoration algorithm
image volume
imaging (also *image; scan; scanner*)
   Adenoscan
   adenosine echocardiography
   adrenal
   aerosol ventilation scan
   A-FAIR (arrhythmia-insensitive flow-sensitive alternating inversion recovery)
   air contrast
   air enema fluoroscopic
   airway fluoroscopy
   Aloka
   Aloka color Doppler real-time 2D blood flow imaging with Cine Memory
   amplitude

imaging *(cont.)*
  AMT-25-enhanced MR
  angiography
  angiography for controlling GI
    bleeding
  angiotensin II, AT_1 receptor
  anisotropic 3D
  annotated
  anterior planar
  anthropometric
  antifibrin antibody
  antegrade
  antegrade pyelography
  aortography
  aperiodic functional MR
  arrhythmia-insensitive flow-
    sensitive alternating inversion
    recovery (A-FAIR)
  arterial flow phase
  arteriovenous shunt
  arthrography
  Artoscan MRI
  A-scan
  ascending contrast phlebography
  Aspire continuous (CI)
  ATL real-time Neurosector scan
  attenuation
  Aurora MR breast
  axial
  axial grade echo
  axial transabdominal
  balloon expulsion
  balloon test occlusion
  barium enema
  barium swallow
  Biad SPECT
  bile duct scan
  biliary tract
  biliary tract CT scan
  binary
  "black blood" T2-weighted
    inversion recovery MR

imaging *(cont.)*
  blood flow
  blood pool
  blood pool phase
  BMIPP SPECT scan
  B-mode
  body coil
  body section radiography
  BOLD
  bolus challenge
  bone age
  bone density
  bone length
  bone mineral content
  bone phase
  bone scintiscan
  brain scan
  breath-hold, contrast-enhanced 3D
    MR angiography scan
  breath-hold T1-weighted MP-GRE
    MR
  breath-hold ungated
  breath-hold velocity-encoded cine
    MR
  bronchial provocation
  bronchography
  B-scan
  bull's eye
  Captopril-stimulated renal
  cardiac
  cardiac blood pool
  cardiac catheterization
  cardiac MRI for function
  cardiac MRI for morphology
  cardiac MRI for velocity flow
    mapping
  cardiac positron emission
    tomography (PET)
  cardiac radiography
  CAT (computerized axial
    tomography)
  cardiac wall motion

imaging *(cont.)*
    cardiokymography (CKG)
    cardiovascular radioisotope scan
      and function
    Cardiolite scan
    CardioTek (Cardiotec) scan
    cardiotocography
    carotid duplex
    carotid sinus
    CathTrack catheter locator system
    CDI (color Doppler imaging)
    celiac and mesenteric
      arteriography
    cephalogram
    cerebral perfusion SPECT
    chemical-selective fat saturation
    chemical shift
    cholangiography
    cine
    cine CT (computed tomography)
    cine gradient-echo
    cine PC (phase contrast)
    cineradiography
    cine view in MUGA scan
    cisternography
    cold spot myocardial imaging
    collimation
    colloid shift on liver-spleen scan
    color amplitude
    color-coded pulmonary blood flow
    color Dopper (CDI)
    color flow
    color-flow duplex
    column mode sinogram
    combined leukocyte-marrow
    combined multisection diffuse-
      weighted and hemodynamically
      weighted echo planar MR
    combined thallium-Tc-HMPAO
    Compuscan Hittman computerized
    computed axial tomography
      (CAT)

imaging *(cont.)*
    computed tomography (CT)
    computed transmission tomog-
      raphy
    chondroitin sulfate iron colloid
      (CSIS)-enhanced MR
    cone-beam
    contiguous
    contrast-enhanced magnetization
      transfer saturation
    contrast material enhanced
    conventional planar (CPI)
    convergent color Doppler
    coronary artery scan (CAS)
    corpus cavernosonography
    correlative diagnostic
    cross-sectional
    CSF-suppressed T2-weighted 3D
      MP-RAGE MR
    CT (computed tomography)
    CTAT (computerized transverse
      axial tomography)
    CT guidance for cyst aspiration
    CT guidance for needle biopsy
    CT guidance for placement of
      radiation therapy fields
    cystography
    cystourethroscopy
    dacryocystography
    delayed
    delayed bone
    DentaScan
    DEXA (dual energy x-ray
      absorptiometry) bone density
      scan
    dexamethasone suppression test
      for Cushing syndrome
    diagnostic
    diffusion and perfusion magnetic
      resonance
    diffusion magnetic resonance
    diffusion-weighted MR

imaging *(cont.)*
    digitally fused CT and
      radiolabeled
    digital radiography
    digital vascular (DVI)
    dipyridamole echocardiography
    dipyridamole handgrip
    dipyridamole infusion
    dipyridamole thallium stress
    dipyridamole thallium-201
    displacement field-fitting MR
    diuretic renal
    Doppler
    Doppler color flow
    Doppler tissue
    Doppler ultrasonography
    Doppler venous
    double contrast
    double-dose gadolinium
    double-helical CT
    double-phase technetium Tc 99m
      sestamibi
    DSC (dynamic susceptibility
      contrast) MR
    dual-echo DIET fast SE (spin
      echo)
    dual energy x-ray absorptiometry
      (DEXA)
    dual isotope
    dual-phase
    duodenography
    duplex
    duplex carotid
    duplex Doppler
    dynamic contrast-enhanced
      subtraction MR
    dynamic scintigraphy
    dynamic susceptibility contrast
      (DSC) MR
    echocardiography (ECG)
      ECG-gated multislice MR
      ECG-gated spin-echo MR

imaging *(cont.)*
    echo-planar (EPI)
    echo-planar FLAIR (fluid attenu-
      ated inversion-recovery)
    echo-planar MRA
    ED (end-diastolic)
    electric joint fluoroscopy
    electrocardiogram-gated MRI
    electrocardiography-gated echo-
      planar
    electrodiagnostic
    electronic portal
    electron radiography
    electromagnetic blood flow
    endoanal MR
    endorectal coil MR
    endoscopic catheterization of
      biliary ductal system
    endoscopic catheterization of
      pancreatic ductal system
    EPI (echo-planar imaging)
    epididymography
    EPR spatial
    equilibrium MUGA
    ERCP (endoscopic retrograde
      cholangiopancreatography)
    esophageal function
    esophagography
    ETL 3D FSE
    excitation-spoiled fat-suppressed
      T1-weighted ST
    excretory urography
    exercise
    exercise thallium-201 stress
    ex vivo MR
    fast cardiac phase contrast cine
    fast Fourier transform (FFT)
    fast low-angle shot (FLASH)
    fast multiplanar spoiled gradient-
      recalled (FMPSPGR)
    fast SE
    fast SE and fast IR (FMPIR)

imaging *(cont.)*
 fast spin-echo MR
 fast spoiled gradient-recalled MR
 fat-suppressed three-dimensional
  spoiled gradient-(FDG)
 FDG myocardial
 FDG PET
 ferumoxides-enhanced MR
 filmless
 511-keV high-energy
 50 msec low resolution
 first-pass myocardial perfusion
 FLAIR (fluid-attenuated inversion-
  recovery)
 FLAIR-FLASH
 FLASH (fast low-angle shot)
 flawed
 flow
 fluid-attenuated inversion-recovery
  (FLAIR)
 FluoroPlus angiography
 FluoroPlus Roadmapper digital
  fluoroscopy
 fluoroscopic
 fluoroscopic localization for transbronchial biopsy or brushing
 fluoroscopy-guided condylar
  lift-off
 flush aortogram
 FMPIR
 FMPSPGR
 Fonar Stand-Up MRI
 four-dimensional (4D)
 four-hour delayed thallium
 frequency domain (FDI) in
  ultrasound
 FS-BURST MR
 fSE (functional SE)
 functional MR (FMR)
 gadolinium (Gd) (see *imaging
  agent*)
 gallbladder

imaging *(cont.)*
 gallium (Ga) (see *imaging agent*)
 gastric emptying
 gastric mucosa
 gastrointestinal motility
 gas ventilation
 gated MR
 gated cardiac blood pool
 gene delivery
 gradient-echo
 gradient-echo phase
 gradient-echo sequence
 gradient-recalled-echo (GRE) MR
 GRASS MR (gradient-recalled
  acquisition in steady state)
 gray-scale
 GRE (gradient-recalled echo)
 GRE breath-hold hepatic
 GRE gadolinium-chelate enhanced
 GRE-in
 GRE-out
 H-1 MR spectroscopic
 half-Fourier, three-dimensional
  technique
 harmonic
 HAT-transformed
 HBCT (helical biphasic computed
  tomography)
 HCTH (helical CT holography)
 Helios diagnostic
 hemodynamically weighted echo
  planar MR
 hepatobiliary scan
 Hewlett-Packard phased-array
 HIDA (hepatoiminodiacetic acid)
 high-definition (HDI)
 high-energy
 high-field-strength MR
 high frequency Doppler ultrasound
 high frequency ultrasound
 high resolution B-mode
 high resolution storage phosphor

imaging *(cont.)*
  HLA (horizontal long axial)
    SPECT scan
  Hologic QDR 1000W dual-energy
    x-ray absorptiometry
  holography
  H-1 CSI (halostatin-1 CSI)
  horizontal long axis (HLA)
    SPECT scan
  hot spot imaging
  hot spot myocardial imaging
  HRCT (high-resolution CT)
  hybrid-RARE
  hydrogen proton
  hypotonic duodenography
  hysterosalpingography
  image acquisition gated scan
  immunoglobulin (Ig), monoclonal
  infarct avid
  infrared
  initial
  in-phase
  in-phase GRE
  intermediate
  interventional
  intracoronary
  intracranial
  intraoperative
  intraperitoneal technetium sulfur
    colloid
  intravenous fluorescein
    angiography (IVFA)
  in vivo
  in vivo He-3 MR
  iodine (see *imaging agent*)
  iodomethylnorcholesterol (^{59}NP)
    scintigraphy
  irreversible compression of MR
  Isocam scintillation
  isotope
  isotope-labeled fibrinogen
  isotope shunt

imaging *(cont.)*
  isotropic 3D
  Judkins coronary arteriography
  kidney function
  kidneys, ureters, bladder (KUB)
  kinematic MR
  kinestatic charge detector (KCD)
  laser-polarized helium MR
  limited
  line
  linear scan
  lipid-polarized helium MR
  lipid-sensitive MR
  liver-spleen
  localizing
  loopogram
  lower extremity
  lower limb venography
  low-field MR
  low-field-strength
  low resolution
  lymphangiography
  macromolecular contrast-enhanced
    MR
  magic-angle spinning
  Magnes 2500 WH (whole head)
  magnetic resonance (MR)
  magnetic resonance angiography
    (MRA)
  magnetic resonance cholangiog-
    raphy with HASTE sequence
  magnetization transfer
  magnetoacoustic
  mammary ductogram
  mammary galactogram
  marker transit
  mass
  Matrix LR3300 laser
  maximum intensity projection
  Meckel ^{99m}Tc pertechnetate
    gastric-mucosa scan
  microwave

imaging *(cont.)*
    middle-field-strength MR
    midsagittal MR
    miniature
    minimum intensity projection
    mirror
    misleading
    M-mode echocardiogram
    monoclonal antibody
    MRA (magnetic resonance angiography)
    MRI (magnetic resonance imaging)
    MUGA (multiple gated acquisition) cardiac blood pool
    multi-echo
    multi-echo coronal
    multimodality
    multiorgan
    multiplanar MR
    multiplanar reformatted radiographic and digitally reconstructed radiographic
    multiple gated acquisition (MUGA) cardiac blood pool
    multipulse
    multisection diffuse-weighted
    multisection MR
    multislice first-pass myocardial perfusion
    multitime point
    multitracer
    MUSTPAC ultrasound
    myelography
    myocardial perfusion
    Myoscint
    native
    navigated spin-echo diffusion-weighted MR
    needle biopsy of intrathoracic lesion with follow-up films
    nephrostogram

imaging *(cont.)*
    nephrotomography
    neurodiagnostic
    neuroradiologic
    noninvasive
    nonsubtraction
    ^{59}NP (iodomethylnorcholesterol) scintigraphy
    nuclear bone
    nuclear gated blood pool
    nuclear perfusion
    oblique axial MR
    off-resonance saturation pulse
    one-dimensional chemical shift (1D-CSI)
    100 msec high resolution
    on-line portal
    opposed GRE
    opposed-phase GRE
    opposed-phase MR
    optical
    oral cholecystogram (OCG)
    Orca fluoroscopic C-arm
    orthopantogram
    orthoroentgenogram
    out-of-phase GRE
    overlapping
    oxygenation-sensitive functional MR
    pancreas ultrasonography
    pancreatography
    panoramic
    parallel hole
    parallel-tag MR
    parathyroid ultrasonography
    PASTA (polarity-altered spectral-selective acquisition)
    PC (phase contrast)
    PDI
    pelvimetry with placental localization
    pelvimetry without placental localization

imaging *(cont.)*
  percutaneous drainage of abscess
  percutaneous intracoronary
    angioscopy
  percutaneous placement of
    enteroclysis tube
  percutaneous placement of
    gastrostomy tube
  percutaneous transhepatic
    cholangiography
  percutaneous transhepatic dilata-
    tion of biliary duct stricture
    with stent placement perfusion
  perfusion and ventilation lung
  perfusion MR
  perfusion-weighted
  perineogram
  peritoneogram
  periorbital Doppler
  peripheral vascular
  Persantine-thallium
  PET (positron emission tomog-
    raphy)
  PET metabolic
  PET myocardial fatty acid
  PET perfusion
  PET perfusion metabolism
  PETT (positron emission trans-
    axial tomography)
  phase
  phase contrast (PC)
  phased-array surface coil MR
  phase encode time reduced
    acquisition sequence
  phase velocity
  pinhole
  PIPIDA hepatobiliary
  plain films
  planar (2D)
  planar spin
  planar thallium
  point

imaging *(cont.)*
  polarity-altered spectral-selective
    acquisition (PASTA)
  positron
  postcontrast MR
  postdrainage
  postexercise
  post-injection
  postmetrizamide CT
  postoperative
  postoperative biliary duct stone
    removal
  postoperative cholangiography
  post-stress
  power Doppler (PDI)
  pre-contrast
  preoperative
  pressure perfusion
  pretherapy
  protodensity MR
  proton density
  proton density-weighted
  pseudodynamic MR
  pullback
  pulmonary perfusion
  pulmonary ventilation
  pulsed electron paramagnetic
  pulsed magnetization transfer MR
  pyelography
  pyelostogram
  PYP (pyrophosphate) technetium
    myocardial
  pyrophosphate (PYP)
  QCT (quantitative computed
    tomography) (for bone loss)
  quantitative
  quantitative fluorescence
  quantitative spirometrically
    controlled CT
  radioactive fibrinogen
  radioactive iodine uptake (RAIU)
  radiographically normal

imaging *(cont.)*
  radioisotope
  radioisotope cisternography
  radioisotope gallium
  radioisotope indium-labeled white blood cell scan
  radioisotope lung scan
  radioisotope technetium
  radioisotope uptake in bone
  radioisotope uptake in vascular brain tumor
  radioisotope voiding cystography
  radionuclide
  radionuclide gated blood pool
  radionuclide milk
  radionuclide renal
  radionuclide renography
  radionuclide thyroid
  rapid axial MR
  rapid-sequence
  RARE MR
  real-time
  real-time echocardiogram
  real-time 2D blood flow
  reconstructed radiographic
  rectilinear bone scan
  redistributed thallium
  redistribution
  redistribution myocardial
  redistribution thallium-201
  regional ejection fraction (REFI)
  registration and alignment of 3D
  renal angiography
  renal computed tomography (CT)
  renal cyst
  renal duplex
  renal ultrasonography
  renal venography
  renogram
  rest (resting)
  rest myocardial perfusion
  rest-redistribution

imaging *(cont.)*
  rest thallium-201 myocardial
  resting MUGA
  retrograde
  retrograde cystography
  retrograde ureteropyelography
  ring-type
  rose bengal sodium ^{131}I biliary
  row mode sinogram
  R-to-R
  sagittal
  sagittal gradient echo
  sagittal oblique
  sagittal T1
  sagittal transabdominal
  saline-enhanced MR
  scanogram
  scintigraphic scan
  scintillation
  scout
  scrambled
  SE (spin echo)
  sector scan echocardiography
  segmented k-space turbo gradient echo breath-hold sequence
  segmenting dual echo MR
  selective
  selenium (^{75}Se)-labeled bile acid
  sequential
  sequential plane
  sequential point
  sequential quantitative MR
  serial
  serial contrast MR
  serial static
  serial duplex
  serialography
  sestamibi stress scan
  shaded surface display (SSD)
  shuntogram
  sialography
  SieScape ultrasound

imaging *(cont.)*
  silhouette
  simultaneous volume
  single-dose gadolinium
  single-voxel proton brain
    spectroscopy (PROBE)
  sinus tract
  sliding-thin-slab maximum
    intensity projection CT
  slip-ring
  small field-of-view (FOV)
  SmartSpot high resolution digital
  Sones coronary arteriography
  source
  SPECT (single photon emission
    CT) thallium
  spine CT with contrast
  spine CT without contrast
  spin-echo (SE)
  spin-echo cardiac
  spin-echo MR
  spin-lock
  spin-lock induced T1rho weighted
  SPIO (superparamagnetic iron
    oxide)
  spirometrically controlled CT
  splanchnic vascular
  spleen ultrasonography
  splenoportography (transsplenic
    portography)
  split-brain
  spot
  spot-film
  SSD (shaded surface display)
  stacked scans
  static
  static 3D FLASH (fast low-angle
    shot)
  stent placement
  stereotactic localization for breast
    biopsy
  STIR (short T1 inversion
    recovery)

imaging *(cont.)*
  stop action
  strain-rate MR
  stress
  stress-redistribution
  stress thallium-201 myocardial
  stroke volume
  subtraction
  superparamagnetic iron oxide-
    enhanced
  SureStart
  survey-view
  susceptibility-weighted MR
  tagging cine MR
  TechneScan MAG3
  technetium (see *imaging agent*)
  thallium (Tl)
    ^{201}Tl exercise
    ^{201}Tl myocardial
    ^{201}Tl SPECT brain
  thallium myocardial perfusion
  thallium rest-redistribution
  thallium scintigraphy
  thallium stress
  thick-slice
  thin-collimation
  thin-slice
  three-dimensional (3D)
    3D Fourier transform (3DFT)
    3DFT GRASS MR
    3DFT SPGR MR
    3D H-1 MR spectroscopic
    3D reformations of MR
    3D turbo SE (spin echo)
  three-phase
  ThromboScan
  thyroid
  thyroid ultrasonography
  time of flight (TOF)
  timed
  TIPS (transjugular intrahepatic
    protosystemic shunt)

imaging *(cont.)*
  tissue Doppler
  TOF (time of flight)
  tomographic
  total body scan
  T1 weighted
  T1 weighted coronal
  T1 weighted sagittal
  Toshiba Aspire continuous
  transabdominal
  transaxial
  transcervical catheterization of
    fallopian tube
  transesophageal Doppler color
    flow
  transluminal atherectomy
  transluminal balloon angioplasty
  triple-dose gadolinium
  triple-phase bone scan
  TSPP (technetium stannous pyro-
    phosphate) rectilinear bone
  T2-QMRI (T2-quantitative
    magnetic resonance imaging)
  T2 weighted
  T2 weighted coronal
  turboFLAIR (fluid-attenuated
    inversion recovery)
  turboFLASH (fast low-angle shot)
  two-dimensional (2D)
    2D Fourier transform
    2D gradient-recalled echo
  two-phase CT
  ultrafast
  ultrafast CT
  ultrasonic tomographic
  ultrasound backscatter microscopy
    (UBM)
  ultrasonography
  unenhanced MR
  unsuppressed
  upper GI and small bowel series

imaging *(cont.)*
  ureteral reflux
  urethrocystography
  urography
  vaginogram
  variance
  vascular flow
  vectorcardiography
  velocity-encoded MR
  venography
  venous
  ventilation
  ventilation-perfusion (V/Q)
  vertical-long axial (VLA)
  vesiculography
  videofluoroscopic
  video radiography
  virtual reality
  Vitrea 3D
  VLA (vertical-long axial)
  voiding cystourethrography
  volume-rendered
  volumetric
  V/Q (ventilation-perfusion)
  wall motion
  water selective SE (spin echo)
  white blood cell
  whole body scan
  whole body thallium
  wide-beam scan
  xenon-133 (^{133}Xe) SPECT
  xeroradiography
  Xillix LIFE-GI fluorescence
    endoscopy
  x-ray sensitive vidicon
imaging agent (including contrast
      media, radioactive drugs,
      radioisotopes, and technetium)
  ABGd
  Adenoscan
  aerosolized technetium Tc DTPA

imaging agent *(cont.)*
  aggregated albumin with technetium
  aggregated iodinated ^{131}I serum
    albumin
  air
  Albunex ultrasound heart
  AMI 121 and 227
  aminopolycarboxylic acid
  Amipaque
  Angio-Conray
  Angiocontrast
  Angiografin
  Angiovist 282, 292, 370
  antifibrin antibody
  antifibrin-MoAb antibody
  antimony
  antimyosin monoclonal (with Fab)
    antibody
  B-19036 chelate
  baby formula with ferrous sulfate
  Baricon
  barium sulfate
  Baro-CAT
  Baroflave
  Barosperse 110
  benzamide
  Biligrafin
  Biliscopin
  Bilivist
  Bilopaque
  Biloptin
  Bis-Gd-mesoporphyrin (Bis-Gd-MP)
  bromospirone (Br)
    ^{76}Br
  bromodeoxyuridine
  bromophenol blue
  bunamiodyl (also buniodyl)
  C (carbon)
  CA15-3 antigen radioimmunoassay
  calcium (Ca)
    ^{45}Ca
    ^{47}Ca

imaging agent *(cont.)*
  carbogen radiosensitizer
  carbon (C)
    ^{11}C acetate
    ^{11}C butanol
    ^{11}C carbon monoxide
    ^{11}C carfentanil
    ^{11}C deoxyglucose
    ^{11}C flumazenil
    ^{11}C-labeled cocaine
    ^{11}C-labeled fatty acids
    ^{11}C L-159
    ^{11}C L-884
    ^{11}C lumazenil
    ^{11}C L-methylmethionine
    ^{11}C methionine
    ^{11}C methoxystaurosporine
    ^{11}C N-methylspiperone
    ^{11}C N-methylspiroperidol (NMS)
    ^{11}C nomifensine
    ^{11}C palmitate
    ^{11}C palmitic acid radioactive
    ^{11}C raclopride
    ^{11}C thymidine
  carbonated saline solution
  carcinoma-specific monoclonal
    antibody
  Cardiografin sodium
  Cardio-Green (indocyanine green)
  Cardiolite
  CardioTec (or Cardiotec)
  CEAker
  CentoRx
  Ceretec radioisotope
  cerium silicate
  cesium chloride (^{137}Cs)
  Cholebrine
  Cholografin
  Cholografin Meglumine
  chromated ^{51}Cr serum albumin

imaging agent *(cont.)*
   fluorocarbon-based ultrasound
   fluorodeoxyglucose (FDG)
   4-azido-2([^{14}C]-methylamino)
     trifluorobenzonitrile
   furosemide
   Ga (gallium)
   gadobenate dimeglumine
   gadobenic acid
   gadobutrol
   gadodiamide
   gadolinium (Gd)
     ^{153}Gd (gadolinium-153)
     Gd-BOPT (benzyloxypropionic-
       tetraacetate)
     Gd-BOPTA/Dimeg
     Gd-DOTA
     Gd-DTPA (diethylenetriamine-
       pentaacetic acid)
     Gd-DTPA/Dimeg
     Gd-DTPA-labeled albumin
     Gd-DTPA-labeled dextran
     Gd-DPTA PGTM
     Gd-DTPA with mannitol
     Gd-EOB-DTPA
     Gd-gadopentetate dimeglumine
     Gd-HIDA chelate
     Gd-Hp-DO3A
   gadolinium oxide contrast medium
   gadoteridol
   gadoversetamide
   gallium (Ga)
     ^{67}Ga bone scan
     ^{67}Ga citrate scan
     ^{68}Ga-EDTA
   Gastrografin (meglumine
     diatrizoate)
   GastroMark oral
   Gastrovist
   Gd (gadolinium)

imaging agent *(cont.)*
   glucagon
   Glucarate ^{99m}Tc hot spot
   gold-195m
   H$_2$ ^{15}O (water O-15) radioactive
   halistatin-1 (H-1)
   hand-agitated
   H-benzapine
   Hedspa
   Hexabrix
   high-density barium
   high osmolar
   Hippuran
   Hipputope
   holmium (Ho)
   holmium-1-66-labeled tetraazacy-
     clododecane tetramethylene
     hybrid
   H-1 (halistatin-1)
   hot spot
   human serum-ABGd
   human serum-albumin
   hydrogen peroxide
   hyoscine butylbromide
   hybrid MRI
   hyoscine butylbromide
   Hypaque
   Hypaque-Cysto
   Hypaque-50
   Hypaque-M
   Hypaque Meglumine
   Hypaque-76
   Hypaque Sodium
   hyperpolarized He-3
   hyperpolarized ^{129}Xe
   I (iodine)
   IBZP (chloro-hydroxy-iodophenyl-
     methyl-tetrahydro-H-benzapine)
   Ig2b kappa monoclonal antibody
   Imagent GI
   Imagopaque

imaging agent *(cont.)*
  imidoacetic acid
  immunoglobuin G (^{111}I-IgG)
  ImmuRAID (CEA Tc99m) antibody
  Immurait (IgG 2A monoclonal
    antibody)
  In (indium)
  Indiclor
  indium (In)
    ^{111}In altumomab pentetate
      monoclonal antibody
    ^{111}In antimyosin antibody
    ^{111}In DTPA (diethylenetriamine
      pentaacetic acid)
    ^{111}In-Fab-DTPA
    ^{111}In-IgG
    ^{111}In imciromab pentetate
    ^{111}In-labeled antimyosin anti-
      body
    ^{111}In-labeled human nonspecific
      immunoglobulin G
    ^{111}In-labeled leukocyte bone
    ^{111}In-labeled white blood cell
    ^{111}In murine anti-CEA mono-
      clonal antibody type ZCE 025
    ^{111}In murine monoclonal anti-
      body Fab to myosin
    ^{111}In pentetreotide (OctreoScan)
    ^{111}In satumomab pendetide
    ^{111}In scintigraphy
    ^{111}In white blood cell imaging
  indocyanine green
  Intropaque
  iobenzamic acid
  iobitridol
  iocarmic acid
  iocetamic acid
  iodamine meglumine
  iodinated
  iodinated ^{131}I human serum albumin
  iodinated ^{125}I radioactive

imaging agent *(cont.)*
  iodine (I)
    ^{123}I ABZM
    ^{125}I brachytherapy
    ^{123}I BMIPP SPECT
    ^{125}I fibrinogen scan
    ^{123}I heptadecanoic acid
    ^{131}I-Hippuran
    ^{123}I IBZM
    ^{123}I IBZP
    ^{192}I high-dose-rate remote
      afterloader
    ^{123}I IMP (iodomethyampheta-
      mine)
    ^{125}I interstitial radiation
      implant
    ^{131}I iodocholesterol
    ^{125}I iodopyracet
    ^{131}I iodopyracet
    ^{131}I iofendylate
    ^{123}I iofetamine HCl
    ^{123}I IPPA (pentylpentadecanoic
      acid)
    ^{131}I-labeled anti-CEA MoAb
      (CC49) and IFN-alpha
    ^{131}I-labeled human MoAb
    ^{131}I labeled monoclonal Fab
      fragment directed against a
      tumor antigen
    ^{131}I-MIBG
  iodipamide meglumine
  iodized oil
  Iodo-gen
  iodohippurate sodium
  iodomethamate sodium
  iodo-phenylated chelates
  iodophthalein sodium
  Iodotope
  iodoxamate meglumine
  iodoxamic acid
  iohexol
  ionic

imaging agent *(cont.)*
    ionic paramagnetic
    iopamidol
    Iopamiron 310; 370
    iopanoic acid
    iopentol
    iopentol nonionic
    iophendylate
    iopydol
    iopydone
    iosefamic acid
    iotetric acid
    iothalamate
    iothalamate meglumine
    iothalamate sodium
    iothalmic acid
    iotrol
    iotroxic acid
    ioversol
    ioxaglate meglumine
    ioxaglate sodium
    ioxilan with iohexol
    ipodate
    ipodate calcium
    ipodate sodium
    Ir (iridium)
    Iriditope radioactive
    iridium (Ir)
        ^{192}Ir (iridium-192)
    isoflurane
    Isopaque
    Isovue nonionic
    Isovue-128; 200; 300; 370
    Isovue-M 200; 300
    K (potassium)
    K4-81
    kinase C antiglioma monoclonal
        antibody
    Kinevac
    Kontrast U
    krypton-81m (^{81m}Kr) radioactive
    LeukaScan

imaging agent *(cont.)*
    Levovist
    Lipiodol
    Lipiodol myelographic
    lipophilic
    Liquipake
    L-methyl ^{11}C-methionine
    L-[1-^{11}C] tyrosine
    long-scale
    low osmolality
    low-osmolar
    lymphangiographic
    L-tyrosine (^{11}C)
    Lymphazurin (isosulfan blue)
    MAA (macroaggregated albumin)
    macromolecular
    Macrotec
    magnetite albumin
    Magnevist
    Mallinckrodt
    mangafodipir trisodium
    manganese (Mn)
        MnCl (manganese chloride)
        Mn DPDP (dipyridoxal
            diphosphate) chelate
        MnPcS4
        Mn-SOD
        Mn TPPS4
    mannitol and saline 1:1 solution
    MD-50; MD-60; MD-76
    MD-Gastroview
    MDP
    meglumine
    meglumine diatrizoate
    meglumine iodipamide
    meglumine iotroxate
    meso-HMPAO
    metabolic 8-hydroxyquinolyl-
        glucuronide
    metaiodobenzylguanidine (MIBG)
    Metastron
    methiodal sodium

imaging agent *(cont.)*
  oxygen (O)
    inhaled (MR contrast)
    ^{15}O (oxygen-15)
    ^{15}O carbon dioxide (inhaled)
    ^{15}O carbon monoxide
    ^{15}O oxygen
    ^{15}O labeled water
    ^{17}O NMR spectroscopy
  P (phosphorus)
  palladium (Pd)
    ^{103}Pd radioactive
  Pantopaque
  paramagnetic
  paramagnetic Cr-labeled red
    blood cells
  ^{212}Pb-labeled monoclonal antibody
  pentagastrin
  pentavalent DMSA
  pentetreotide ^{111}I
  Pentreotide
  peppermint oil (with barium
    enema)
  peptide
  Perchloracap
  perflubron
  perfluoro-1H,-1H-neopentyl
  perfluorocarbon
  perfluorocarbon ^{19}F
  perfluoroctylbromide (PFOB)
  perfluoro-1H,-1H-neopentyl
  pertechnetate sodium
  phenobarbital
  Phentetiothalein
  phosphoric acid
  phosphorus (P)
    ^{32}P chromic phosphate
    ^{32}P sodium phosphate
  PMT (pyridoxyl-5-methyl
    tryptophan)
  polygelin colloid

imaging agent *(cont.)*
  potassium (K)
    ^{43}K (potassium-43)
      ^{81}Kr-m (krypton-81m) radio-
        active
  Priodax
  ProHance (gadoteridol) nonionic
    gadolinium
  propyliodone
  Prostascint diagnostic
  Prostascint monoclonal antibody
  P623-Gd (gadolinium)
  pSV-b-Gal plasmid
  QW 3600
  Racobalamin-57 radioactive agent
  radioactive iodinated serum
    albumin (RISA)
  radioactive isotope
  radiolabeled MoAb
  radiolabeled peptide alpha-M2
  radiopaque
  Rb (rubidium)
    ^{82}Rb-based cardiac
  Re (rhenium)
  Reno-M-Dip
  Reno-M-30
  Reno-M-60
  Renografin
  Renografin-60
  Renografin-76 microbubbles
  Reno-M
  Reno-M-Dip
  Renotec
  Renovist
  Renovist II
  Renovue-Dip
  Renovue-65
  residual
  reticuloendothelial
  rhenium (Re)
    ^{186}Re hydroxyethylidene
      diphosphate (HEDP)

imaging agent *(cont.)*
    RIGScan CR49
    Robengatope radioactive agent
    rose bengal sodium ^{131}I radioactive
        biliary agent
    rubidium chloride (^{82}Rb)
        ^{82}Rb (rubidium-82)
        ^{86}Rb (rubidium-86)
        ^{86}Rb-35S-33P
    Rubratope-57 radioactive agent
    Salpix
    samarium (Sm)
        ^{153}Sm ethylene diamine tetra-
            methylene phosphoric acid
    satumomab pendetide (OncaScint
        CR/OV)
    selenium (Se)
        ^{75}Se (selenium-75)
    sestamibi
    Sethotope radioactive
    7E3 monoclonal antiplatelet
        antibody
    7-methoxy ^{11}C methoxystauro-
        sporine
    SHU 454 (Echovist)
    SHU 508A (Levovist)
    Sinografin
    Skiodan
    Sm (samarium)
    SmartPrep
    sodium bicarbonate solution
    sodium chloride 0.9%
    sodium diatrizoate
    sodium diatrizoate with
        Menoquinon
    sodium iodide
    sodium iodide ring
    sodium iodipamide
    sodium iodohippurate
    sodium iodomethamate
    sodium iothalamate

imaging agent *(cont.)*
    sodium ipodate
    sodium methiodal
    sodium pertechnetate Tc99m
    sodium thorium tartrate
    sodium tyropanoate
    Solu-Biloptin
    Somatostatin
    sonicated
    sonicated meglumine sodium
    sonicated Renografin-76
    sorbitol 70%
    SPIO (superparamagnetic iron
        oxide)
    spontaneous echo
    SPP (superparamagnetic particle)
    sprodiamide
    Sr (strontium)
    Sterling
    strontium (Sr)
        ^{82}Sr (strontium-82)
        ^{85}Sr (strontium-85)
        ^{89}Sr (strontium-89)
    sucrose polyester
    sulfobromophthalein (BSP)
    sulfur colloid labeled with Tc 99m
    superparamagnetic iron oxide
        (SPIO)
    suppo-cire C
    tantalum (Ta)
        ^{183}Ta
    Tc (technetium)
    TcHIDA (technetium HIDA)
    Tc O$_4$
    teboroxime
    Techneplex
    TechneScan MAG3 (^{99m}Tc mertia-
        tide) renal diagnostic
    TechneScan Q-12
    technetated aggregated human
        albumin

imaging agent *(cont.)*
  technetium (Tc, ^{99m}Tc)
    ^{99m}Tc albumin
    ^{99m}Tc albumin aggregated
    ^{99m}Tc albumin colloid
    ^{99m}Tc albumin microaggregated
    ^{99m}Tc albumin microspheres
    ^{99m}Tc anti-granulocyte mono-
      clonal murine antibody Fab
      fragments
    ^{99m}Tc antimelanoma murine
      monoclonal antibody
    ^{99m}Tc antimony-trisulfide
      colloid
    ^{99m}Tc biciromab
    ^{99m}Tc bicisate (Neurolite)
    ^{99m}Tc BIDA
    ^{99m}Tc colloid
    ^{99m}Tc DIEDA
    ^{99m}Tc dimercaptosuccinic acid
    ^{99m}Tc DISIDA
    ^{99m}Tc disofenin
    ^{99m}Tc DMSA
    ^{99m}Tc DTPA
    ^{99m}Tc DTPA aerosol
    ^{99m}Tc DTPA-galactosyl-human
      serum-albumin
    ^{99m}Tc ECD
    ^{99m}Tc etidronate
    ^{99m}Tc exametazine
    ^{99m}Tc Fab fragment of anti-
      CEA antibody IMMU-4
    ^{99m}Tc ferpentetate
    ^{99m}Tc furifosmin
    ^{99m}Tc GH (glucoheptonate)
    ^{99m}Tc GHP
    ^{99m}Tc Glucarate hot spot
    ^{99m}Tc gluceptate
    ^{99m}Tc GSA
    ^{99m}Tc HDP
    ^{99m}Tc HIDA
    ^{99m}Tc HMPAO (hexamethyl-
      propylamine oxime)

imaging agent *(cont.)*
  technetium *(cont.)*
    ^{99m}Tc human serum albumin
    ^{99m}Tc IDA (iminodiacetic acid)
    ^{99m}Tc IMMU-4 monoclonal
      antibody
    ^{99m}Tc iron-ascobate-DTPA
    ^{99m}Tc labeled A.C. (albumin
      colloid)
    ^{99m}Tc labeled anti-alpha-
      fetoprotein
    ^{99m}Tc labeled anti-CEA MoAb
    ^{99m}Tc labeled antifibrin DD-
      3B6/22 Fab monoclonal
      antibody fragments
    ^{99m}Tc labeled antigranulocyte
      antibodies
    ^{99m}Tc labeled fibrinogen
    ^{99m}Tc labeled red blood cells
    ^{99m}Tc labeled stannous methyl-
      ene diphosphonate
    ^{99m}Tc lidofenin
    ^{99m}Tc MAA (macroaggregated
      albumin)
    ^{99m}Tc MAG3 (mercaptoacetyl-
      triglycerine)
    ^{99m}Tc MDP
    ^{99m}Tc mebrofenin
    ^{99m}Tc medronate
    ^{99m}Tc medronate disodium
    ^{99m}Tc mertiatide
    ^{99m}Tc MIBI uptake
    ^{99m}Tc MISO
    ^{99m}Tc murine monoclonal anti-
      body IgG2a to B cell
    ^{99m}Tc murine monoclonal anti-
      body to human alpha-feto-
      protein
    ^{99m}Tc murine monoclonal anti-
      body to human chorionic
      gonadotropin
    ^{99m}Tc oxidronate

imaging agent *(cont.)*
    technetium
       ^{99m}Tc pentetate sodium
       ^{99m}Tc pentetate calcium tri-
          sodium
       ^{99m}Tc pentetic acid
       ^{99m}Tc PIPIDA
       ^{99m}Tc PMT
       ^{99m}Tc polyphosphate
       ^{99m}Tc PYP (pyrophosphate)
       ^{99m}Tc RBC (red blood cells)
       ^{99m}Tc SC (sulfur colloid)
       ^{99m}Tc sestamibi
       ^{99m}Tc siboroxime
       ^{99m}Tc sodium
       ^{99m}Tc sodium gluceptate
       ^{99m}Tc sodium pertechnetate
       ^{99m}Tc SPP (stannous pyrophos-
          phate)
       ^{99m}Tc succimer
       ^{99m}Tc sulfur colloid
       ^{99m}Tc sulfur microcolloid
       ^{99m}Tc teboroxime
       ^{99m}Tc tetrofosmin
       ^{99m}Tc tin-pyrophosphate
       ^{99m}Tc triisocyanide
       ^{99m}Tc trimetaphosphates
    technetium antimony trisulfide
       colloid
    technetium bound to DTPA
    technetium bound to serum
       albumin
    technetium bound to sulfur colloid
    technetium ethylene cysteine
       diethylester
    technetium pertechnetate sodium
    technetium-tagged RBCs
    Telepaque
    Tesuloid
    thallium (Tl)
       ^{201}Tl (thallium-201)
    thallous chloride

imaging agent *(cont.)*
    TheraSeed (palladium 103) active
       isotope in titanium capsule
    Thixokon
    thorium dioxide
    Thorotrast
    ThromboScan
    tissue
    Tl (thallium)
    TmDOTP-5
    Tomocat
    triisocyanide ^{99m}Tc
    triiodinated
    Tru-Scint AD
    TSPP (technetium stannous
       pyrophosphate)
    tyropanoate
    tyropanoate sodium
    Tyropaque
    U (uranium)
       ^{235}U (uranium-235)
    ultrasmall particle superpara-
       magnetic iron oxide
    Ultravist (iopromide)
    uniphasic
    Urografin
    Urografin-76
    Urografin 290
    urokinase
    Urovist Cysto
    Urovist Meglumine
    Urovist Sodium
    USPIO (ultrasmall superparamag-
       netic iron oxide)
    Vascoray
    visualization of
    water-soluble
    water-soluble iodinated
    water-soluble nonionic positive
    whole blood monoclonal antibody
    Xe (xenon)

imaging agent *(cont.)*
  xenon (Xe)
    ^{127}Xe (xenon-127)
    ^{133}Xe (xenon-133)
  xylenol orange
  ZK44012
imaging anatomic correlation
imaging-based stereotaxis in tumor
  neurosurgery
imaging-directed 3D volumetric
  information on intracranial lesion
imaging pathologic correlation
imaging plane
imaging renogram
imaging system (see *scanner*)
imaging workstation
Imagopaque contrast media
Imatron C-100 ultrafast CT scanner
Imatron C-100 scanner
Imatron C-100XL CT Scanner
Imatron C-150L EBCT scanner
Imatron Fastrac C-100 cine x-ray CT
  scanner
Imatron Ultrafast CT scanner
imbalance of phase or gain artifact
imbricate
imbrication
  capsular
  facetal
IMED intravenous infusion device
IMI (inferior myocardial infarction)
imidoacetic acid radioactive agent
immediate intervention
immediate post-ictal period
immersion B-scan ultrasound
imminent death
imminent demise
immobilization
immobilized
immune electron microscopy
immuno-lymphoscintigraphy
immunoblastic

immunocompetency
immunocompromised patient
immunoelectrophoresis
Immunomedics system
immunoreactive parathyroid hormone
  (iPTH)
immunoscintigraphy
immunoscintimetry
ImmuRAID (CEA-Tc 99m) antibody
  imaging agent
Immurait (IgG 2A monoclonal antibody)
IMPA cephalometric measurement
IMP SPECT scan
impacted fracture
impacted subcapital fracture
impacted urethral stones
impacted valgus fracture
impaction
  fecal
  stone
impaired renal function
impaired venous return
impaired ventilation-perfusion
impairment
  circulatory
  functional
  inspiratory muscle function
  motor
  renal function
  sensory
ImpaxPACS system
impedance phlebography
impedance plethysmography (IPG)
impede filling
impediment
impending myocardial infarction
imperfect regeneration
imperforate aneurysm
imperforate anus
impinge
impinged upon

indium (In)
    ^{111}In (indium-111, In-111)
    ^{111}In antimyosin antibody
    ^{111}In DTPA (diethylenetriamine
        pentaacetic acid)
    ^{111}In-Fab-DTPA
    ^{111}In-IgG
    ^{111}In imciromab pentetate
    ^{111}In-labeled antimyosin anti-
        body
    ^{111}In-labeled human nonspecific
        immunoglobulin G
    ^{111}In-labeled leukocyte bone
    ^{111}In-labeled white blood cell
    ^{111}In murine monoclonal anti-
        body Fab to myosin
    ^{111}In pentetreotide (OctreoScan)
    ^{111}In scintigraphy
    ^{111}In white blood cell imaging
indocyanine dilution curve
indocyanine green angiography
indocyanine green dye for detection
    of intracardial shunt
indocyanine green dye method for
    cardiac output measurement
indolent radiation-induced rectal ulcer
indolent ulcer
induced thrombosis of aortic
    aneurysm
inducibility basal state
inducible
inductance
induction anesthesia
indurated mass
indurated tissue
induration
indurative pleurisy
indwelling catheter
indwelling Foley catheter
indwelling nonvascular shunt
indwelling stent
inelastic collision

inelastic pericardium
inequality, limb-length
inexorable progression
in extremis
Inf (infarction)
infant, profoundly obtunded
infantile hydrocephalus
infantile lobar emphysema
infantile-onset spinocerebellar ataxia
infantile pneumonia
infantile syndrome
infantile thoracic dystrophy
infarct (see *infarction*)
infarcted heart muscle
infarcted lung segment
infarct expansion
infarct size limitation
infarction (also infarct)
    acute myocardial (AMI)
    age indeterminate
    anemic
    anterior communicating artery
        distribution
    anterior myocardial (AMI)
    anterior-wall myocardial
    anteroinferior myocardial
    anterolateral myocardial
    anteroseptal myocardial
    apical myocardial
    arrhythmic myocardial
    atherothrombotic
    atherothrombotic brain
    atrial
    bicerebral
    bland
    bone
    brain stem
    capsular
    capsulocaudate
    capsuloputaminal
    capsuloputaminocaudate
    cardiac

infarction *(cont.)*
  cerebellar
  cerebral
  cerebral artery
  concomitant
  cortical
  diaphragmatic myocardial (DMI)
  dominant-hemisphere
  embolic
  evolving myocardial
  extensive anterior myocardial
  focal skin
  frontal lobe
  full-thickness
  gyral
  healing
  hemispheric
  hemorrhagic
  high lateral myocardial
  hippocampal
  hyperacute myocardial
  impending
  impending myocardial
  inferior myocardial (IMI)
  inferolateral myocardial
  inferoposterolateral myocardial
  intestinal
  intraoperative myocardial
  ischemic brain stem
  lacunar brain
  lateral myocardial
  livedo reticularis, digital
  medullary
  mesencephalic
  mesenteric
  multifocal
  multiple cortical
  myocardial (MI)
  nonarrhythmic myocardial
  nonembolic
  nonfatal myocardial

infarction *(cont.)*
  non-Q wave myocardial
  nonseptic embolic brain
  nontransmural myocardial
  occipital lobe
  old myocardial
  papillary muscle
  paramedian
  parenchymal
  pituitary
  pontine
  posterior cerebral territory
  posterior myocardial
  posteroinferior myocardial
  postmyocardial
  pulmonary
  Q wave myocardial
  red
  recent myocardial
  renal
  right ventricular
  segmental bowel
  septal myocardial
  septic pulmonary
  severe
  silent myocardial
  sinoatrial node
  spinal cord
  subacute myocardial
  subcortical
  subendocardial (SEI)
  subendocardial myocardial
  temporal lobe
  testicular
  thalamic
  thrombotic
  transmural myocardial
  uninfected
  ventral pontine
  watershed
  white matter

infarct avid imaging (hot spot scan,
  technetium pyrophosphate scan)
infarctoid cardiomyopathy
infected thrombosed graft
infectious disease
infective thrombosis (or thrombus)
inferior basal segment
inferior border
inferior cerebellar peduncle
inferior dorsal radioulnar ligament
inferior epigastric artery
inferior facet
inferior frontal gyrus
inferior ligaments
inferior lobe of lung
inferior margin of superior rib
inferior mediastinum
inferior mesenteric artery
inferior parietal lobule
inferior pubic ramus (pl. rami)
inferior pulmonary ligament
inferior pulmonary vein
inferior quadriceps retinaculum
inferior temporal gyrus
inferior temporal lobule
inferior thyroid vein
inferior tip of scapula
inferior vena cava (IVC) orifice
inferior vena cava syndrome
inferior vena caval filter
inferior wall akinesis
inferior wall hypokinesis
inferior wall MI (myocardial
  infarction)
inferiormost
inferoapical wall
inferobasal
inferolateral displacement of apical
  beat
inferolateral wall myocardial
  infarction
inferolaterally

inferomedial
inferomedially
inferoposterior wall myocardial
  infarction
inferoposterolateral
INFH (ischemic necrosis of femoral
  head)
infiltrate (also infiltration)
  active
  aggressive interstitial
  aggressive perivascular
  alveolar
  apical
  basilar
  basilar zone
  bilateral interstitial pulmonary
  bilateral upper lobe cavitary
  bronchocentric inflammatory
  butterfly pattern of
  calcareous
  calcium
  cavitary
  circumscribed
  confluent
  consolidated
  diffuse
  diffuse aggressive polymorphous
  diffuse alveolar interstitial
  diffuse bilateral alveolar
  diffuse interstitial
  diffuse perivascular
  diffuse reticulonodular
  eosinophilic
  epituberculous
  fatty
  fibronodular
  fluffy
  focal interstitial
  focal perivascular
  ground glass
  hazy

inflammatory adhesions
inflammatory bowel disease (IBD)
inflammatory disease
inflammatory fracture
inflammatory lesion
inflammatory polypoid mass
inflammatory process
inflammatory reaction
inflammatory response syndrome
inflammatory response, whole body
inflate
inflation
   air
   balloon
   sequential balloon
   simultaneous balloon
inflow
   aortic
   blood
inflow cuff
inflow disease progression
inflow tract of left ventricle
influenza
information, hierarchical
infra-apical
infra-auricular
infracardiac type total anomalous
   venous return
infraclavicular pocket
infracolic midline
infracristal ventricular septal defect
infradiaphragmatic vein
infragastric
infragenicular popliteal artery
infragenicular position
infrageniculate artery
infraglenoid tuberosity
infragluteal crease
infrahepatic vena cava
infrainguinal bypass stenosis
infrainguinal revascularization
infrainguinal vein bypass graft

inframammary crease
inframammary syndrome
inframyocardial
infrapatellar contracture syndrome
   (IPCS)
infrapatellar fat pad
infrapopliteal artery occlusion
infrapopliteal vessel
infrapulmonary position
infrared imaging
infrared light-emitting diode
infrarenal abdominal aortic aneurysm
infrarenal aorta
infrarenal stenosis
infrascapular
infraspinous fossa
infrasternal angle
infratemporal fossa
infratentorial approach
infratentorial compartment
infratentorial Lindau tumor
infraumbilical mound
infravesical obstruction
infundibular atresia
infundibular chamber
infundibular pulmonary stenosis
infundibular septum
infundibular stalk
infundibular subpulmonic stenosis
infundibuloventricular crest
infundibulum
   bile duct
   cerebral
   gallbladder
   hypophysis
   os
   right ventricular
   tumor of
Infuse-a-port catheter
infusion line, peripheral intravenous
infusion transcatheter therapy

Ingram-Bachynski classification of
    hip fracture
ingrowth, bone
inguinal bulge
inguinal crease
inguinal floor
inguinal fold
inguinal hernia
inguinal ligament syndrome
inguinal node
inguinal region
inguinal ring
inguinal trigone
inhalation by slow inspiration
inhalation of krypton-77 to measure
    cerebral blood flow on PET scan
inhalation of radioactive xenon gas
inhalation pneumonia
inhalation study
inhalation technique
inhalation tuberculosis
inhaled oxygen brain MR contrast
    agent
inhaled radionuclide
inherently unstable condition
inhomogeneity correction
inhomogeneity, off-axis dose
inhomogeneous distribution
inhomogeneous echo pattern
inhomogeneous image
inhomogeneous tracer distribution
inion bump
initial delay in appearance time of
    contrast material
initial shock
initial staging evaluation
initiation
injection
    air
    barium (through colostomy)
    bolus
    contrast medium

injection *(cont.)*
    double
    hand (done by hand)
    intra-amniotic
    intra-arterial
    intramuscular (I.M., IM)
    intramuscular fetal
    intraperitoneal fetal
    intrathecal
    intravascular
    intravenous (I.V., IV)
    intravenous bolus
    intravenous fetal
    machine (done by machine)
    manual
    Omnipaque (iohexol) intrathecal
    opacifying
    percutaneous ethanol
    power
    rest
    sclerosing
    selective arterial
    serial
    straight AP pelvic
    venous
injection port
injection test for pneumoperitoneum
injector
    auto
    Hercules power
    Medrad power angiographic
    power
    pressure
    PulseSpray
injury (pl. injuries)
    acute stretch
    axial compression (of spine)
    ballistic
    barked
    bilateral incomplete ureteral
    blunt
    brachial plexus

injury *(cont.)*
  burst
  cervical spine
  closed head (CHI)
  cocking
  compression flexion
  compression-plus-torque theory of
    cervical
  compressive hyperextension
  concomitant tracheal
  crush
  crushing
  decelerative
  degloving
  discoligamentous
  distraction hyperflexion
  Erb (to brachial plexus)
  Erb-Duchenne-Klumpke
  extension (of spine)
  extensive head
  flexion-distraction
  flexion-rotation
  forced flexion
  growth plate
  head (HI)
  high-caliber, low-velocity handgun
  hyperextension
  hyperflexion
  hyperflexion/hyperextension
    cervical
  hypertension
  hypoxic
  hypoxic/ischemic
  iatrogenic ureteral
  immunologic
  intercostal nerve
  intraperitoneal
  inversion
  ischemic
  Klumpke (to brachial plexus)
  lateral bending (of spine)
  Lisfranc

injury *(cont.)*
  low back
  matrix
  meniscal
  mild head
  motor vehicle (MVI)
  nerve
  obstetrical
  penetrating lung
  perinatal
  peripheral nerve
  physeal
  plexus
  postnatal
  prenatal
  pronation-external rotation (P-ER)
  pulmonary parenchymal
  radial vascular thermal
  radiation-induced skin
  rapid deceleration
  repetitive strain (RSI)
  repetitive stress (RSI)
  seat belt
  severe head
  skier's
  soft tissue
  softball sliding
  spinal cord (SCI)
  straddle
  strain-sprain
  subendocardial
  supination-outward rotation
  three-column (spinal column)
  through-and-through
  throwing-arm
  transcutaneous crush
  traumatic
  traumatic brain (TBI)
  traumatic head
  two-column
  ultrasonic assessment of
  vesical

injury *(cont.)*
   weight-bearing rotational
   whiplash
   windup
Injury Scale, Abbreviated
Injury Severity Score (ISS)
injury to nerve roots
inlay graft
inlet
   esophageal
   pelvic
   thoracic
inner adrenal cortex
inner stripe of Baillinger (in brain)
inner table
innermost intercostal muscles
Innervision MR scanner
innocuous
innominate (*not* innominant)
innominate aneurysm
innominate angiography
innominate artery buckling
innominate artery kinking
innominate artery stenosis
innominate bone
innominate vein
Innovator Holter system
inoperable brain tumor
inoperable disease
Inoue balloon catheter
in-phase GRE imaging
in-phase image
in-phase sequence
in-plane vessels
Inrad HiLiter ultrasound-enhanced
   stylet
insertion
   anomalous
   Bosworth bone peg
   ligamentous
   percutaneous (via femoral vein)
   percutaneous pin
   tendinous

insidious onset
insidious progression
in situ
in situ bypass
in situ grafting
in situ pinning
insonation, Doppler
insonifying wave field
inspiration, inhalation by slow
inspiration phase
inspiratory effort
inspiratory flow
inspiratory flow rates
inspiratory flow-volume, tidal
inspiratory increase in venous
   pressure
inspiratory phase
inspiratory reserve volume (IRV)
inspiratory retraction
inspiratory spasm
inspired air
inspissated mucus
inspissation of feces
instability
   anterolateral rotary knee
   articular
   atlantoaxial
   chronic functional
   dorsal intercalary segment (DISI)
   first ray
   hindfoot
   inversion
   joint
   lateral rotatory ankle
   ligamentous
   osseous
   postlaminectomy
   rotary
   rotary ankle
   rotational
   rotatory
   shoulder joint

instability *(cont.)*
  spinal
  subtalar
  truncal
  varus-valgus
  volarflexed intercalated segment
    (VISI)
instantaneous enhancement rate
instantaneous gradient
InstaScan scanner
in-stent balloon redilation
instillation, subarachnoid
insufficiency
  acute cerebrovascular
  acute coronary
  aortic (AI)
  aortic valve
  arterial
  autonomic
  basilar
  basilar artery
  brachial-basilar
  cardiac
  cardiopulmonary
  cerebrovascular
  chronic venous
  congenital pulmonary valve
  coronary
  gastric
  hepatic
  hypostatic pulmonary
  ileocecal
  mitral (MI)
  muscular
  myocardial (MI)
  nonocclusive mesenteric arterial
  nonrheumatic aortic
  parathyroid
  postirradiation vascular
  post-traumatic pulmonary
  pulmonary (PI)
  pulmonary arterial flow

insufficiency *(cont.)*
  pulmonary valve
  pyloric
  renal
  respiratory
  Sternberg myocardial
  thyroid
  transient ischemic carotid
  tricuspid (TI)
  uterine
  valvular
  valvular aortic
  velopharyngeal
  venous
  vertebrobasilar arterial
insufficiency fracture
insufflation
  air
  CO_2
  gas
  tubal
insular gyrus
insular lobe
insula, roof of
insular region of brain
insulative development
insulinoma
insult
  aortic
  bihemispheral
  cerebrovascular
  infectious
  mechanical (to spine)
  myocardial
  occlusive cerebrovascular
  toxic
intact valve cusp
intact ventricular septum
integral, Choquet fuzzy
integral dose
integrated bipolar sensing
integration, telecom

Integris 3000 scanner
Integris V3000 imager
integrity, spinal
integrity and alignment
Intel PC Link2 board
Intel Plink Ethernet card
intensified radiographic imaging
    system (IRIS)
intensifier, image
intensifying screen artifact
intensity
    angina with recent increase in
    beam
    CIDNP signal
    decreased
    equal in
    fat-signal
    low signal
    maximal
    radiation
    signal (SI)
    variable
intensity-modulated photon beams
intensity windowing
intensive care unit (ICU)
intentional reversible thrombosis
interactive electronic scalpel
interactive MR-guided biopsy
interactive visual approach
interarticular disk
interarticularis, pars
interatrial baffle
interatrial communication
interatrial groove
interatrial septal defect
interatrial septum, lipomatous
    hypertrophy of the
interatrial transposition of venous
    return
interbody fusion
interbronchial mass
intercalary defect

intercarpal articulation
intercarpal coalition
intercarpal joints
intercaudate distance
intercaval band
intercavernous anastomosis
intercellular adhesive molecule
    (ICAM-1)
intercellular edema
intercellular space
interchondral joint
interchordal space fenestration
interclavicular notch
intercollicular groove
intercom, noise reduction
intercomparison measurement
    technique
intercondylar eminence
intercondylar fossa
intercondylar fracture
intercondylar groove
intercondylar notch
intercondyloid eminence
intercondyloid fossa
intercondyloid notch
intercoronary anastomosis
intercoronary collateral flow
intercoronary steal syndrome
intercostal artery
intercostal muscle
intercostal nerve injury
intercostal retraction on inspiration
intercostal space (ICS)
intercostal vein
intercostal vessels
intercostobrachial nerve
intercristal diameter
interdigital clavus
interdigital ligament
interdigital neoplasm
interdigital neuroma
interdigitating coil stent

internal femoral rotation
internal iliac artery
internal intercostal muscles
internal intermuscular septum
internal jugular approach for cardiac
    catheterization
internal jugular bulb
internal jugular triangle
internal jugular vein
internal jugular venous cannula
internal mammary artery (IMA)
internal pudendal artery
internal retention mechanism
internal rotation in extension (IRE)
internal rotation in flexion (IRF)
internal snapping hip syndrome
internal thoracic artery
internal thoracic vein
internal tibial torsion (ITT)
internal tibiofibular torsion
internuclear distance
interopercular distances
interorbital distance
interosseous ligament
interosseous membrane
interosseous muscle groups of hand
interosseous nerve
interosseous space
interosseous talocalcaneal ligament
interparietal bone
interpedicular distance
interpediculate
interpeduncular cistern
interpeduncular notch
interpeduncular space
interperiosteal fracture
interphalangeal (IP)
interphalangeal dislocation
interphalangeal fusion
interphalangeal joint
interpleural space
interpolate cues

interpolation
    color space
    cubic convolution
    linear
    nearest neighbor
    prism
    trilinear
interpolation algorithm
interpolation kernel
Interpore bone replacement material
interposed colon segment
interposition graft
interposition, soft tissue
interpretive criteria
interpretive variability
interpulse time
interrenal stenosis
interrogation
    color-duplex
    pulse Doppler
    radiation
    transtelephonic ICD
interruption, aortic arch
intersection gap
intersegmental aberration
interseptal region
intersesamoid ligament
intersigmoid recess
interslice distance
interslice gap
interspace
    ballooning of vertebral
    disk
    vertebral disk
    wedging of vertebral
intersperse
intersphincteric abscess
interspinal ligament
interspinous distance
interspinous ligament
interspinous process
interspinous widening

interstices, bone
interstitial boost
interstitial brachytherapy
interstitial changes
interstitial diffuse pulmonary fibrosis
interstitial edema
interstitial emphysema
interstitial fibrosis
interstitial fluid
interstitial heat generating source
interstitial hyperthermia treatment
interstitial implant
    permanent
    temporary
interstitial infiltrate
    diffuse alveolar
    invasive angiomatous
interstitial insertion of temperature
    sensors
interstitial laser photocoagulation
    (ILP)
interstitial lung disease (ILD)
interstitial markings, increased
interstitial meniscal tear
interstitial nonlobar infiltrates
interstitial pneumonia air leak
interstitial prematurity fibrosis
interstitial probe
interstitial prominence
interstitial pulmonary edema
interstitial pulmonary fibrosis
interstitial radioactive colloid therapy
interstitial radioelement application,
    ultrasonic guidance for
interstitial radiotherapy
interstitial scarring
interstitial shadowing
interstitial space
interstitial template irradiation
interstitial thermoradiotherapy
interstitial tissues
intertarsal

interthalamic bridge
intertrabecular hemorrhage
intertrabecular soft tissue
intertrochanteric plate
intertubercular diameter
interval
    acromiohumeral (AHI)
    atlantoaxial
    atlantodens (ADI)
    supracricoid
interval change
interval development
interval improvement
interval intra-atrial conduction
interval progression
interval resolution
intervention
    immediate
    surgical
    therapeutic
interventional limb salvage
interventional neuroradiology
interventional procedure
interventional radiography
interventional radiology
interventricular (IV)
interventricular foramen
interventricular groove
interventricular septal defect
interventricular septum
interventricular sulcus, posterior
interventricular vein, posterior
intervertebral disk narrowing
intervertebral disk space
intervertebral foramen
intervertebral joint
intervertebral ligament
interzone
intestinal atresia
intestinal diverticulum
intestinal emphysema
intestinal follicle

intestinal hypoperistalsis syndrome
intestinal infantilism
intestinal malrotation
intestinal ureter, construction of
intestinal villous architecture
intestinal web
intestine
   blind
   coils of
   kink in
   large
   malrotation of
   small
"in the magnet" (in magnetic
   resonance imaging)
intima
   arterial
   diffuse thickening of arterial
   friable thickened degenerated
   hypertrophied
   tunica
intimal attachment of diseased
   vessel
intimal atherosclerotic disease
intimal debris
intimal dissection
intimal flap
intimal irregularity
intimal proliferation
intimal remodeling
intimal tear
intimal thickening
intimal-medial dissection
intimomedial thickness
in toto
intra-abdominal arterial bypass graft
intra-abdominal fat
intra-acetabular
intra-acinar pulmonary arteries
intra-alveolar fibrosis
intra-aneurysmal thrombus
intra-aortic balloon assist

intra-aortic balloon counterpulsation
intra-aortic balloon double-lumen
   catheter
intra-aortic balloon pump(ing) (IABP)
intra-arterial chemotherapy
intra-arterial digital subtraction
   angiography (IADSA)
intra-arterial DSA
intra-arterial filling defects
intra-arterial injection of water-
   soluble iodinated contrast agent
intra-arterial intracerebral thrombolysis
intra-arterially
intra-arterial superselective
   nimodipine
intra-arterial thrombosis
intra-arterial thrombus
intra-articular adhesion
intra-articular body
intra-articular calcaneal fracture
intra-articular fracture
intra-articular ligament
intra-articular loose body
intra-articular radiopharmaceutical
   therapy
intra-atrial baffle
intra-atrial filling defect
intra-atrial reentry
intra-atrial thrombi
intra-axial brain tumor
intra-axial cyst
intra-axial varix
intra-orbital air
intra-pixel sequential processing
   (IPSP)
intracanalicular
intracapsular fracture
intracardiac baffle
intracardiac calcium
intracardiac echocardiography (ICE)
intracardiac mass

intracardiac pressure in Doppler
  echocardiogram
intracardiac right-to-left shunt
intracardiac shunt(ing)
intracardiac thrombus
Intracath catheter
intracatheter
intracaval endovascular ultrasonography (ICEUS)
intracavitary afterloading applicators
intracavitary brachytherapy
intracavitary clot formation
intracavitary extension of tumor
intracavitary filling defect
intracavitary hyperthermia treatment
intracavitary prostate ultrasonography
intracavitary radiation source
intracavitary radioactive colloid
  therapy
intracavitary radioelement application
intracavitary radiotherapy
intracellular DNA double-strand
intracerebral hematoma
intracerebral hemorrhage
  basilar
  bulbar
  cerebellar
  cerebral
  cerebromeningeal
  cortical
  internal capsule
  intrapontine
  pontine
  subcortical
  ventricular
intracerebral lesion
intracerebral lymphoma
intrachondrial bone
intracompartmental ischemia and
  edema
intracondyloid
intracoronary imaging

intracoronary stent placement
intracoronary stenting
intracoronary ultrasound (ICUS)
intracortical osteogenic sarcoma
intracranial air
intracranial aneurysm
  arteriosclerotic
  congenital
  dissecting
  mycotic
  traumatic
intracranial berry aneurysm
intracranial calcification
intracranial circulation
intracranial cyst
intracranial electroencephalography
intracranial fat proplase
intracranial glioma
intracranial hemorrhage
intracranial imaging
intracranial malformation
intracranial mass
intracranial neoplasm
intracranial sinus thrombosis
intracranial tuberculoma
intracranial tumor
intracranial vascular lesion
intracranial vascular occlusion
intracranial vessel
intractable bleeding disorder
intractable heart failure
intractable ulcer
intradermal injection of Tc-HSA
intradiaphragmatic aortic segment
intradiskal
intraductal mucin-producing tumor
intraductal pressure
intradural abscess
intradural anastomosis
intradural arteriovenous fistula
intradural extramedullary tumor of
  spinal cord

intradural nerve root
intradural retromedullary arteriovenous fistula
intradural vessels
intraesophageal stent
intraforaminal approach
intrahepatic atresia (IHA)
intrahepatic biliary drainage catheter
intrahepatic biliary duct dilatation
intrahepatic biliary radicles
intrahepatic biliary tract dilatation
intrahepatic biliary tree
intralabyrinthine
intralaminar thalamus
intralobular fibrosis
intraluminal air
intraluminal brachytherapy
intraluminal defect
intraluminal dilation
intraluminal dimension
intraluminal duodenal diverticulum
(IDD)
intraluminal filling defect
intraluminal flow
intraluminal foreign bodies
intraluminal low dose rate
brachytherapy
intraluminal mass
intraluminal membranes
intraluminal Silastic esophageal stent
intraluminal sutureless prosthesis
intraluminal thrombus, laminated
intramammary
intramedullary epidermoid cyst
intramedullary fixation
intramedullary rod (rodding)
intramedullary spinal cord tumor
intramedullary spinal lesion
intramural air in colon
intramural arterial hemorrhage
intramural clot
intramural colonic air

intramural coronary artery aneurysm
intramural diverticulum
intramural gas
intramural hematoma
intramural portion of the distal ureter
intramural thrombus
intramural tunnel
intramuscular aortic segment
intramuscular hemangioma
intramyocardially
intraneural ganglion cyst
intraneuronal neurofibrillary tangles
intranodal architecture
intranuclear diskogram
intraoperative arteriography
intraoperative digital subtraction
angiography (IDSA)
intraoperative electrocortical stimulation (IOECS) mapping
intraoperative gamma probe
intraoperative high dose rate
(IOHDR) brachytherapy
intraoperative imaging
intraoperative laser ablation
intraoperative laser photocoagulation
of ventricular tachycardia
intraoperative myocardial infarction
intraoperative pancreatography
intraoperative radiation therapy
(IORT)
intraoperative radiography
intraoperative radiolymphoscintigraphy
intraoperative radiotherapy (IORT)
intraoperative scanning technique
intraoperative ultrasound
intraoperative x-ray visualization of
fixation devices
intraoral periapical radiograph
intraosseous ganglia
intraosseous vascular malformations
intraosseous venography

intraosseous wiring
intrapapillary terminus
intraparenchymal cyst
intrapedicular fixation
intrapericardial bleeding
intrapericardial pressure
intraperiosteal fracture
intraperitoneal air
intraperitoneal cavity
intraperitoneal exposure
intraperitoneal fluid
intraperitoneal injury
intraperitoneal rupture
intraperitoneal Tc-sulfur colloid scan
intrapleural hemorrhage
intrapleural pressure
intrapleurally
intrapontine intracerebral hemorrhage
intraportal endovascular ultrasonography (IPEUS)
intrapulmonary barotrauma
intrapulmonary disease
intrapulmonary hemorrhage
intrapulmonary pressure
intrapulmonary shunt(ing)
intrarenal collecting system
intrarenal hematoma
intrarenal pelvis
intrarenal reflux
intrasellar Rathke cleft cyst (RCC)
intrasellar tumor
intraspinal adenoma
intraspinal lesion
intraspinal tumor
intrastitial afterloading nylon tubes
intrastitial radiation source
intratendinous fluid collection
intratentorial lipoma
intrathecal imaging
intrathecal injection of metrizamide
intrathecal injection of radiopharmaceutical

intrathecal ionics
intrathecal roots
intrathecal space
intrathoracic airways obstruction
intrathoracic dimension
intrathoracic dislocation of shoulder
intrathoracic goiter
intrathoracic Kaposi sarcoma
intrathoracic pressure
intrathoracic stomach
intrathoracic thyroid
intrathoracic upper airway
  obstruction
intratracheal
intratumoral agent
intratumoral necrosis
intratumoral structure
intrauterine cardiac failure
intrauterine cytomegalic inclusion
  disease
intrauterine fetal transfusion, ultrasonic guidance for
intrauterine fracture (of fetus)
intrauterine growth retardation
  (IUGR)
intrauterine heart failure
intrauterine pregnancy
intrauterine sac
intravascular clotting process
intravascular coagulation of blood
  (ICD), disseminated
intravascular contents, secondary
  extravasation of
intravascular filling defect
intravascular guide wire
intravascular mass
intravascular prosthesis
intravascular radiopharmaceutical
  therapy
intravascular sickling, lung
intravascular space
intravascular stenting

intravascular thrombosis
intravascular tumor thrombus
intravascular ultrasound (IVUS)
intravascular ultrasound catheter
intravascular volume depletion
intravascular volume status
intravenous (I.V. or IV)
intravenous bolus injection of con-
    trast medium
intravenous cholangiography (IVC)
intravenous coronary thrombolysis
intravenous DSA (digital subtraction
    angiography)
intravenous fetal injection
intravenous fluorescein angiography
    (IVFA)
intravenous infusion line, peripheral
intravenous injection of isotope as
    bolus
intravenous line
intravenous pyelogram (IVP)
intravenous pyelography
    excretory
    rapid-sequence
intravenous urogram (IVU)
intravenous urography
intravenously enhanced CT scan
intraventricular aberration
intraventricular conduction block
intraventricular conduction defect
intraventricular conduction delay
intraventricular cryptococcal cyst
intraventricular hemorrhage (IVH)
intraventricular meningioma
intraventricular right ventricular
    obstruction
intraventricular systolic tension
intravesical obstruction
intravesical stone
intravesical ureter
Intrepid PTCA catheter
intrinsic deflection
intrinsic disease

intrinsic foot muscles
intrinsic lesion
intrinsic minus deformity (clawhand)
intrinsic minus hallux
intrinsic plus deformity
intrinsic pulmonary disease
intrinsic sick sinus syndrome
intrinsic stenotic lesions
intrinsic vein graft stenosis
introducer
    Becton-Dickinson
    Bentson
    Check-Flo
    Cook
    Desilets-Hoffman catheter
    Hemaquet catheter
    Hemaquet sheath
    Littleford-Spector
    LPS Peel-Away
    Pacesetter
    peel-away
    Schwartz
    Terumo sheath
    Tuohy-Borst
introducer sheath
introitus
Intropaque contrast medium
intubated small bowel series
intubation
    endotracheal
    esophagogastric (EG)
    nasal
    nasogastric (NG)
    nasotracheal
    oral
    orotracheal
intussusception
    appendiceal
    bowel
    intestinal
    retrograde
    vein
    venous

ischemic area
ischemic brain damage
ischemic changes, persistence of
ischemic contracture
ischemic decompensation
ischemic disease
ischemic episode
ischemic event
ischemic heart disease (IHD)
ischemic hypoxia
ischemic infarction
ischemic injury
ischemic instability
ischemic necrosis
ischemic-reperfusion injury
ischemic segment (on echocardio-
    gram)
ischemic time
ischemic ulcer, hypertensive
ischemic viable myocardium
ischemic zone
ischial bone
ischial spine
ischial tuberosity
ischioacetabular fracture
ischiogluteal bursa
ischiorectal abscess
ischiorectal fossa plane
ischium
    ascending ramus of
    ramus of
ISDN connection
ISG medical imaging workstation
ISIS spectroscopy
island
    bone
    bony
    mucosal
    tissue
    Reil
Isocam scintillation imaging system
Isocam SPECT imaging system

isocapnic hyperventilation-induced
    bronchoconstriction
isocenter placement error
isocenter shift method
isocenter, single
isoclosed curve
isodense appearance
isodense enhancement
isodense mass
isodensity
isodose contour
isodose plan
isodose width
isoechoic
isoeffective bronchial mucosa
isoelectric at J point
isoelectric line
isoelectric period
isointense soft tissue on MRI
isolated clustered calcifications of
    breast
isolated dislocation of semilunar bone
isolated heat perfusion of extremity
isolated ventricular inversion
isomerism, atrial
isometric exercise stress test
isometric heart contraction
Isopaque contrast medium
isoperistaltic ileal reservoir
isoproterenol infusion
isosulfan blue contrast medium
isotope
isotope bone scan
isotope cisternography
isotope injected intravenously as bolus
isotope meal
isotope scan (scanning)
isotope, stable
isotope venogram
isotopic bone scanning
isotopic cisternography
isotopic dilution

isotopic ratio
isotopic skeletal survey
isotropic 3D or volume study
isotropic imaging
isotropic lung scan
isotropic voxels
isovolumetric contraction
isovolumetric period
isovolumic contraction time
isovolumic period
isovolumic relaxation
Isovue (iopamidol, injectable) nonionic contrast agent
Isovue contrast series (128, 200,
300, 370), parenteral injection
Isovue-M contrast series (200, 300),
intrathecal injection
Israel camera
ISS (inferior sagittal sinus)
ISS (Injury Severity Score)
ISSI (interspinous segmental spinal
instrumentation)
isthmic coarctation, congenital
isthmus
aortic
stenotic
temporal
isthmus aneurysm
isthmus of aorta
isthmus of femur
isthmus of Vieussens
IT (iliotibial) band
ITA (internal thoracic artery) graft
ITC (Interventional Therapeutics
Corporation)
ITC balloon catheter
ITC radiopaque balloon catheter

iterative algorithm
iterative gradient optimzation
iterative halftoning
IUdR (idoxuridine, iododeoxyuridine)
halogenated thymidine analogue, a
radiosensitizer
IUGR (intrauterine growth retarda-
tion)
IV (interventricular) septum
IV, I.V. (intravenous)
IV bolus
Ivalon embolization
Ivalon particles
Ivalon sponge
IVB (intraventricular block)
IVC (inferior vena cava)
IVC (intravenous cholangiogram)
IVC filter, percutaneous
IVDSA (intravenous digital subtrac-
tion angiography)
Ivemark syndrome
IVFA (intravenous fluorescein
angiography)
IVH (intraventricular hemorrhage)
IVP (intravenous pyelogram)
IVR (idioventricular rhythm)
IVS (interventricular septum)
IVSD (interventricular septal defect)
IVST (interventricular septal thick-
ness)
IVU (intravenous urogram)
IVUS (intravascular ultrasound)

J, j

J (joule)
jackknife position
Jackman orthogonal catheter
Jackson-Pratt catheter
Jaffe-Lichtenstein disease
jagged bone fragments
jagged osteophytes
Jahss classification of metatarso-
    phalangeal joint dislocation
Janeway lesion
Jansen disease
Janus syndrome
Jarcho-Levin syndrome
jaw bone
JB1 catheter
JB3 catheter
J-coupled spins
J-curve movable core guide wire
Jefferson burst fracture
Jefferson cervical fracture
Jefferson fracture of atlas
Jeffery classification of radial fracture
jejunal loop interposition of Henle
jejunal motility
jejunoileal bypass (JIB)
Jelco intravenous catheter
jeopardize

jet area (JA)
jet, high-velocity
jet length (JL)
jet lesion
jet nebulizer
Jeune-Tommasi syndrome
J guide wire
J-hook deformity of distal ureter
JIB (jejunoileal bypass)
JL (jet length)
JL4 (Judkins left 4) catheter
JL5 (Judkins left 5) catheter
J loop technique on catheterization
Jobert fossa
Jod-Basedow phenomenon
Johnson-Jahss classification of
    posterior tibial tendon tear
joint
    AC (acromioclavicular)
    atlantoaxial
    bail-lock knee
    ball-and-socket
    basal
    calcaneocuboid
    capitate hamate
    capitolunate
    carpometacarpal (CMC)

joint *(cont.)*
    carpophalangeal
    Charcot
    Chopart
    chronic recurrent dislocation of
    condyloid
    costochondral
    costotransverse
    costovertebral
    cubonavicular
    cuneiform
    distal interphalangeal (DIP)
    distraction of
    ellipsoid
    facet
    flail
    free knee
    Gaffney
    Gillette
    glenohumeral
    gliding
    hallux interphalangeal (IP)
    hinge
    hip capsule
    hyperextensibility of
    immovable
    intercarpal
    interchondral
    intermetatarsal (IM)
    interphalangeal (IP)
    intervertebral
    lesser metatarsophalangeal
    Lisfranc
    lunotriquetral (LT)
    Luschka
    manubriosternal
    metacarpal-phalangeal (MCP, MP)
    metacarpophalangeal (MCP, MP)
    metatarsal-phalangeal (MTP)
    metatarsocuneiform (MC)
    metatarsophalangeal (MPJ, MTP)
    midcarpal

joint *(cont.)*
    midtarsal
    mortise
    naviculocuneiform
    neuropathic tarsal-metatarsal
    occipital-axis
    proximal interphalangeal (PIP)
    pisotriquetral
    pivot
    radiocapitellar
    radiocarpal
    radioscaphoid
    radioulnar
    Regnauld degeneration of MTP
    sacroiliac (SI)
    saddle
    scaphocapitate
    scapholunate
    scaphotrapezoid-trapezial (STT)
    secondary cartilaginous
    sesamoidometatarsal
    SI (sacroiliac)
    Silastic finger
    SL (scapholunate)
    sternal
    sternoclavicular
    sternocostal
    STT (scaphotrapezoid-trapezial)
    subtalar
    surgeon's tarsal joint
    Swanson finger
    synovial
    talocalcaneal
    talocrural
    talofibular
    talonavicular
    tarsal-metatarsal
    tarsometatarsal
    temporomandibular
    thoracic
    tibiofibular
    tibiotalar

joint *(cont.)*
   transverse tarsal
   trapeziometacarpal
   trapezioscaphoid
   trapeziotrapezoid
   triquetrohamate
   uncovertebral
   unstable
   weightbearing
   xiphisternal
joint arthrography
joint capsule
joint congruency
joint congruity
joint debris
joint depression fracture
joint dislocation
joint effusion
joint fracture
joint fulcrum
joint hyperextendability
joint incongruity
joint interface
joint kinematics
joint laxity
joint mice (or mouse)
joint morphology
joint photographic experts group
   (JPEG) algorithms
joint play, excessive
joint segment
joint space
   cartilage
   narrowed
   widened
joint survey
joint swelling
Joliot method for sorption studies
Jones classification of diaphyseal
   fractures
Jones fracture
joule (J)

joule radiation absorbed dose
joule shocks
JPEG (joint photographic experts
   group) algorithms
J pouch, two-loop ileal
J-shaped tube
J-shaped ureter
Jude pelvic x-ray
Judkins cardiac catheterization
Judkins coronary angiography
Judkins coronary arteriography
Judkins 4 diagnostic catheter
Judkins left 4 coronary catheter (JL4)
Judkins right 4 coronary catheter
   (JR4)
Judkins selective coronary
   arteriography
Judkins USCI catheter
jugular bulb, internal
jugular catheter
jugular foramen syndrome
jugular triangle, internal
jugular vein distention (JVD)
jugular veins filled from above
jugular veins filled from below
jugular venous distention (JVD)
jugular venous excursions
jugular venous impulse
jugular venous pressure (JVP)
jugular venous pressure collapse
jugular venous pulsation (pulse)
jugulodigastric chain
jugulodigastric node
jugulovenous distention (JVD)
jump vein graft
jumped facet
jumper's knee
junction
   anorectal
   aortic sinotubular
   atriocaval
   atrioventricular

junction *(cont.)*
   cardioesophageal (CE)
   cardiophrenic
   caval-atrial
   cervicomedullary
   cervicothoracic
   choledochopancreatic ductal
   chondrosternal
   corticomedullary
   costochondral
   craniocervical
   craniovertebral
   cystic-choledochal
   duodenojejunal
   esophagogastric (EG)
   fundic-antral
   gastrocnemius-soleus
   gastroesophageal (GE)
   gray-white matter
   ileocecal
   J
   meniscosynovial
   metaphyseal-diaphyseal
   mucocutaneous
   musculotendinous
   myoneural
   myotendinous
   neuromuscular
   occipitocervical
   pancreaticobiliary ductal
   pelviureteral
   phrenovertebral
   pontomedullary
   pontomesencephalic
   pyloroduodenal
   saphenofemoral
   sinotubular

junction *(cont.)*
   squamocolumnar
   sternoclavicular
   sylvian/rolandic
   temporal-occipital
   tracheoesophageal (TE)
   ureteropelvic
junctional defect
junctional focus (pl. foci)
junction separation, costochondral
juvenile ossifying fibroma
juvenile Paget disease
juvenile Tillaux fracture
juxta-anastomotic stenoses
juxta-arterial ventricular septal defect
juxta-articular osteoid osteoma
juxta-articulation
juxtacortical chondroma
juxtacortical sarcoma
juxtacrural
juxtaductal coarctation of aorta
juxtapapillary diverticulum
juxtaphrenic peak
juxtaposed leftward
juxtaposed rightward
juxtaposition
juxtapyloric ulcer
juxtarenal aortic aneurysm
juxtarenal aortic atherosclerosis
juxtarenal cava
juxtatricuspid ventricular septal defect
juxtavesical
JVD (jugulovenous or jugular venous
   distention)
JVP (jugular venous pressure)
J wire

K, k

Kager triangle
Kahler disease
Kalamchi-Dawe classification of
  congenital tibial deficiency
Kalman filter
Kaplan-Meier method
Kaposi sarcoma
  endobronchial
  epicardial
  intracolonic
  intrathoracic
  myocardial infiltration by
  pulmonary
Karplus sign of pleural effusion
Kartagener syndrome
Kartagener triad
Kasabach-Merritt phenomenon
Kashin-Bek disease
Kast syndrome
Katayama syndrome
Katzman infusion of radionuclide
  cisternography
Katz-Wachtel phenomenon
Kawai bioptome
Kawasaki disease
Kayexalate enema
k-capture

KCD (kinestatic charge detector)
KDA profile
Kearns-Sayre syndrome
keel of glenoid component
keel-like ridge
keeled chest
Keith bundle of fibers in heart
Keith-Flack sinoatrial node
Kellock sign of pleural effusion
Kellogg-Speed lumbar spinal fusion
Kelly-Goerss Compass stereotactic
  system
keloid scar
Kemp-Elliot-Gorlin syndrome
Kennedy area-length method
Kennedy ligament technique
Kennedy method for calculating
  ejection fraction
Kensey atherectomy catheter
Kent-His bundle
keratocyst
Kerckring fold
Kerckring nodule
Kerley A lines
Kerley B lines
Kerley C lines
kernel size

Kernig sign
Kernohan classification of astro-
    cytomas and glioblastomas
Kernohan notch phenomenon
Keshan disease
Kety equation
keV or kev (kiloelectron volt)
keV gamma ray
Key-Conwell classification of pelvic
    fracture
keyboard, Cherry
keyhole deformity
keystone of calcar arch
kg (kilogram)
kHz (kilohertz)
kick, atrial (AK)
kidney arteriovenous fistula
kidney
    abdominal
    arteriosclerotic
    atrophic
    cicatricial
    congenital absence of
    congested
    contracted
    contralateral
    cortical scarring of
    crush
    cyanotic
    cystic
    disk
    distended
    double
    doughnut
    duplication of left
    duplication of right
    dysfunctional
    ectopic
    edematous
    enlarged
    fatty
    fibrotic

kidney *(cont.)*
    floating
    Formad
    fused
    Goldblatt
    granular
    hilum of
    hilus of
    horseshoe
    hydronephrotic
    hypermobile
    infundibulum of
    irregular
    lobe of
    lobulated
    long axis of
    lumbar
    medullary sponge
    movable
    multicystic dysplastic
    mural
    myeloma
    nonfunctioning
    pelvis of
    polycystic
    porous
    ptotic
    Rose-Bradford
    sacciform
    scarred
    sclerotic
    shriveled
    sigmoid
    sponge
    supernumerary
    suspension of
    thoracic
    wandering
kidney function study
kidney-pancreas transplant
kidney rest
kidney scan

knee view
knife, roentgen
knob, blurring of aortic
knobby process
knock-knee (genu valgum) deformity
knuckle bone
knuckle of colon
knuckle-shaped
knuckle sign
Knuttsen bending roentgenograms
Kocher anastomosis
Kocher fracture
Kocher lateral J approach
Kocher-Lorenz classification of
    capitellum fracture
Kocher maneuver
Koch sinoatrial node
Koch triangle, apex of
Kock pouch
Kodak software
Koerber-Salus-Elschnig syndrome
Köhler disease
Köhler-Pellegrini-Stieda disease
Kohlrausch fold
Kohn, pores of3334
Komai stereotactic head frame
Kommerell diverticulum
Konica scanner
Konstram angle
Kontrast U radiopaque contrast
    medium
Kontron balloon catheter
Kopans needle
Korányi-Grocco sign
Korányi-Grocco triangle
Korotkoff method in Doppler
    cerebrovascular examination
Korsakoff syndrome

Korotkoff test for collateral circulation
Kouchoukos method
Kr-81m (krypton) imaging agent
Krabbe diffuse sclerosis
Krukenberg tumor
krypton (^{81m}Kr) imaging agent
k-space
k-space matrix
k-space velocity mapping
KUB (kidneys, ureters, and urinary
    bladder)
Kubelka-Munk theory
Kugel anastomosis
Kugel artery
Kugel collaterals
Kugelberg-Welander juvenile spinal
    muscle atrophy
Kumeral diverticulum
Kümmell disease
Kurtz-Sprague-White syndrome
Kussmaul-Maier disease
Kveim test
kVp (kilovolts peak) meter
Kyle fracture classification system
kyllosis (clubfoot)
kymography
kyphoscoliosis
kyphoscoliotic heart disease
kyphosis
    Cobb method of measuring
    loss of
    lumbar
    lumbosacral
    postlaminectomy
    Scheuermann juvenile
    thoracic
kyphotic angulation
kyphotic pelvis

L, l

L (liter)
L (lumbar vertebra)
LA (left atrium)
LAA (left atrial appendage)
LAA (left auricular appendage)
LA/AR (left atrium/aortic root) ratio
LABA (laser-assisted balloon
   angioplasty)
Labbé triangle
Labbé, vein of
label
   double
   long wavelength photolabel
   radioactive
   radionuclide
   single
   triple
labeled antibodies
labeled fibrinogen
labeled positron
labeled RBCs
labeled red blood cell sequestration
labeling
   antibody
   [111]In (indium-111) WBCs
   in vitro
   in vivo

labeling *(cont.)*
   in vivo/in vitro
   microglobulin
   radioactive
   radioisotope
   site-specific
   technetium Tc-human serum
     albumin
   Tc-tagged RBCs
   white blood cell
labile blood pressure
labral injury
labral variant
labrum
   acetabular
   articular
   glenoid
   glenoidal
labyrinth
   artery of
   bony
   cochlear
   ethmoidal
   Ludwig
   membranous
   osseous
   renal

labyrinth (*cont.*)
    Santorini
    vestibular
labyrinthine artery
labyrinthine hydrops
labyrinthine structures
LACD (left apexcardiogram,
    calibrated displacement)
laciniate ligament of ankle
lack of clear-cut cerebral dominance
lacrimal bone
lacrimal canaliculus obstruction
lactulose enema
lacuna (pl. lacunae)
    bone
    cartilage
    intervillous
    osseous
    penis
    resorption
lacunar abscess
lacunar infarct
lacunar ligament
lacunar stroke
LAD (left anterior descending)
    coronary artery
Ladder diagram
LAE (left atrial enlargement)
LAID (left anterior internal diameter)
LAIS excimer laser for coronary
    angioplasty
Laitinen CT guidance system
Laitinen stereotactic head frame
lake
    bile
    capillary
    mucous
    lipid
    venous
Laks method
lambdoid suture
Lambert projection

lamella (pl. lamellae)
    articular
    circumferential
    concentric
    enamel
lamellar body density (LBD) count
lamellated bone
lamina
    medullary
    osseous spiral
lamina propria
laminar flow
laminated calcification
laminated intraluminal thrombus
lamination of gyrus
laminography, cardiac
Lancisi muscle
landmark
    anatomic
    bony
    bony skull
landmark registration
Landolfi sign
Landsmeer ligament
Lane disease
Lane kink
Lanex medium screen
Langenbeck triangle
Langer line
Lanier clinical reporting system
lanthanide-induced shifts
Lanz point
LAO (left anterior oblique)
    LAO position
    LAO projection
    LAO view
LAP (left atrial pressure)
laparoscopic contact ultrasonography
    (LCU)
laparoscopic Doppler probe
laparoscopic intracorporeal ultrasound
    (LICU)

laterally displaced fracture
lateral opposed beam
lateral position
lateral projection
lateral spring ligament of foot
lateral sulcus
lateral tomography
lateral ventricle
lateral view
lateral web
lateral wedge fracture of vertebral
   body
lateroconal fascia
late systolic posterior displacement on
   echocardiogram
LaTeX device-independent
latissimus dorsi muscle
LATS (long-acting thyroid stimulator)
lattice, fibrovascular
lattice model
lattice relaxation time
lattice vibrations
latticework
Laubry-Pezzi syndrome
Laue pattern
Laue photographic technique
Lauge-Hansen classification of ankle
   fracture
Laurence-Moon-Biedl-Bardet
   syndrome
Laurin angle
Laurin x-ray view
Lausanne stereotactic robot
law
   Bragg
   Courvoisier
   Hilton
Law view
laxity
   joint
   ligament
   varus stress

layer
   bright
   circumferential echodense
   echodense
   echo-free
   hypoechoic
   inner bright
   sonolucent
layering calcification
layering effusion
layering of contrast material
layering of gallstones
lazaroid U74389G
LBA (laser balloon angioplasty)
L/B (lesion-to-brain) ratio
LBBB (left bundle branch block)
LBCD (left border of cardiac
   dullness)
LBP (low back pain)
LC-DCP (low-contact dynamic
   compression plate)
LCA (left coronary artery)
LCF or LCX (left circumflex)
   coronary artery
LCL (lateral collateral ligament)
LCP (Legg-Calvé-Perthes disease)
LCT (liquid crystal contact
   thermography)
LCU (laparoscopic contact ultrasonography)
LDF (laser-Doppler flowmetry) probe
lead apron
lead eye shield
lead-pipe colon
lead-pipe fracture
lead-pipe rigidity
lead pellet marker
lead points
leaflet
leaf of diaphragm
leak
   air
   aortic paravalvular

leak *(cont.)*
  baffle
  blood
  capillary
  cerebrospinal fluid (CSF)
  chyle
  contained (of aortic aneurysm)
  current
  generalized capillary
  interatrial baffle
  light
  mitral
  paraprosthetic
  paravalvar
  paravalvular
  periprosthetic
  perivalvular
leakage
  blood-tumor-barrier
  cerebrospinal fluid (CSF)
  contrast media
leaking abdominal aortic aneurysm
leaking vein
leaky valve
lean mass
least-squares (LS) algorithms
leather bottle stomach
leaves of diaphragm
leaves of mesentery
Le Fort (I, II, or III) fracture
left anterior descending (LAD) artery,
  superdominant
left anterior oblique (LAO) projection
left atrial active emptying fraction
left atrial end-diastolic pressure
left atrial enlargement
left atrial maximal volume
left atrial pressure (LAP)
left atrium, giant
left auricle
left auricular appendage (LAA)
left border of heart

left bundle branch block (LBBB)
left bundle branch hemiblock
left circumflex (LCX) coronary artery
left common femoral artery
left coronary artery arising from
  pulmonary artery
left coronary cusp
left coronary plexus (of heart)
left heart failure
left heart pressure
left iliac system
left internal mammary artery (LIMA)
left Judkins catheter
left main coronary artery (LMCA)
left main stem bronchus
left mid lung
left posterior oblique (LPO) position
left pulmonary artery
left pulmonary cusp
left respiratory nerve (phrenic)
left-right asymmetry
left-sided heart failure
left-side-down decubitus position
left sternal border
left-to-right shift
left-to-right ventricular shunt
left ventricle
  double-inlet
  hypoplastic
  morphologic
left ventricular afterload
left ventricular assist device (LVAD),
left ventricular chamber
left ventricular ejection fraction
  (LVEF)
left ventricular ejection fraction by
  acoustic quantification
left ventricular end-diastolic pressure
  (LVEDP)
left ventricular end-diastolic volume
left ventricular end-systolic volume
left ventricular hypertrophy (LVH)

left ventricular hypoplasia
left ventricular loading
left ventricular maximal volume
left ventricular outflow tract
left ventricular preload
left ventricular pressure
left ventricular regional wall motion
   abnormality
left ventricular segmental contraction
left ventricular stroke work (LVSW)
left ventricular stroke work index
   (LVSWI)
left ventricular systolic pump function
left ventricular systolic time interval
   ratio
left ventriculogram
left ventriculography
leg
   baker
   bayonet
   postphlebitic
Legg-Calvé-Perthes disease
Legg-Calvé-Waldenström disease
Lehman ventriculography catheter
Leiner disease
Leitner syndrome
Leksell D-shaped stereotactic frame
Leksell-Elekta stereotactic frame
Leksell stereotaxic device used with
   CT scanner
length
   crown-heel
   crown-rump
   echo-train
   limb
   track cone
LENI (lower extremity noninvasive)
LENT (late effects of normal tissues)
   scoring system
lenticular bone of hand
lenticular nucleus
lenticulostriate artery

lentiform nucleus
LEOPARD syndrome
leptomeningeal cyst
leptomeningeal disease
leptomeninges
Leriche syndrome
LEs (lower extremities)
LES (lower esophageal sphincter)
Lesgaft hernia
Lesgaft triangle
lesion
   acute cerebellar hemispheric
   adrenal
   afferent nerve
   angulated
   annular
   anterior parietal
   anterochiasmatic
   aortic arch
   apical
   apple core
   Armanni-Ebstein
   atheromatous
   atherosclerotic
   atrophic
   Baehr-Lohlein
   Bankart shoulder
   Bennett
   bifurcation
   bilateral
   biparietal
   bird's nest
   blastic
   bleeding
   Blumenthal
   Bracht-Wachter
   brain stem
   Brown-Séquard
   bull's-eye
   calcified
   callosal
   cardiac valvular

lesion (*cont.*)
  cartilaginous
  cavernous sinus
  caviar
  cavitary
  central
  cerebral
  cervical cord
  chiasmal
  chiasmatic
  circular
  circumscribed
  coin (of lungs)
  cold
  complete nerve
  complex
  concentric
  constricting esophageal
  constrictive
  conus medullaris
  coronary artery
  cortical
  corticospinal pathway
  critical
  culprit
  cyclops
  cystic
  deep
  de nov
  deep-seated
  dendritic
  desmoid
  destructive
  Dieulafoy
  diffuse
  discrete
  disk
  dominant hemisphere
  dorsal root entry zone
  doughnut
  DREZ (dorsal root entry zone)
  dumbbell

lesion (*cont.*)
  Duret
  Ebstein
  eccentric
  eccentric restenosis
  echogenic
  ellipsoid
  endobronchial
  enhancing
  epicortical
  epileptogenic
  esophageal
  excitatory
  expansile lytic
  extra-axial
  extrinsic
  fibro-osseous
  fibromuscular
  fingertip
  florid duct
  flow-compromising
  flow-limiting
  focal
  focal hemispheric
  focal ischemic
  frank
  frontal lobe
  geographic
  Ghon primary
  gross
  hamartomatous
  hemodynamically significant
  hemorrhagic
  high cervical spinal cord
  high-density
  high-grade obstructive
  high pontine
  high-signal
  Hill-Sachs shoulder
  homogeneous
  hot
  hourglass-shaped

lesion (*cont.*)
    hyperintense
    hypodense
    hypothalamic
    impaction
    indiscriminate
    infiltrating
    infranuclear
    intra-axial brain
    intracerebral
    intracranial vascular
    intramedullary spinal
    intrasellar
    intraspinal
    intrinsic stenotic
    invasive
    irregular-shaped
    irregularly shaped
    ischemic
    isointense
    Janeway
    jet
    Kidner
    lateral temporal epileptogenic
    left lower lobe (LLL)
    left upper lobe (LUL)
    lipomatous
    local
    localized
    Löhlein-Baehr
    low-density
    lower motor neuron
    lytic (osteolytic) bone
    malignant
    Mallory-Weiss
    mass
    medial longitudinal fasciculus
        (MLF)
    median nerve
    mesenteric vascular
    mesial temporal epileptogenic
    metabolic

lesion (*cont.*)
    metastatic bone
    midbrain
    midline
    mixed
    mongolian spot-like
    Monteggia
    multifocal
    multiple focal
    muscular
    nail bed
    napkin-ring annular
    necrotic
    neoplastic
    neurogenic
    neurologic bladder
    nidus of
    nodular
    nondominant hemisphere
    nonenhancing
    noninvasive
    nucleus basalis
    obstructive (of the CSF pathways)
    occipital
    occlusive
    occult
    onion scale
    onionskin
    organic
    osseous
    osteoblastic
    osteocartilaginous
    osteochondral (of the talus)
    ostial
    outcropping of
    papillary
    papular
    papulonecrotic
    parasagittal
    parasellar
    parietal cortex
    parietal lobe

lesion *(cont.)*
- parieto-occipital
- partial
- pedunculated
- periapical
- peripheral
- peripheral nerve
- periventricular
- permeative
- Perthes-Bankart
- photon-deficient
- plaquelike
- polyostotic bone
- polypoid
- pontine
- posterior column
- posterior compartment
- posterior fossa-foramen magnum
- posterior language area
- pretectal
- primary
- pulmonary
- purulent
- questionable
- radial sclerosing
- radiofrequency
- radiographic stability of
- radiopaque
- rectal
- rectosigmoid polypoid
- recurrent
- regurgitant
- renal mass
- resectable
- retrochiasmal
- retrochiasmatic
- rheumatic
- rib
- right lower lobe (RLL)
- right upper lobe (RUL)
- ring-enhancing (on CT)
- root

lesion *(cont.)*
- root entry-zone
- satellite
- secondary
- segmental
- serial
- sessile
- sharply demarcated circumferential
- signal characteristics of
- skip
- SLAP (superior labrum anterior posterior)
- slowly developing
- solitary
- sonolucent
- space-occupying
- spherical
- spinal cord
- spontaneous
- stacked ovoid
- Stener
- stenotic
- striatal
- structural
- subchondral
- subcortical intracranial
- submucosal
- subtentorial
- subtotal
- superficial
- supranuclear
- suprasellar
- supratentorial
- suspicious
- synchronous
- systemic
- tandem
- target
- tectal
- telangiectatic
- temporal
- temporal lobe

Lhermitte sign
LHV (left hepatic vein)
Lian-Siguier-Welti venous thrombosis
    syndrome
Libman-Sacks endocarditis disease
LICS (left intercostal space)
LICU (laparoscopic intracorporeal
    ultrasound)
Liddle syndrome
lidocaine
Lido-Pen Auto-Injector
lie
    horizontal
    longitudinal
    posterior
    transverse
Liebel-Flarsheim CT 9000 contrast
    delivery system
Lieberkühn crypt
lienography
LiF (lithium fluoride)
LiF thermoluminescence dosimeter
Life-Pack 5 cardiac monitor
ligament
    accessory
    acromioclavicular
    acromiocoracoid
    alar
    annular
    anococcygeal
    apical (of dens)
    Arantius
    arcuate
    arterial
    atlantal
    attenuated
    auricular
    avulsed
    axis
    Bardinet
    Barkow
    beak

ligament *(cont.)*
    Bellini
    Berry
    Bertin
    Bichat
    bifurcated
    Bigelow
    Botallo
    Bourgery
    broad (of uterus)
    Brodie
    Burns
    calcaneoclavicular
    calcaneocuboid
    calcaneofibular (CF)
    calcaneonavicular
    calcaneotibial
    Caldani
    Campbell
    Camper
    capsular
    Carcassonne
    cardinal
    caroticoclinoid
    carpometacarpal
    Casser
    casserian
    caudal
    ceratocricoid
    cervical
    check
    check rein
    cholecystoduodenal
    chondroxiphoid
    ciliary
    Civinini
    Clado
    Cleland
    Cloquet
    collateral
    Colles
    congenital laxity of

ligament *(cont.)*
  conjugate
  conoid
  conus
  coracoacromial
  coracoclavicular
  coracohumeral
  corniculopharyngeal
  coronary
  costoclavicular
  costocolic
  costotransverse
  costoxiphoid
  cotyloid
  Cowper
  cricopharyngeal
  cricosantorinian
  cricothyroid
  cricotracheal
  cross
  crucial
  cruciate
  cruciatum cruris
  cruciform
  Cruveilhier
  cuboideonavicular
  cuneocuboid
  cuneonavicular
  cystoduodenal
  deep collateral
  deltoid (of shoulder, of ankle)
  Denonvilliers
  dentate
  denticulate
  Denucé
  diaphragmatic
  Douglas
  duodenal
  duodenorenal
  epihyal
  extracapsular
  falciform

ligament *(cont.)*
  fallopian
  femoral
  Ferrein
  fibular collateral
  fibulotalar
  fibulotalocalcaneal
  flaval
  floating
  Flood
  fundiform
  gastrocolic
  gastrodiaphragmatic
  gastrohepatic
  gastrolienal
  gastropancreatic
  gastrophrenic
  gastrosplenic
  genital
  genitoinguinal
  Gerdy
  Gillette suspensory
  Gimbernat
  gingivodental
  glenohumeral
  glenoid
  glossoepiglottic
  Grayson
  Günz (Guenz)
  Günzberg (Guenzberg)
  Haines-McDougall medial
  hammock
  Helmholtz axis
  Henle
  Hensing
  hepatic
  hepatocolic
  hepatocystocolic
  hepatoduodenal
  hepatoesophageal
  hepatogastric
  hepatogastroduodenal

ligament *(cont.)*

    hepatophrenic
    hepatorenal
    hepatoumbilical
    Hesselbach
    Hey
    Holl
    Hueck
    Humphry
    Hunter
    Huschke
    hyalocapsular
    hyoepiglottic
    iliofemoral
    iliolumbar
    iliopectineal
    iliopubic
    iliotibial (of Maissiat)
    iliotrochanteric
    infrapatellar
    infundibulo-ovarian
    infundibulopelvic
    inguinal
    intercapital
    intercarpal
    interclavicular
    interclinoid
    intercornual
    intercostal
    intercuneiform
    interdigital
    interfoveolar
    intermetatarsal
    internal collateral
    interosseous
    intersesamoid
    interspinal
    interspinous
    intertransverse
    intervertebral
    intra-articular
    intrascapular

ligament *(cont.)*

    ischiocapsular
    ischiofemoral
    Jarjavay
    jugal
    Krause
    laciniate
    lacunar
    Landsmeer
    Lannelongue
    lateral arcuate
    lateral collateral (LCL)
    Lauth
    lienophrenic
    lienorenal
    limited proteoglycan matrix of
    Lisfranc
    Lockwood
    longitudinal
    LTC (lateral talocalcaneal)
    lumbocostal
    lunotriquetral
    Luschka
    Mackenrodt
    macroscopic hemorrhage
    Maissiat
    Mauchart
    Meckel
    medial collateral (MCL)
    median arcuate
    meniscofemoral
    meniscotibial
    metacarpoglenoidal
    metacarpophalangeal
    microscopic hemorrhage of
    mucosal suspensory
    natatory
    naviculocuneiform
    nuchal
    occipital-atlas-axis
    occipitoaxial
    odontoid

ligament *(cont.)*
    orbicular
    ovarian
    palmar
    pectinate
    pectineal
    peridental
    periodontal
    peritoneal
    Petit
    Pétrequin
    petroclinoid
    phalangeal glenoidal
    phrenicocolic
    phrenicoesophageal
    phrenicolienal
    phrenicosplenic
    phrenoesophageal
    phrenogastric
    phrenosplenic
    pisohamate
    pisometacarpal
    pisounciform
    pisouncinate
    plantar
    posterior cruciate (PCL)
    posterior longitudinal (PLL)
    posterior oblique (POL)
    Poupart
    pterygomandibular
    pterygospinal
    pterygospinous
    pubocapsular
    pubocervical
    pubofemoral
    puboprostatic
    pubovesical
    pulmonary
    quadrate
    radial collateral
    radial metacarpal
    radiate sternocostal

ligament *(cont.)*
    radiocarpal
    radiolunotriquetral
    radioscaphocapitate
    radioscaphoid
    radioscapholunate
    reflected inguinal
    reflecting edge of
    retinacular
    Retzius
    rhomboid
    right triangular
    ring
    Robert
    round
    Rouviere
    sacrodural
    sacrospinous
    sacrotuberous
    Santorini
    Sappey
    scapholunate
    Schlemm
    serous
    sesamoid
    sesamophalangeal
    sheath
    Simonart
    Soemmerring
    sphenomandibular
    spinoglenoid
    spiral
    splenocolic
    splenorenal
    spring
    Stanley cervical
    stellate
    sternoclavicular
    sternopericardial
    stretched out
    Struthers
    stylohyoid

ligament *(cont.)*
  stylomandibular
  stylomaxillary
  superficial dorsal sacrococcygeal
  superficial posterior sacrococcygeal
  superficial transverse metacarpal
  superficial transverse metartarsal
  superior costotransverse
  superior pubic
  superior transverse scapular
  suprascapular
  supraspinous
  suspensory
  sutural
  syndesmotic
  synovial
  talocalcaneal
  talofibular
  talonavicular
  tarsal
  tarsometatarsal
  tectoral
  temporomandibular
  Teutleben
  Thompson
  thyroepiglottic
  thyrohyoid
  tibial collateral
  tibial sesamoid
  tibiocalcaneal
  tibiofibular
  tibionavicular
  torn meniscotibial
  transverse atlantal
  transverse carpal
  transverse crural
  transverse genicular
  transverse humeral
  transverse intertarsal
  transverse metacarpal
  transverse metatarsal
  transverse perineal

ligament *(cont.)*
  transverse tibiofibular
  trapezoid
  Treitz
  triangular
  triquetrohamate
  Tuffier inferior
  ulnar collateral (UCL)
  ulnocarpal
  ulnolunate
  ulnotriquetral
  umbilical
  urachal
  uterine
  uterosacral
  uterovesical
  vaginal (of fingers and toes)
  venous
  ventral sacrococcygeal
  ventral sacroiliac
  ventricular
  vertebropelvic
  vesicoumbilical
  vesicouterine
  vestibular
  vocal
  volar
  volar carpal
  Walther oblique
  Weitbrecht
  Winslow
  Wrisberg
  xiphicostal
  xiphoid
  Y-shaped
  Zaglas
  Zinn
ligament laxity
ligamentous bouncing
ligamentous box
ligamentous complex
ligamentous disruption

line *(cont.)*
   raster
   reference
   resonance
   Schoemaker
   semilunar
   Shenton
   soleal
   subcutaneous fat
   subpleural curvilinear
   Ullman
   vertebral body
   Wagner
   white (linea alba)
linea alba
linear absorption coefficient
linear accelerator isocenter motion
linear accelerator (LINAC, linac)
   radiosurgery
linear amplifier
linear and depressed skull fracture
linear array
   Acuson 5 MHz
   convex
   high-density
linear-array-hydrophone assembly
linear artifact
linear attenuation coefficient
linear band of maximal radiolucency
linear defect
linear density
linear fracture
linear infiltrate
linear interpolation
linearity
linearization, perceptual
linear lucency
linear markings
linear opacity
linear phased arrays
linear scanning
linear shadow

linear skull fracture
linear streaks en face
linear tomography
line imaging
line placement
line saturation
   gaussian
   Lorentzian
line scanning
line shadow
line-shape sensitivity
line width
lingual bone
lingual thyroid
linguine sign in breast
lingula pulmonis
lingular artery
lingular bronchus
lingular mandibular bony defects
   (LMBD)
lingular nodule
lingular orifice
link, musculotendinous-osseous
Linton shunt
Linx exchange guide wire
lipid-laden plaque
lipid-lowering therapy
lipid-rich material
lipid-sensitive MR
lipid signal
lipid zone
Lipiodol (iodized poppy seed oil)
   myelographic imaging agent
liplike projections of cartilage
lipofibroma
lipoid pneumonia
lipoma
   cardiac
   filar
   intratentorial
lipomatous hypertrophy of interatrial
   septum

liponecrosis
lipophilic contrast agents
lipophilic sequestration system
liposarcoma of heart
liposomes, antibody-conjugated
    paramagnetic (APCLs)
lipping, osteophytic
liquefactive emphysema
liquid crystal contact thermography
    (LCT)
liquid crystal thermogram
liquid pleural effusion
liquid scintillation analysis
liquid scintillation spectrometer
Liquipake contrast medium
Lisfranc dislocation
Lisfranc fracture
Lisfranc joint
Lissauer column
lissencephaly, cobblestone
list mode data collection
Lister tubercle
liters per minute per meter squared
    (L/min./m^2)
lithiasis, renal (also renolithiasis)
lithium
lithogenic bile
litholysis
Lithostar nonimmersion lithotriptor
lithotripsy
    laser
    ultrasonic
lithotriptor (also lithotripter)
lithotriptor with fluoroscopic and
    ultrasound localization
LITT (laser-induced thermotherapy)
Litten diaphragm phenomenon
Littre hernia
Litzmann obliquity
liver
    alcoholic fatty
    biliary cirrhotic

liver *(cont.)*
    capsule of
    caudate lobe of
    centrilobular region of
    cirrhosis of
    cirrhotic
    degenerative
    degraded
    diaphragmatic surface of
    dome of
    duodenal impression on
    echogenic
    enlarged
    fatty
    floating
    frosted
    hobnail
    infantile
    large-droplet fatty
    left lobe of
    metastasis to
    nodular
    noncirrhotic
    polycystic
    polylobar
    potato
    prominent
    pyogenic
    quadrate lobe of
    renal impression on
    right lobe of
    shrunken
    small-droplet fatty
    stasis (in cirrhosis)
    undersurface of
    visceral surface of
    wandering
    waxy
liver/aorta (L/A) peak ratio
liver bed
liver coil
liver edge

liver flap
liver function
liver hydatid disease
liver-jugular sign
liver, kidneys, and spleen (LKS)
liverlike lung
liver/liver peak (L/LP) ratio
liver parenchyma
liver scan, radionuclide
liver scintiphotograph
liver span
liver-spleen scan
Livingston triangle
LKS (liver, kidneys, and spleen)
LLD (leg length discrepancy)
LLD (limb length discrepancy)
LLE (left lower extremity)
LLQ (left lower quadrant)
L-loop heart
L-looping
L-loop ventricular situs
L/LP (liver/liver peak) ratio
L-malposition of aorta
LMCA (left main coronary artery)
L/min./m^2 (liters per minute per
    meter squared)
LMP (last menstrual period)
LMR (localized magnetic resonance)
LNV (last normal vertebra)
loading
    differential
    peripheral
    spike
    uniform
loading dose
lobar bronchus (pl. bronchi)
lobar cavitation
lobar consolidation
lobar emphysema
lobar lung atrophy
lobar pneumonia

lobe
    anterior tip of temporal
    azygos vein
    caudate (of liver)
    collapsed
    cuneiform
    falciform
    fetal
    flocculonodular (of cerebellum)
    frontal
    inferior
    insular
    left
    limbic
    lower
    medial temporal
    middle
    occipital
    orbital aspect of frontal
    parietal
    polyalveolar
    pulmonary
    pyramidal
    quadrate
    Riedel
    right
    sequestered (lung)
    superior
    temporal
    thyroid
    uncus of temporal
    upper
lobe of azygos vein
lobectomy
lobster-claw deformity
lobular architecture of liver
lobulated border
lobulated filling defect
lobulated saccular appearance
lobule
local compression fracture

localization
   autoradiographic
   CT-directed hook wire
   off-axis point
   wire
localization grid
localized H1 spectroscopy
localized magnetic resonance (LMR)
localized mass effect
localized obstructive emphysema
localizer, breast
localizing images
lock washer configuration
loco-regional hyperthermia
locomotor pattern
loculated effusion on chest x-ray
loculated fluid collection
loculated pleural effusion
locus, scanning
Loeffler (Löffler)
Loeffler endocarditis
Loehr-Kindberg syndrome
Löffler (Loeffler)
Löfgren syndrome
Lohlein diameter
LOM (low osmolar media)
L1-L5 (five lumbar vertebrae)
L1-APo cephalometric measurement
L1-L6 intervertebral disks
L1-NB cephalometric measurement
long ACE fixed-wire balloon catheter
long-acting thyroid stimulator (LATS)
long axial oblique view
long axis acquisition
long axis parasternal view
long axis slice
long axis view
Long Beach stereotactic robot
long bone
long bone fracture
long bore collimator
long fibers of the posterior talofibular
   ligament

long segment narrowing
Long Skinny over-the-wire balloon
   catheter
long taper/stiff shaft Glidewire
   (coronary artery imaging)
long TR, short TE
long TR/TE (T2 weighted image)
long tract signs
long wavelength photolabel
long-standing
Longdwel Teflon catheter
longitudinal arch of foot
longitudinal arteriography
longitudinal B-mode
longitudinal blood supply to ulnar
   nerve
longitudinal fasciculus, medial (MLF)
longitudinal fissure
longitudinal fracture
longitudinal lie
longitudinally
longitudinal magnetization
longitudinal muscles
longitudinal narrowing
longitudinal relaxation
longitudinal taenia musculature
longitudinal ultrasonic biometry
loop
   afferent
   air-filled
   alpha sigmoid
   bowel
   capillary
   cervical
   closed
   closed conducting
   colonic
   contiguous
   diathermic
   dilated bowel
   double reverse alpha sigmoid
   duodenal

loop *(cont.)*
    efferent
    flow-volume
    gamma transverse colon
    Gerdy interatrial
    Gerdy interauricular
    Henle
    intestinal
    J (on catheterization)
    jejunal
    lenticular
    Meyer
    Meyer-Archambault
    N-shaped sigmoid
    P (on vectorcardiography)
    peduncular
    pressure-volume
    puborectalis
    reentrant
    rubber vessel
    sentinel
    sigmoid
    small-bowel
    Stoerck
    subclavian
    T (on vectorcardiography)
    transverse colon
    vector
    ventricular
    vessel
    Vieussens
loop ostomy bridge
loopogram (ileostogram)
loose fracture
loose joint body
Looser-Milkman syndrome
Lo-Por tracheal tube
Lo-Profile and Lo-Profile II balloon
    catheter
Lorad M-II D mammographic system
Lorad StereoGuide stereotactic breast
    biopsy system

lordosis
    cervical
    lumbar
    reversal of
    thoracic
lordotic curve
lordotic position
lordotic view
Lorentzian line saturation
loss, electron equilibrium
loss of definition
loss of sigmoid curve
loss of thoracic kyphosis
lossy algorithm
Louis, sternal angle of
low angle scattering
low angle shot (flash) technique
low attenuation pulsation artifact
Low-Beers view
low cardiac output syndrome
low-contrast film
low-contrast structure
low-density lesion
low-density structure
low-dose film mammographic
    technique
low-dose folinic acid
low-dose screen-film technique
low-dose mammography
low-energy collimator
low-energy photon attenuation
    measurement
low-energy radiofrequency conduction
    hyperthermia treatment
lower esophageal sphincter (LES)
lower extremity noninvasive (LENI)
lower left sternal border
lower lobe lung mass
lower lung field
lower pole collecting system
lower pole of kidney
lower pole of patella

lower pole ureter
Lower (Richard Lower)
Lower rings
Lower tubercle
low-field MR angiography
low-field MR imaging
low-field-strength MR imaging
low-flow syndrome
low-intensity laser irradiation (LILI)
low-intensity pulsed ultrasound
low-level echo
low osmolality
low-osmolar contrast media
low-output heart failure
low-pressure cardiac tamponade
low signal intensity
low-speed rotational angioplasty
    catheter
low temperature diffraction
low urethral pressure (LUP)
low-velocity flow
Lown-Ganong-Levine syndrome
    (LGL)
LPA (left pulmonary artery)
LPO (left posterior oblique) position
LPS balloon catheter
LPS Peel-Away introducer
LPV (left pulmonary vein)
LRA (low right atrium)
LS (lumbosacral) spine
LSB (lower sternal border)
LSC background prediction
LSCVP (left subclavian central
    venous pressure)
LSD-image (line scan diffusion
    imaging)
L-transposition (levotransposition)
    of great arteries
L-tyrosine (^{11}C) imaging agent
lucency
    interspersed
    linear

lucent defect
Lucey-Driscoll syndrome
lucite beam spoiler
Ludovici angle
Ludwig angle
luetic aortitis
luetic arteritis
Lugol solution
Lukes-Collins classification of
    lymphoma
Lumaguide catheter
lumbar artery
lumbar pneumencephalography
lumbar scoliosis
lumbar spine view
lumbar transverse process
lumbar vertebra
lumbarization
lumbosacral kyphosis
lumbosacral series
lumbosacral spine
lumen (pl. lumens, lumina)
    aortic
    arterial
    attenuated
    bile duct
    bowel
    bronchial
    clot-filled
    cloverleaf-shaped
    crescentic
    cystic duct
    D-shaped vessel
    double-barrel
    duct
    duodenal
    eccentrically placed
    elliptical
    esophageal
    false
    gastroduodenal
    intestinal

lumen *(cont.)*
   occluded
   patent
   slitlike
   slit-shaped vessel
   star-shaped vessel
   true
   vascular
lumen-intimal interface
lumenogram
lumina (pl. of lumen)
luminal area
luminal caliber
luminal configuration, scalloped
luminal contour, irregular hazy
luminal cross-sectional area
luminal diameter
luminal dimension
luminal encroachment
luminal irregularity
luminal narrowing
luminal plaquing
luminal silhouette
luminal stenosis
luminal thrombosis
luminance
luminogram, air
luminol
Lumiscan scanner
lumpy appearance of lung
Lunar DPX densitometer
Lunar Expert densitometer
Lunar scanner
lunate bone
lunate dislocation
lunatomalacia
lung
   acquired unilateral hyperlucent
   air-conditioner
   airless
   arc welder's
   artificial
   atelectatic

lung *(cont.)*
   bauxite
   bird breeder's
   bird fancier's
   bird handler's
   black
   brown
   bubbly
   budgerigar-fancier's
   cardiac
   cheese handler's
   cheese washer's
   coal miner's
   coal worker's
   coffee worker's
   collapsed
   consolidated
   cork handler's
   cork worker's
   corundum smelter's
   dark and mottled
   drowned
   dynamic
   emphysematous
   empty collapsed
   eosinophilic
   expanded
   farmer's
   fibrinoid
   fibroid
   fibrosis of
   fish-meal worker's
   fissures of
   fresh
   furrier's
   gangrene of
   grain handler's
   hardened
   harvester's
   hemorrhagic consolidation of
   hen worker's
   hilum of
   honeycomb

lung *(cont.)*
  humidifier
  hyperlucent
  hypogenetic
  hypoplastic
  light pink
  liverlike
  malt worker's
  maple bark-stripper's
  mason's
  meat wrapper's
  miller's
  mottled gray
  mushroom worker's
  pigeon-breeder's
  pigeon-fancier's
  premature infant's
  pump
  rheumatoid
  root of
  rudimentary
  septic
  shock
  shrunken
  silicotic
  silo-filler's
  silver finisher's
  silver polisher's
  smoker's
  static
  stiff noncompliant
  stretched
  subsegment of
  thatched roof worker's
  thresher's
  tropical eosinophilic
  underventilated
  unilateral hyperlucent
  vanishing
  welder's
  well-inflated
  wet
  white

lung abscess
lung agenesis
lung air spaces
lung apex (pl. apices)
lung architecture
lung base
lung calculus
lung carcinoma
lung cirrhosis
lung collapse
lung consolidation
lung count curve
lung disease, interstitial
lung expansion
lung field
lung fissure
lung/heart ratio of thallium 201
    activity
lung hemangioma
lung hepatization
lung hypoplasia
lung infiltrate (infiltration)
lung inflammation
lung injury, penetrating
lung lobule
lung lymphoid hyperplasia
lung markings
lung mass with mediastinal invasion
lung necrosis
lung opacity
lung overexpansion
lung overinflation
lung parenchyma consolidation
lung periphery
lung reexpansion
lung scan, perfusion and ventilation
lung segment, infarcted
lung segmentation
lung stiffness
lung transplantation
lung underinflation
lung washout

lung zone
lunula (pl. lunulae)
LUP (low urethral pressure)
LUQ (left upper quadrant)
Luque rod used in spinal fusion for scoliosis
Luque sublaminar wire used in spinal fusion for scoliosis
LUS (laparoscopic ultrasound)
Luschka crypts of gallbladder mucosa
Luschka, joint of
Luschka muscle
Lutembacher complex
Lutembacher syndrome
luxated bone
luxation
Luxtec fiberoptic system for diagnostic and surgical visualization
luxury perfusion
LV (left ventricular) function pressure
LV (left ventricular) function wall motion
LVAD (left ventricular assist device), HeartMate
LVAS (left ventricular assist system), Novacor
LVdd (left ventricular diastolic dimension)
LVD (left ventricular dysfunction)
LVEDD (left ventricular end-diastolic dimension)
LVEDI (left ventricular end-diastolic volume index)
LVEDP (left ventricular end-diastolic pressure)
LVEF (left ventricular ejection fraction)
LVESD (left ventricular end-systolic dimension)
LVESVI (left ventricular end-systolic volume index)
LVET (left ventricular ejection time)

LVFS (left ventricular functional shortening)
LVFW (left ventricular free wall)
LVG (left ventriculogram)
LVH (left ventricular hypertrophy) with strain
LVID (left ventricular internal diameter) (or dimension)
LVIDd (left ventricular internal dimension at end-diastole)
LVIDD (left ventricular internal diastolic dimension)
LVIDs (left ventricular internal dimension at end-systole)
LVIV (left ventricular inflow volume)
LVM (left ventricular mass)
LVMI (left ventricular mass index)
LVOT (left ventricular outflow tract)
LVOTO (left ventricular outflow tract obstruction)
LVOV (left ventricular outflow volume)
LVP (left ventricular pressure)
LVP1 and LVP2 (left ventricular pressure on apex cardiogram)
LVPW (left ventricular posterior wall)
LVs (left ventricular systolic) dimension
LVS (left ventricular support) system
LVS (left ventricular systolic) pressure
LVSW (left ventricular stroke work)
LVSWI (left ventricular stroke work index)
LVW (left ventricular wall)
lym-1 monoclonal antibody labeled with iodine-131 (^{131}I)
Lyme carditis
Lyme disease
lymphangiographic contrast
lymphangiography
lymphangioma, cardiac

lymphangitic carcinomatosis
lymphangitic metastasis
lymphatic cachexia
lymphatic channels
lymphatic drainage
lymphatic duct
lymphatic malformation (LM)
lymphaticovenous malformation
   (LVM)
lymphatic system
lymphatic vessel
Lymphazurin (isosulfan blue) contrast
   medium
lymph capillaries
lymph gland
lymph node (see *node*)
lymph node enlargement
lymph node metastases
lymph node syndrome
lymphoblastoma
lymphocytic infiltrate
lymphocytic interstitial pneumonitis
   (LIP)
lymphocytic splenomegaly,
   postcardiotomy
lymphogenous dissemination
lymphogenous metastasis
lymphography, time-lapse quantitative
   computed tomography
lymphoid interstitial pneumonia
lymphoma
   adult T-cell
   African
   B-cell
   B-cell monocytoid
   Burkitt
   centrocytic
   cleaved cell
   diffuse
   diffuse large cell
   diffuse mixed small and large cell
   diffuse small cleaved cell

lymphoma *(cont.)*
   follicular center cell
   follicular mixed small cleaved
   follicular predominantly large cell
   follicular predominantly small cell
   giant follicle
   granulomatous
   histiocytic
   Hodgkin
   infiltrative
   intermediate lymphocytic
   large cell, immunoblastic
   large cleaved cell
   large noncleaved cell
   Lennert
   lymphoblastic
   lymphocytic plasmacytoid
   lymphocytic poorly differentiated
   lymphocytic well differentiated
   malignant
   mantle zone
   Mediterranean
   mixed lymphocytic-histiocytic
   multifocal
   nodular
   noncleaved cell
   non-Hodgkin
   pleomorphic
   polypoid
   primary of central nervous system
   small B-cell
   small cleaved cell
   small lymphocytic
   small noncleaved cell
   T-cell
      convoluted
      cutaneous
      small lymphocytic
   U-cell (undefined)
   ulcerative
   undefined
   undifferentiated

lymphonodular hyperplasia
lymphoproliferative disorder,
   intrathoracic
lymphosarcoma
LymphoScan nuclear imaging system
lymphoscintigraphy, radiocolloid
lymph vessels of thymus gland

Lynch and Crues Type 2 lesion on
   MRI scan
lyoluminescence
lytic (osteolytic) lesion
lytic area
lytic bone lesion
lytic change

M, m

m (meta-stable) (in technetium ^{99m}Tc)
m (meter)
m/sec (meters per second)
mA (milliampere)
mA/kV (milliamperes per kilovolt)
MAA (^{99m}Tc MAA) (macroaggregated albumin)
Mab-170 monoclonal antibody
MAC (mitral annular calcium)
Macalister muscle
machine, parallel virtual
Machlett collimator
Mackenzie point
MacLean-Maxwell disease
Macleod syndrome
macroadenoma, prolactin-secreting pituitary
macroaggregated albumin
macrocolon
macrofistulous AV (arteriovenous) communications
macromolecular contrast-enhanced MR imaging
macromolecular drugs
macronodular pattern
macroscopic magnetization vector
Macrotec imaging agent

MacSpect real-time NMR station
Maddahi method of calculating right ventricular ejection fraction
Madelung deformity
Maffucci syndrome
Magendie, foramen of
magic angle artifact
magic angle spinning NMR
Magna-SL scanner
Magnes biomagnetometer system
magnet
    doughnut
    GE Signa 1.5T
    Magnex
    non-enclosed
    open
    Oxford
    pancake MRI
    passively shimmed superconducting
    shim
    shimmed
    superconducting
    tubular
    2T large bore
magnet mode
magnet rate
magnet response

malignancy *(cont.)*
  high-grade
  low-grade
  metastatic
  primary
  secondary
  staging of
malignancy threshold
malignant acetabular osteolysis
malignant airway obstruction
malignant degeneration
malignant fibrous histiocytoma
malignant hemangioendothelioma
malignant lymphoma
malignant mesothelioma
malignant mixed tumor
malignant nephrosclerosis
malignant osteoid
malignant osteopetrosis
malignant pleomorphic adenoma
malignant pleural implants
malignant pleural mesothelioma
malignant teratoma
malleolar
malleolus (pl. malleoli)
  lateral
  medial
malleolus fibulae
malleolus tibiae
mallet finger
Mallinckrodt angiographic catheter
Mallinckrodt imaging agent
Mallinckrodt scanner
Mallory-Weiss mucosal tear
malperfused
malperfusion
malpighian vesicle
malposition of heart
malpositioned fetus
malrotation of intestine
malt worker's lung

malum coxae senile
malum perforans pedis
malunion of fracture fragments
malunited
Mamex DC mammography
mamillary body
mammalation
mammary-coronary artery bypass
mammary ductogram
mammary galactogram
mammary implant
Mammo QC
mammogram (see *mammography*)
mammographic features
mammographic-histopathologic
  correlation
mammographic measurement
mammographic parenchymal patterns,
  Wolfe
mammography
  baseline
  computed tomographic
  contoured tilting compression
  CT laser (CTLM)
  digital
  Egan
  high-resolution CT
  low-dose
  magnetic resonance (MRM)
  magnification
  Mamex DC
  Mammo QC
  Mammomat B
  microfocal spot
  radionuclide
  screen-film
  screening
  ultra-high magnification (UHMM)
  ultrasound augmented
  xero-
  x-ray (XMG)
Mammotest breast biopsy system

mandible
  alveolar border of
  angle of
mandibular canal
mandibular incisor angle, Frankfort
mandibular notch
mandibulofacial dysostosis
maneuver (pl. maneuvers)
  Adson
  costoclavicular
  flexion
  Heineke-Mikulicz
  hyperabduction
  Kocher
  Müller (Mueller)
  Osler
  Rivero-Carvallo
  scalene
  squatting
  transabdominal left lateral
    retroperitoneal
  Valsalva
mangafodipir trisodium imaging agent
manganese (Mn)
  Mn Cl (chloride) imaging agent
  Mn-DPDP (dipyridoxal diphos-
    phate) imaging agent
  Mn PcS4 imaging agent
  Mn-SOD
  Mn-TPPS
Mani catheter
manifest
manifestations, extrapulmonary
Mann-Bollman fistula
Mannkopf sign
Mann-Whitney test
manofluorography (MFG)
manometer-tipped cardiac catheter
manometric pattern
manometry
  anal
  aneroid

manometry *(cont.)*
  anorectal
  biliary
  ERCP
  esophageal
  rectosigmoid
  sphincter of Oddi
Mansfield Atri-Pace catheter
Mansfield orthogonal electrode
  catheter
Manson schistosomiasis-pulmonary
  artery obstruction syndrome
mantle
  anechoic
  hypoechoic
mantle block
mantle complex
mantle field
manual computed method
manual pressure over carotid sinus
manual subtraction films
manubriosternal joint
manubriosternal syndrome
manubrium
map
  acceleration
  bull's-eye
  bull's-eye polar
  color flow
  cylindrical
  cylindrical projection
  decimalized variance
  end-diastolic polar
  end-systolic polar
  sestamibi polar
  spherical
MAP (mean arterial pressure)
map-guided partial endocardial
  ventriculotomy
maple bark stripper's lung
maple bark worker's suberosis
maple syrup urine disease

mapper, brain
mapping
  activation-sequence
  body surface
  body surface potential
  brain
  catheter
  Doppler color flow
  electrophysiologic
  endocardial activation
  endocardial catheter
  epicardial
  FMRI
  homology
  ice
  intramural
  intraoperative electrocortical
    stimulation
  K-space velocity
  MR (magnetic resonance) velocity
  MRI (magnetic resonance imaging)
  pace
  parallel analog
  phase-shift velocity
  precordial
  retrograde atrial activation
  sinus rhythm
  spatial
  straight-line Hough transform (HT)
  2D pulsatility index
  2D resistance index mapping
mapping algorithms
mapping of cerebral sulci
mapping probe, hand-held
Marable syndrome
marantic clot
marantic thrombus
Marathon guiding catheter
march foot (fracture)
Marex MRI system
Marfan syndrome
marfanoid hypermobility syndrome

margin
  cardiac
  colon
  convex
  cortical
  costal
  disk
  obtuse
  scapular
  stomach
marginal artery of Drummond
marginal branch
marginal circumflex bypass
marginal osteophyte formation
marginal placenta
marginal serration
marginal spur
marginal ulcer
marginal vein
Marie-Bamberger disease
Marie-Tooth disease
Marie-Strümpell disease
Marine-Lenhart syndrome
markedly accentuated pulmonic
  component
marker
  implanted imaging opaque
  lead pellet
  nipple
  radioactive string
  radiopaque
marker-channel diagram
marker transit study
markings
  bronchovascular
  bronchovesicular
  coarse bronchovascular
  haustral
  increased pulmonary vascular
  linear
  peribronchial
  pulmonary vascular
  vascular

Markov chain Monte Carlo technique
Markov random field
Markov source model
Maroteaux-Lamy syndrome
marrow, bone
marrow edema pattern
Marshall, vein of
Martin disease
Martorell aortic arch syndrome
Martorell-Fabre syndrome
Martorell hypertensive ulcer
Mary Allen Engle ventricle
MAS (Morgagni-Adams-Stokes)
  syndrome
masculinizing tumor
mask (pl. masks)
  convolution
  ISAH stereotactic immobilizing
  Orfit
mask-based approach
masking
mask ventilation
mason's lung
masquerading effect
mass
  abdominal
  adnexal
  airless
  appendiceal
  apperceptive
  calcified
  cavitary
  conical
  cordlike
  cystic
  discrete
  doughy
  echogenic
  elongated
  encapsulated
  enhancing
  exophytic

mass *(cont.)*
  expansile
  extraovarian
  firm
  fixed
  fleecy
  fluctuant
  fluid
  fluid-filled
  focal
  high signal
  hilar
  hyperdense
  hyperintense
  hypodense
  ill-defined
  injection
  interbronchial
  intermediate signal
  intra-abdominal
  intracardiac
  intracavity
  intraluminal
  intraventricular
  irregular
  left ventricular (LVM)
  lobulated
  low attenuation
  low-density
  lower lobe lung
  low signal
  mediastinal
  mixed echogenic solid
  mixed signal
  molar
  nodular
  nonpulsatile abdominal
  paracardiac
  perirenal
  polypoid calcified irregular
  pulsatile
  relativistic

mass *(cont.)*
   right ventricular (RVM)
   saccular
   signal
   soft tissue
   solid
   solitary
   space-occupying
   spherical
   stony
   suspicious
   ventricular
mass attenuation coefficient
mass balance
mass effect
mass lesion
mass-like configuration
Massachusetts (General Hospital)
   Utility Multiprogramming System
   (MUMPS)
massage, carotid sinus
masseter muscle
massive ascites
massive edema
massive effusion
massive embolism (embolization)
Master syndrome
Master two-step exercise stress test
masticator muscle
masticator space
mastoid polytomography
mastoid sinus
match
   non-transmural
   transmural
   triple
match-line wedge
Match 35 PTA catheter
matched V/Q defect
matching
   atlas
   electron-photon field
   general pattern

mater (not *matter*)
   dura
   pia
material
   atheromatous
   contrast
   inspissated
matrix (pl. matrices)
   bone
   calcific
   cartilage
   chondroid
   germinal
   image
   solid
   transformation
Matrix LR3300 laser imaging
matter
   cortical gray
   cortical white
   gray
   white
maturation, disk
mature pseudocyst of pancreas
Maugeri syndrome
Max Plus MR scanner
maxillary sinus
maxillary spine
maximal volume (of left atrium)
maximal voluntary ventilation (MVV)
maximum amplitude constants
maximum diameter to minimum
   diameter ratio
maximum intensity pixel (MIP)
maximum intensity projection (MIP)
maximum intensity projection and
   source images
maximum likelihood algorithms
maximum predicted heart rate
   (MPHR)
maximum slew rate ramps
Maxwell 3D Field Simulator

Mayer view
Mazer stent
mazoplasia, cystic
MBF (myocardial blood flow)
MBIH catheter
MBq (megabecquerel)
McArdle syndrome
MCAT (myocardial contrast
    appearance time)
McBurney point
McCort sign
MCE (myocardial contrast
    echocardiography)
McGoon coronary perfusion catheter
mCi (millicurie)
McIntosh double-lumen catheter
MCL (midclavicular line)
MCLS (mucocutaneous lymph node
    syndrome)
MCP (metacarpophalangeal) joint
MCS (middle coronary sinus)
MCTC (metrizamide CT
    cisternogram)
MD-Gastroview contrast medium
MD-50 contrast medium
MD-60 contrast medium
MD-76 contrast medium
MEA syndromes IIa and IIb
Meadows syndrome
meal
    barium
    Boyden test
    double contrast barium
    Ewald test
    fatty
    isotope
    motor
    motor test
    opaque
    retention
    small bowel
    test

mean aortic pressure
mean arterial pressure (MAP)
mean atrial pressure
mean blood pressure
mean cardiac vector
mean circulatory filling pressure
mean circumferential fiber shortening
    rate (MCFSR)
mean free path
mean left atrial pressure
mean maximal expiratory flow
    (MMEF)
mean mitral valve gradient
mean pulmonary artery (MPA)
    pressure
mean pulmonary capillary pressure
    (MPCP)
mean pulmonary transit time
mean rate of circumferential
    shortening
mean right atrial pressure
mean-square error
mean time
mean vectors
mean venous pulsation
measurable endpoint
measure
    Hausdorff metric
    linear
    prophylactic
    root-mean-squared gradient
measurement
    attenuation (of photon)
    cardiac output
    cerebrospinal fluid flow
    Cerenkov
    diode
    excitation function
    4 T
    high-sensitivity
    intercomparison
    low-energy photon attenuation

measurement *(cont.)*
  mammographic
  morphometric
  nutation angle
  polarographic needle electrode
  rocking curve
  semiquantitative
  topographic
measurement and depiction in vivo
meatal segment
meat wrapper's lung
metacarpal-phalangeal (or metacarpophalangeal) (MCP) joint
mechanical augmentation
mechanical counterpulsation
mechanical dottering effect
mechanical insufflation
mechanical small bowel obstruction
mechanical thrombolysis
mechanical valve
mechanics, intramural
mechanism
  check-valve
  deglutition
  flap-valve
  Frank-Starling
  humeral
  internal retention
  pinchcock
  propulsive
  sphincteric
  swallowing
Meckel cave
Meckel diverticulitis
Meckel diverticulum
Meckel scan (scanning)
meconium plug
MEDDARS analysis system for
  cardiac catheterization
media (see *medium*)
media-adventitia interface
medial compartment

medially
medial rotation of viscera to right of
  midline
median arcuate ligament of diaphragm
median lethal dose
median level echos
median line
median sacral artery
mediastinal air
mediastinal border
mediastinal emphysema
mediastinal fat
mediastinal fibrosis
mediastinal fistula
mediastinal hernia
mediastinal invasion
mediastinal lung surface
mediastinal lymph node
mediastinal mass
mediastinal neoplasm
mediastinal node
mediastinal pleura
mediastinal prominence
mediastinal septum
mediastinal shift
mediastinal structures
mediastinal thickening
mediastinal tumor
mediastinal wedge
mediastinal widening
mediastinodiaphragmatic pleural
  reflection
mediastinum
  anterior
  deviated
  inferior
  middle
  posterior
  superior
  widened (or widening of)
mediastinum cerebelli
mediastinum cerebri

mediastinum displacement
medical cyclotron
medical linear accelerator
medication (see also *bowel prep*;
  imaging agents)
  ACE inhibitor
  AMI 227
  bromodeoxyuridine
  bromophenol blue
  Captopril
  Colonlite bowel prep
  CoLyte bowel prep
  dextrose 5% in water
  diazepam
  dihydroxyphenylalanine [DOPA]
  Dulcolax bowel prep
  EDTMP
  Emulsoil bowel prep
  enalaprilat ACE inhibitor
  etanidazole
  Ethiodol
  Evac-Q-Kit bowel prep
  Evac-Q-Kwik bowel prep
  ferric ammonium citrate-cellulose
    paste
  15-NH3
  5-chlorodeoxycytidine
  Fleet bowel prep
  furosemide
  glucagon
  GoLytely bowel prep
  indomethacin
  iophendylate
  isoflurane
  K4-81
  methyl methacrylate
  naloxone
  nicotinamide
  nimodipine
  nitrous oxide
  nonsteroidal antiphlogistics
  OCL bowel prep

medication *(cont.)*
  olsalazine
  P-32
  pentagastrin
  phenobarbital
  radiopharmaceutical
  Sincalide
  6FD
  somatostatin
  suppo-cire C
  tetramethylene
  Tridrate bowel prep
  U-235
  urokinase
  X-Prep bowel prep
  xylenol orange
medicine, photonic
Medigraphics analyzer
MedImage scanner
mediolateral oblique view
mediolateral stress
mediopatellar
MediPort implanted vascular access
  device
Medison scanner
Medi-Tech balloon catheter
medium (pl. media)
  contrast
  high osmolar (HOM)
  ionic contrast
  low osmolar (LOM)
  nonionic contrast media
  radiopaque
  tunica
Medrad contrast medium injector
Medrad Mrinnervu endorectal colon
  probe coil
medronate scan
Medspec MR imaging system
Medtronic balloon catheter
Medtronic Minix

Medtronic radiofrequency (RF)
  receiver
medulla (pl. medullas, medullae)
  adrenal
  lymphatic
  ovarian
  renal
  spinal
medulla oblongata
medullaris, conus
medullary canal
medullary nephrocalcinosis
medullary pyramids
medullary sponge kidney
medulloblastoma
Medweb clinical reporting system
MEDX gamma camera
Mees lines
MEG (magnetoencephalography)
megacolon
  acquired
  congenital
  idiopathic
  toxic
megacystis
megaduodenum
megaesophagus of achalasia
megahertz (MHz)
megalocystis
megaloureter
megarectum
megaureter
megavolt (MV)
megavoltage grid therapy
megavoltage radiation therapy
megavoltage treatment beams
meglumine diatrizoate imaging agent
meglumine imaging agent
meglumine iodipamide imaging agent
meglumine iothalamate imaging agent
meglumine iotroxate imaging agent
Meige lymphedema

Meigs capillaries
Meigs-Cass syndrome
Meigs disease
Meigs syndrome
Meissner plexus
melanin, leptomeningeal
melanoma, metastatic
melanosarcoma
melanosis, parenchymal neurocutaneous
melorheostosis of Leri
Melrose solution
Meltzer sign
membrane
  microporous
  mucous
  premature rupture of
  synovial
membranous septum
membranous subvalvular aortic
  stenosis
membranous urethra
membranous ventricular septal defect
memory-intensive algorithms
Memory-Vu angiographic catheter
MEN (multiple endocrine neoplasia)
Ménétrier disease
Mengert index in pelvimetry
meningeal hemorrhage
meningeal myelomatosis
meningioma
  cerebellopontine angle
  clival
  convexity
  cystic
  falcine
  falx
  fibroblastic
  fibrous
  malignant
  meningotheliomatous
  parasagittal

meningioma *(cont.)*
  posterior fossa
  suprasellar
  tentorial
  transitional
meniscal injury
meniscus
  articular
  diverging
meniscus (crescent) of contrast-saline
  mixture
meniscus articularis
meniscus lateralis
meniscus medialis
meniscus sign on upper GI study
meniscus (pl. menisci)
menses
menstrual age
menstrual date
mensuration algorithm
mental spine
mentoanterior
mentoposterior
mentum
Mercator projection
Mercedes Benz sign, reversed
mercury artifact
mercury-in-Silastic strain gauge
Meridian echocardiography
Merkell cell carcinoma cell lines
meroacrania
mesenchymoma
mesenteric angiography
mesenteric apoplexy
mesenteric arterial thrombosis
mesenteric artery occlusion
mesenteric infarction
mesenteric ischemia
mesenteric node
mesenteric rupture
mesenteric sclerosis

mesenteric tear
mesenteric venous thrombosis
mesenterium commune
mesentery
  fan-shaped
  fatty
  leaves of
  root of
  small intestine (SIM)
  ventral
mesial aspect
mesial hyperperfusion
mesial temporal sclerosis
meso-HMPAO
mesoappendix
mesoblastic nephroma
mesocardia
mesocaval anastomosis
mesocaval H-graft shunt
mesocolon
mesocolonic fat
mesocolonic vessels
mesocuneiform bone
mesoderm
  extraembryonic
  gastral
mesoderma
meson
mesorectum
mesosigmoid colon
mesosternum
mesothelial
mesothelioma
mesoversion of heart
Mester test for rheumatic disease
meta-analysis
metabolic 8-hydroxyquinolyl-glu-
  curonide
metabolic rate of oxygen
metabolic response
metabolic tracer uptake

metabolism
  cerebral
  fat
  fatty acid
  myocardial
metabolite
  $CMRO_2$ glucose
  phosphorus
metacarpal bone
metacarpophalangeal (or metacarpal-phalangeal) (MCP) joint
metaiodobenzylguanidine (MIBG)
  imaging agent
metal technetium target
metallic foreign body
metallic stent
metalloporphyrins
metaphyseal dysostosis
metaphyseal-epiphyseal angle
metaphyseal lucent bands
metaphysis (pl. metaphyses)
  agnogenic myeloid
  apocrine (of breast)
  autoparenchymatous
  celomic
  columnar
  fundic
  intestinal
  metaphyseal
  myeloid
  primary myeloid
  secondary myeloid
  squamous
metaplasia
  cartilaginous
  osteocartilaginous
metapneumonic empyema
metastasis (pl. metastases)
  air-space
  calcareous
  CX-1
  drop

metastasis *(cont.)*
  hematogenous
  local
  lymph node
  lymphangitic
  lymphatic
  micronodular
  neuroendocrine hepatic
  nodal
  osteoblastic
  osteolytic
  pulsating
  satellite
  white
  widespread
metastatic abscess
metastatic disease
metastatic tumor
metasynchronous tumor
metatarsal-phalangeal (or metatarso-phalangeal) (MTP) joint
metatarsal bone
metatarsal head
metatarsocuneiform joint
metatarsophalangeal (or metatarso-phalangeal) (MTP) joint
metatarsus adductocavus deformity
metatarsus adductus deformity
metatarsus atavicus deformity
metatarsus latus deformity
metatarsus primus varus deformity
metatarsus varus deformity
meter (m), rate
meter per second (m/sec; also mps)
  velocity
methionine
method (see also *technique*)
  Born
  calibration
  CHESS
  column extraction
  computer

method *(cont.)*
  DIET
  Dixon
  empirical
  Enhance deblurring
  error diffusion
  FBP (filtered back-projection)
  fixed grid stereologic
  fractal-based
  GLF lymphography
  in vivo
  IPSP neuron evaluation
  isocenter shift
  Joliot
  Kaplan-Meier
  manual computed
  multiple line scanning
  multiple sensitive point
  multisection
  NEUGAT (neutron/gamma
    transmission)
  neutron/gamma transmission
    (NEUGAT)
  PASTA
  Pfeiffer-Comberg
  phase-unwrapping
  radiotracer foil
  segmentation
  selective excitation
  selective saturation
  shock-monitoring
  spin-label
  stereologic
  sum-peak
  surface coil
  Syed-Neblett brachytherapy
  thresholding
  transvaginal US-guided drainage
    with trocar
method/projection
  full-scan (FS)
  full-scan with interpolation (FI)

method/projection *(cont.)*
  half-scan (HS)
  half-scan with extrapolation (HE)
  half-scan with interpolation (HI)
  simulated annealing
  under-scan (US)
methoxy polyethylene glycol-L-lysine-
  DTPA imaging agent
methyl methacrylate
methyl protons
metrizamide cisternography
metrizamide computed tomographic
  cisternogram (MCTC)
metrizamide contrast material
metrizamide myelography
metrizoate acid contrast material
metrizoate sodium contrast medium
metrology
metroperitoneal fistula
"mets" (metabolic equivalents)
"mets" (slang for *metastases*)
MeV (megaelectron) dose
Mevatron 74 linear accelerator
MEVH (multiple exposure volumetric
  holography)
MFG (magnetic field gradients)
MFG (manofluorography)
mGy/MBq (milligray per megabecquerel)
MHC-2 (major histocompatibility
  complex class II antigen)
MHV (middle hepatic vein)
MHz (megahertz)
MI (mitral insufficiency)
MI (myocardial infarction)
MI adenosine thallium imaging
MIBG (metaiodobenzylguanidine)
  imaging agent
  MIBG scintigraphy
  MIBG SPECT scan
micelle
microabscess

microadenoma
microaneurysm
microbubble contrast imaging agent
microbubbles, Renografin-76
microcalcification, clustered
microcardia
Micro-CAST collimator
microcatheter (see also *catheter*)
   flow-directed
   UroLume flow-directed
   Wanderer
microcavitation
microcirculation, pulmonary
microculatory blood flow
microclusters, biodegradable magnetic
microcolon
microcurie
microcyst
microdactylia
microdistribution, heterogeneous
microdosimetry
microemboli
microencapsulated cisplatin
microerosion
microfiche
microfistulous AV (arteriovenous)
   shunt
microfluidization
microfocal spot mammogram
microfracture
microglobulin labeling
Micro-Guide catheter
microimaging
microinfarct
microlithiasis
micromanometer-tip catheter
micromelena
micronodular infiltrates
micronodular metastases
micronodular pattern
micronodule, centrilobular
microperforation

microporous membrane
microscope, scanning electron (SEM)
microscopic cortical dysplasia
microscopic imaging
microscopy
   differential interference contrast
     (DIC)
   electron
   in vivo
   light
   three-dimensional magnetic
     resonance (3D MR)
   ultrasound backscatter (UBM)
microsecond pulsed flashlamp pumped
   dye laser
Microsoft Access program
microsphere
   trisacryl gelatin
   ytterbium-90 (^{90}Yb)
microsphere perfusion scintigraphy
microtomography
Microtron, MM50 Racetrack
microvascular anastomosis
microvascular circulation
microvascular retrieval
microvasculature
Microvasive Rigiflex TTS balloon
   catheter
microvenoarteriolar fistula
microvesicular fat
microvillus (pl. microvilli)
microwave hyperthermia treatment
microwave imaging
microwave thermal balloon
   angioplasty
MID (multi-infarct dementia)
midabdominal wall
midaortic arch
midaortic syndrome
midaxillary line
midbody
MIDCAB (minimally invasive direct
   coronary artery bypass) procedure

midcircumflex
midclavicular line (MCL)
midcolon
mid-diastole
mid-distal
middle aortic syndrome
middle cardiac vein
middle lobe syndrome
middle third of the thoracic esophagus
middle-field-strength MR imaging
middorsal
midepigastrium
midesophageal diverticulum
midesophagus
midface, fetal
midface retrusion
midfemur
midfoot
midget MRI scanner
midgraft stenosis
mid-groove portion of lumina
midgut volvulus with malrotation
midlateral course
mid-left sternal border
midline, infracolic
midline mucosa-sparing blocks
midline shift
midline structures
midlung field
midlung zone
midmarginal branch of artery
midpelvis
midpole
midportion
midriff
midsagittal MR image
midscapular line
midshaft fracture
midshunt peak velocities (MSPv)
midsternum
midsystolic notching of velocity
    spectrum

mid-ventricular short-axis slice
midzone
migrational anomaly
migratory patchy infiltration
Mikro-tip micromanometer-tipped
    catheter
Mikulicz angle
Mikulicz syndrome
miliary lung disease
miliary pattern
miliary tuberculosis
milieu, therapeutic
milk leg syndrome
Milkman syndrome (also Looser-
    Milkman)
milky effusion
Millar catheter-tip transducer
Millar MPC-500 catheter
Miller-Abbott tube
Miller-Dieker syndrome
Miller disease
miller's lung
milliampere (mA)
millicurie (mCi)
millijoule (mJ)
Millikan-Siekert syndrome
millimeter (mm)
millimeters of mercury (mm Hg)
Millenia balloon catheter for percuta-
    neous transluminal coronary angio-
    plasty
milliroentgen
milliseconds (ms, msec)
millivolt (mV)
Milroy disease
Milton angioedema disease
mimic
mimicked
mimicking
mineral oil contrast
mineralization, bone
miner's lung

Ming classification of gastric
   carcinoma
Mini C-arm device
minimal luminal diameter (MLD)
minimally displaced fracture
minimal volume
minimum blood pressure
minimum intensity projection (MIP)
   image
mini-PACS
minipapillotome
Mini-Profile dilatation catheter, USCI
Minot–von Willebrand syndrome
minuscule
minute-sequence study
minute vessels
minute volume
MION (monocrystalline iron oxides)
   MION-gene complex
MIP (maximum intensity pixel)
MIP (maximum intensity projection)
   algorithms
MIPcor (coronal maximum-intensity
   projection)
Mirage over-the-wire balloon catheter
MIRI (myocardial infarction recovery
   index)
mirror image reversal
mirror, polygon
MIS (minimally invasive surgery)
misalign
misery perfusion
misleading images
mismatch
   perfusion-metabolism
   ventilation-perfusion (V/Q)
misonidazole (radiosensitizer)
missile wound
mitochondrial uncoupler CCCP
mitral annular calcification
mitral annulus
mitral apparatus

mitral arcade
mitral atresia
mitral configuration of cardiac shadow
mitral deceleration slope
mitral inflow velocities
mitral insufficiency
mitral leaflets
mitral leak
mitral orifice
mitral regurgitant signal area
mitral regurgitation
   congenital
   pansystolic
mitral regurgitation artifact
mitral regurgitation-chordal elongation
   syndrome
mitral ring calcification
mitral stenosis
   congenital
   relative
   true
mitral valve
   billowing
   cleft
   hammock
   parachute
   prosthetic
mitral valve atresia
mitral valve calcification
mitral valve commissures
mitral valve configuration, fishmouth
mitral valve echogram
mitral valve leaflet tip
mitral valve myxomatous degeneration
mitral valve prolapse, holosystolic
mitral valve regurgitation
mitral valve replacement
mitral valve septal separation
mitral valve stenosis (MVS)
Mitsubishi angioscopic catheter
mixed connective tissue disease
mixed echogenic solid mass

mixed lesion
mixed petal-fugal flow
mixed restrictive-obstructive lung
    disease
mixed signal mass
mixed tumor
mixed venous saturation
ml/min/100 g (milliliters per minute
    per 100 grams)
MLC (multileaf collimator)
MLD (minimal luminal diameter)
mm (millimeter)
mm Hg (millimeters of mercury)
MM50 Racetrack Microtron
MMCM (macromolecular contrast
    medium)
M-mode Doppler echocardiography
M-mode echocardiogram
M-mode echophonocardiography
M-mode transducer
M-mode ultrasound
mmol (millimoles)
mmol/kg (millimoles per kilogram)
mmol/L (millimoles per liter)
Mn (manganese)
MnCl2 (manganese chloride 2)
    imaging agent
MNP10 protocol
MO (mitral orifice)
MOAB, MoAb (monoclonal anti-
    body), radiolabeled
Mobetron electron beam system
mobile magnetic resonance (MR)
    imager
mobile thrombus
mobility
mode
    A-
    AAI (noncompetitive atrial
        demand)
    AAI rate-responsive
    active
    asynchronous transfer (ATM)

mode *(cont.)*
    atrial triggered and ventricular
        inhibited
    atrial-burst
    atrioventricular dual-demand
    B-
    bipolar pacing
    blink
    byte
    cine (high frame-rate)
    committed
    DDD pacing
    dual-demand pacing
    DVI (digital vascular imaging)
    fixed rate
    full-to-empty VAD
    inactive
    inhibited pacing
    M-mode
    multiplanar
    noncommitted
    pacing
    road-mapping
    semicommitted
    sequential
    64 x 64 byte
    stimulation
    triggered pacing
    underdrive
    unipolar pacing
    VAD (ventricular assist device)
    VVI (noncompetitive demand
        ventricular)
mode abandonment
model
    figure-of-eight
    lattice
    leading circle
    Markov source
    Renkin
    ring
    Shames
    xerography

MPF catheter
MPGR (multiplanar gradient-recalled) echo
MPHR (maximum predicted heart rate)
MPPv flow
MPR (multiplanar reformation)
MPR (myocardial perfusion reserve)
mps (meters per second)
MR (magnetic resonance), 3D
MR (mitral regurgitation)
MRA (magnetic resonance angiography)
MRC (magnetic resonance cholangiography)
MRE (magnetic resonance elastography)
MRI (see *magnetic resonance imaging*; also *imaging*)
MRM (magnetic resonance mammography)
MRM (magnetic resonance myelogram)
MRN (magnetic resonance neurography)
MRS (magnetic resonance spectroscopy)
MRSA (pronounced "mer-suh") (methicillin-resistant MRU, magnetic resonance urography)
MRU (molecular recognition unit)
ms (milliseconds)
MS (mitral stenosis)
MS (morphine sulfate)
MS (multiple sclerosis) plaquing
MS Classique balloon dilatation catheter
MS-325 imaging agent
MSA (multiple system atrophy) syndrome
MSAD (multiple scan average dose)
MSAFP (maternal serum alpha fetoprotein)

msec (millisecond)
M-shaped pattern of mitral valve
MSI (magnetic source imaging), 3D
MSO_4 (morphine sulfate)
MT (magnetization transfer)
MTEs (main timing events)
MTP (metatarsophalangeal) joint
MTR (magnetization transfer ratio)
MTT (mean pulmonary transit time)
mu (μ) rhythm (μ, twelfth Greek letter)
mucinous tumor
mucocele
mucoid degeneration
mucoid impaction
mucoid plugging of airways
mucosa
   "burned out"
   cobblestone
   friable
   frothy
   isoeffective
   muscularis
mucosal abnormality
mucosal crinkling
mucosal folds
mucosal inflammation
mucosal island
mucosal pattern
mucosal relief
mucosa-sparing blocks
mucous fistula
mucous lake of stomach
mucous membrane
mucus hypersecretion
mucus plugging
Mueller (Müller) fibers
MUGA (multiple gated acquisition) blood pool radionuclide scan
mulberry gallstones
mulberry-type calcification
Müller (Mueller) fibers

Müller sign (aortic regurgitation)
multangular bone, accessory
multangular ridge fracture
multangulum
multiagent chemotherapy
multiangle, multislice acquisition magnetic resonance imaging
multibreath washout study
multicentric lytic lesions
multicentricity
multicolor flow cytometry
multicompartment clearance
multicoupled loop-gap resonator
multicrystal gamma camera
multicystic
multidetector system
multiecho axial
multiecho coronal image
multiecho image
multiecho sequence
multielemental neutron activation analysis
multiexponential relaxation
multifiber catheter
multifield beam
multifocal lesions
multifocal lymphoma
multifocal short stenosis
multiform ventricular complexes
multiforme, glioblastoma
multigated pulsed Doppler flow system
multigravida
multi-interval
multi-illuminant color correction
multi-infarct dementia (MID)
multilaminar bodies
multileaf collimator (MLC)
multilesion angioplasty
multilocular cyst
Multi-Med triple-lumen infusion catheter

multimodal image fusion technique
multimodality imaging
multinodular goiter
multinuclear magnetic resonance imaging
multiorgan imaging
multipara
multiparametric color composite display
multiparous
multiparticle cyclotron
multiphasic multislice magnetic resonance imaging technique
multiphasic renal computerized tomography (CT)
multiplanar gradient-recalled (MPGR) echo
multiplanar magnetic resonance imaging
multiplanar mode
multiplanar reformation (MRP) view
multiplanar reformatted radiographic and digitally reconstructed images
multiplanar transesophageal echocardiography
multiplane dosage calculations
multiple-beam interface spacing
multiple chord, center-line technique in echocardiogram
multiple endocrine neoplasia (MEN)
multiple exposure volumetric holography (MEVH)
multiple fractures
multiple gated acquisition (MUGA) blood pool radionuclide scan
multiple-gated acquisition (MUGA) scan
multiple jointed digitizer
multiple organ failure
multiple plane imaging
multiple scan average dose (MSAD)
multiple sclerosis plaquing

multiple slice acquisition
multiple trauma
multipulse nuclear magnetic resonance (NMR) imaging
multipurpose catheter
Multipurpose-SM catheter
multirod collimator
multisectional dose-volume histogram
multisection diffuse-weighted magnetic resonance imaging
multisection magnetic resonance imaging
multisection multirepetition acquisition
multisensor structured light range digitizer
multiseptate appearance
multishot echoplanar imaging
multislab magnetic resonance angiography
multislice first-pass myocardial perfusion imaging
multislice FLASH 2D
multislice mode
multislice multiphase spin-echo imaging technique
multislice spin echo sequence
multispin relaxation
multitracer study
multivessel angioplasty
MUMPS (Massachusetts [General Hospital] Utility Multiprogramming System)
Münchmeyer disease
mural aneurysm
mural architecture
mural clot
mural degeneration
mural dilatations
mural endomyocardial fibrosis
mural infiltration
mural leaflet of mitral valve
mural nodule

mural thrombosis
mural thrombus formation
muscle (pl. muscles)
   accessory
   adductor magnus
   Aeby
   Albinus
   anterior
   auricular
   axillary
   bipennate
   Bochdalek
   Bovero
   Bowman
   Braune
   Brücke
   bulbocavernosus
   canine
   cardiac
   Casser
   casserian
   cervical
   Chassaignac
   chin
   circular
   Coiter
   conal papillary
   Crampton
   deep
   detrusor
   digastric
   dorsal
   Dupré
   Duverney
   electrically conditioned and driven skeletal
   external
   fixation
   fixator
   Folius
   fused papillary
   Gantzer

muscle *(cont.)*
   gastrocnemius
   Gavard
   greater
   Guthrie
   Hilton
   Horner
   Houston
   iliococcygeal
   iliocostal
   inferior
   intercostal
   internal
   interosseous
   interspinal
   intertransverse
   intra-auricular
   ischiocavernosus
   Jung
   Klein
   Lancisi
   lateral
   latissimus dorsi
   left ventricular
   lesser
   levator
   longitudinal
   Luschka
   Macalister
   major
   Marcacci
   masticator
   medial
   medial papillary
   Merkel
   middle
   minor
   Müller (Mueller)
   multipennate
   nonstriated
   oblique
   Ochsner

muscle *(cont.)*
   Oddi
   Oehl
   omohyoid
   opposing
   organic
   papillary
   pectoralis major
   pectoralis minor
   peroneal
   peroneus quartus
   Phillips
   plantaris
   platysma
   posterior
   Pozzi
   pubococcygeal
   quadrate
   Reisseisen
   rhomboideus major
   ribbon
   rider
   Riolan
   Rouget
   round
   Ruysch
   sacrospinalis
   Santorini
   sartorius
   Sebileau
   semimembranous
   semispinal
   semitendinous
   serratus anterior
   short
   Sibson
   skeletal
   smaller
   Soemmerring
   soleus
   somatic
   sphenomandibularis

myeloma
  indolent
  localized
  multiple
  sclerosing
  solitary
myenteric plexus of Auerbach
Myler catheter
mylohyoid ridge
myoblastoma, granular cell
myocardial blood flow (MBF)
myocardial blush
myocardial bridging
myocardial contractile dysfunction
myocardial contractility
myocardial contrast appearance time
  (MCAT)
myocardial contusion
myocardial degeneration
myocardial depression
myocardial dysfunction
myocardial fibers degeneration
myocardial fibrosis
myocardial granulomatous disease
myocardial hibernation
myocardial hypoperfusion, resting
  regional
myocardial incompetency
myocardial infarct imaging
myocardial infarction
myocardial infiltration by Kaposi
  sarcoma
myocardial injury
  lethal
  nonlethal
myocardial insufficiency, Sternberg
myocardial ischemia, exercise-induced
  transient
myocardial muscle
myocardial necrosis
myocardial oxygen consumption
myocardial oxygen demand

myocardial perfusion defect
myocardial perfusion scan
myocardial perfusion tomography
myocardial preservation
myocardial protection
myocardial recovery
myocardial reperfusion injury
myocardial revascularization
myocardial rupture
myocardial scan
myocardial shortening, fractional
myocardial-specific marker
myocardial stunning
myocardial tagging
myocardial thickening
myocardial tissue viability
myocardial tumor, metastatic
myocardial uptake of thallium
myocardial work
myocardium
  asynergic
  calcification of
  dilated
  hibernating
  hypertrophied
  ischemic reperfused
  ischemic viable
  jeopardized
  noninfarcted
  nonperfused
  perfused
  reperfused
  rupture of
  senile
  stunned
  ventricular
  viable
myofibril volume fraction
myofibroma
myoma
  pedunculated subserous
  submucous
  uterine

myometrium
Myoscint (monoclonal antibody Fab to
  myosin, labeled with indium-111)
myositis ossificans (MO)
myotendinous junction
Myoview imaging drug in scintigraphy
myxofibroma
myxoma
  atrial
  biatrial
  cardiac

myxoma *(cont.)*
  familial (of the heart)
  heart
  left atrial
  pedunculated
  vascular
  ventricular
myxomatous degeneration
myxomatous proliferation
myxomatous valve leaflet

N, n

N (nitrogen)
NAA metabolite signal
Nagele obliquity
Nagele pelvis
naloxone
nanoparticles
nanoparticulate contrast agent
napkin-ring annular stenosis
napkin-ring annular tumor
Narco esophageal motility machine
naris (pl. nares)
narrow-band spectral-selective 90 RF
    pulse
narrow gating tolerance
narrowing
    arterial
    atherosclerotic
    diffuse
    disk space
    focal
    high-grade
    joint space
    large airway
    luminal
    neural foramen
    residual luminal
    subcritical

nasal sinus
nasal spine
nasion recession
nasobiliary drainage catheter
nasogastric (NG) tube
nasolabial cyst
nasopharyngeal atresia
nasopharyngeal carcinoma (NPC)
nasopharyngeal craniopharyngioma
nasotracheal tube
National Institutes of Health (NIH)
    catheter
native aortic valve, preservation of
native atherosclerosis
native coronary artery
native images
native kidney
native ventricle
native vessel
natural neon gas
Naughton-Balke treadmill protocol,
    modified
Navarre interventional radiology
    devices
navel string
navicular
    carpal
    tarsal

navicular view
naviculocapitate fracture
navigable echo signal
navigated spin-echo diffusion-weighted
  MR imaging
navigating heart structures
navigator echo-based real-time
  respiratory gating and triggering
navigator echo motion correction
  technique
navigator pulse
navigator shifts
NCC (normalized cross-section)
NCL-Arp monoclonal antibody
  imaging agent
NCL-ER-LHZ monoclonal antibody
  imaging agent
NCL-PGR monoclonal antibody
  imaging agent
NCPF (noncirrhotic portal fibrosis)
Nd:YAG (neodymium:yttrium-
  aluminum-garnet) laser
near anatomic position of joint
near field
near-infrared spectroscopy
near-resonance spin-lock contrast
nearest neighbor interpolation
neck
  aneurysmal
  bone
  dental
  femoral
  Madelung
  pancreatic
  surgical
  uterine
  wry
neck vessel engorgement
necroscopy, perinatal
necrosed tissue
necrosis
  acute sclerosing hyaline (ASHN)
  acute tubular

necrosis *(cont.)*
  alveolar septal
  aorta idiopathic
  arteriolar
  aseptic
  avascular
  bilateral cortical
  biliary piecemeal
  bloodless zone of
  bowel
  bridging
  caseous
  centrilobular
  coagulation
  colliquative
  colonic
  contraction band
  cystic medial
  diffuse
  embolic
  epiphyseal
  epiphyseal ischemic
  Erdheim cystic medial
  fat
  fatty
  fibrinoid
  fibrosing piecemeal
  focal
  focal hepatic
  frank
  heart muscle
  hemorrhagic
  hepatic
  hyaline
  indurative
  intestinal
  ischemic
  liquefaction
  localized
  lung
  massive
  massive hepatic

necrosis *(cont.)*
  medial cystic
  midzonal
  mucosal
  myocardial
  Paget quiet
  pancreatic
  papillary
  peripheral
  piecemeal
  postoperative
  postpartum pituitary
  pressure
  progressive emphysematous
  radiation
  renal cortical
  renal tubular
  septic
  strangulation
  stromal
  subacute hepatic
  subcutaneous fat
  subendocardial
  submassive
  submassive hepatic
  superficial
  total
  tracheobronchial mucosal
  ventricular muscle
  Zenker
necrotic myocardium
necrotizing emphysema
necrotizing pneumonia
necrotizing respiratory granulomatosis
necrotizing thrombosis
needle
  nonferromagnetic
  Quincke spinal
  stabilization
  Whitacre spinal
needle biopsy, CT-scan directed
needle hydrophone

needle tracking, real-time biplanar
Neer shoulder fractures (I, II, III
  classification)
NEFA (non-esterified fatty acid)
  scintigraphy
negative contrast agent
negative image
negative predictive value
negligible pressure gradient
Nélaton dislocation
Nélaton fold
NEMD (nonspecific esophageal
  motility disorder)
neoadjuvant chemotherapy
neoadjuvant hormonal therapy
neoaorta
neoaortic valve
neocerebellum
neocholangiole
neodymium:yttrium-aluminum-garnet
  (Nd:YAG) laser
neointimal hyperplasia
neointimal proliferation
neonatal adrenal ultrasound
neonatal cystic pulmonary emphysema
neonate
neon particle protocol
neopallium
neoplasia, multiple endocrine (MEN)
neoplasm
  benign
  encapsulated
  firm
  functioning
  gonadal
  lethal
  low-grade
  malignant
  ovarian
  primary
  spherical
  well-circumscribed

neoplastic fracture
neoplastic stenosis
Neoprobe radioactivity detector
neorectum
neovascularity
nephroblastoma
nephrogram
nephrographic phase (NP)
nephrolithiasis
nephroptosis
nephrosclerosis
   arterial
   senile
nephrosis
nephrotic
nephrostogram
nephrotic edema
nephrotomogram
nephrotomography
nephrotoxic contrast medium
nephrotoxicity
Neptune trident appearance
Nernst equation
nerve root compression
nerve root edema
nerve root sheath
nervous heart syndrome
net magnetization factor
net tissue magnetization
network
   articular
   lymphatic
   neural
   venous
network architecture
NEUGAT (neutron/gamma
   transmission) method
neural arch
neural crest origin
neural evaluation algorithm
neural foramen (pl. foramina)
neural network

neural tube defect
neurenteric cyst
neurinoma
neuritic plaque
neuritic plaquing
neuroangiography
neuroblastoma
neuroblockage
neurodiagnosis
NeuroEcho software
neuroendocrine carcinoma
neurofibrillary tangles
neurofibromatosis
neurogenic bladder
neurogenic dysfunction of the bladder
neurogenic fracture
neurogenic pulmonary edema
neurogenic sarcoma
neurogenic tumor
neurography, magnetic resonance
   (MRN)
neuroholography
neuroimaging
neurointerventional radiology
neuroleptic
Neurolite (technetium Tc 99m
   bicisate) imaging agent
Neuro Lobe software
neurologic signs, focal
neuroma
   Morton
   multicystic acoustic
neuromorphometry
neuromuscular blockade
Neuropac
neuropathic bladder
neuroradiologic examination
neuroradiology
   interventional
   pediatric
neuroreceptor ligand
NeuroScan 3D imager

NeuroSector ultrasound system
neurosonogram
neurosonology
Neuro SPGR software
neurosurgery, stereotactic
neurotoxic effect
neurotropic MR imaging contrast
　agents
neurovascular bundle
neurovascular compression
neutron activation analysis
neutron capture therapy
neutron/gamma transmission
　(NEUGAT) method
neutron
　slow
　thermal
neutron-deficient nuclei
neutron irradiation
neutron-rich biomedical tracer
neutron therapy
nevus (pl. nevi)
NEX (number of excitations) (on MRI
　scan)
NG (nasogastric) tube
NH region of AV (atrioventricular)
　node
Nicaladoni-Branham sign
niche
　Barclay
　Haudek
Nicolet NMR spectrometer
nicotinamide radiosensitizer
nidus demarcation
nidus, thrombus
Niemann-Pick disease
Niemeier gallbladder perforation
NIH (National Institutes of Health)
Nikolsky sign
nimodipine, intraarterial superselective
ninety-degree (or 90°) RF pulse (on
　MR spectroscopy)

91-41 MeV proton
Niopam contrast medium
nipple marker
NIPS (noninvasive programmed
　stimulation)
NIRS (near-infrared spectroscopy)
Nishimoto Sangyo scanner
Nissen antireflux operation
nitinol stent
nitrogen, body
nitrogen washout
nitrogen (N)
　^{13}N ammonia radioactive tracer
　^{13}N ammonia uptake on PET scan
nitrogen-nipple sign, aortic
nitrous oxide synthetase
NMIS (nuclear medicine information
　system)
NMR (nuclear magnetic resonance)
　imaging (see *imaging*)
no discernible findings
no therapy zone
NO (nitrous oxide)
no-carrier-added fluorine-18 imaging
　agent
no-gap technique
no-reflow phenomenon
nociceptive
nodal conduction
nodal contractions
nodal escape
nodal impulse
nodal metastases
nodal point
nodal premature contraction
nodal rupture
node
　abdominal lymph
　accessory lymph
　anorectal lymph
　aortic lymph
　aortic window

node *(cont.)*
  apical lymph
  appendicular lymph
  Aschoff
  Aschoff-Tawara
  atrioventricular (AV, AVN)
  auricular lymph
  AV (atrioventricular)
  axillary lymph
  bifurcation lymph
  Bouchard
  brachial lymph
  bronchopulmonary lymph
  buccal lymph
  buccinator lymph
  cardiac
  caval lymph
  celiac lymph
  central lymph
  cervical lymph
  cervical paratracheal lymph
  Cloquet inguinal lymph
  common iliac lymph
  companion lymph
  coronary
  cubital lymph
  cystic lymph
  Delphian lymph
  deltopectoral lymph
  diaphragmatic lymph
  Dürck
  epicolic lymph
  epigastric lymph
  epitrochlear lymph
  Ewald
  external iliac lymph
  facial lymph
  fibular lymph
  Flack
  Flack sinoatrial
  foraminal
  gastric lymph

node *(cont.)*
  gastroduodenal lymph
  gastroepiploic lymph
  gastro-omental lymph
  gluteal lymph
  gouty
  Haygarth
  Heberden
  hemal
  hemolymph
  Hensen
  hepatic lymph
  hilar lymph
  ileocolic lymph
  iliac circumflex lymph
  iliac lymph
  infraclavicular
  infrahyoid lymph
  inguinal lymph
  intercostal lymph
  interiliac lymph
  interpectoral lymph
  intramammary
  jugular lymph
  jugulodigastric lymph
  jugulo-omohyoid lymph
  juxtaintestinal
  Keith
  Keith-Flack sinoatrial
  Koch sinoatrial
  lacunar
  lumbar lymph
  lymph
  malar lymph
  mandibular lymph
  mastoid lymph
  medial supraclavicular
  mediastinal lymph
  mesenteric lymph
  Meynet
  nasolabial lymph
  NH region of AV (atrioventricular)

node *(cont.)*
- obturator lymph
- occipital lymph
- Osler
- pancreatic lymph
- pancreaticoduodenal lymph
- pancreaticolienal lymph
- pancreacticosplenic
- paracardial lymph
- paracolic lymph
- paramammary lymph
- pararectal lymph
- parasternal lymph
- paratracheal lymph
- parauterine lymph
- paravaginal lymph
- paravesicular lymph
- parietal lymph
- parotid lymph
- Parrot
- pectoral lymph
- pelvic lymph
- peribronchial
- pericardial lymph
- peroneal
- phrenic lymph
- popliteal lymph
- postaortic lymph
- postcaval lymph
- posterior mediastinal
- postvesicular lymph
- preaortic lymph
- precaval lymph
- prececal lymph
- prelaryngeal
- prepericardial lymph
- pretracheal lymph
- prevertebral lymph
- prevesicular lymph
- pulmonary juxtaesophageal lymph
- pulmonary lymph
- pyloric lymph

node *(cont.)*
- Ranvier
- rectal lymph
- regional lymph
- retroaortic lymph
- retroauricular lymph
- retrocecal lymph
- retropharyngeal lymph
- retropyloric
- retrorectal lymph node
- Rosenmüller
- Rotter
- SA (sinoatrial)
- sacral lymph
- satellite
- scalene
- Schmorl
- sentinel
- shotty lymph
- sick sinus
- sigmoid lymph
- signal
- singer
- sinoatrial (SAN)
- sinoauricular
- sinus
- Sister Mary Joseph
- solitary lymph
- splenic lymph
- subcarinal
- submandibular lymph
- submental lymph
- subpyloric
- subscapular lymph
- superficial inguinal lymph
- supraclavicular lymph
- suprapyloric
- supratrochlear lymph
- syphilitic
- Tawara
- teacher
- thyroid lymph

node *(cont.)*
  tibial
  tracheal lymph
  tracheobronchial lymph
  Troisier
  vesicular lymph
  vestigial left sinoatrial
  Virchow
  visceral lymph
nodo-Hisian (nodohisian) bypass tract
nodosum
  erythema
  polyarteritis (PAN)
nodoventricular bypass fiber
nodoventricular bypass tract
nodoventricular pathway
nodoventricular tachycardia
nodular aneurysm
nodular density
nodular enhancement
nodular fibrosis
nodular goiter
nodular-like
nodular lymphoid hyperplasia (NLH)
nodular mass
nodularity
  calcified
  coarse
  noncalcified
  surface
  vein
nodule (pl. nodules)
  air-space
  Albini
  aortic valve
  Arantius
  Aschoff
  autonomous
  Bianchi
  cold
  cortical
  Cruveilhier

nodule *(cont.)*
  cutaneous
  Dalen-Fuchs
  discordant
  enhancing
  fibrous
  Fraenkel typhus
  functioning
  Gamna
  Gamna-Gandy
  Gandy-Gamna
  Hoboken
  hot
  hypermetabolic
  Kerckring
  Koeppe
  Morgagni
  mural
  non-enhancing
  noncavitary
  nondelineated
  nonfunctioning thyroid
  ossific
  peripheral
  Picker
  regenerative
  rheumatic
  rheumatoid
  Schmorl
  semiautonomous
  siderotic
  silicotic
  singer's
  Sister Mary Joseph
  solitary
  surfer's
  teacher's
  tobacco
  toxic
  tuberculous
  typhoid
  typhus
  warm

nodulus Arantii (pl. noduli Arantii)
nodus arcus venae azygos
noise
   lesion-to-cerebrospinal fluid
   lesion-to-white matter
   pixel
   respiratory
   subtractive
   white
noise distribution, spectral
noise reduction intercom
NOMOS correction factor
nonablative heating
nonarticular radial head fracture
nonasbestos pneumoconiosis
noncalcified mitral leaflets
noncalcified nodule
noncardiac pulmonary edema
noncardiogenic pulmonary edema
noncaseating granuloma
noncaseating tubercles
noncavitary nodule
noncircularity degree
noncoaxial catheter tip position
noncollagenous pneumoconiosis
noncommunicating cyst
noncommunicating hydrocephalus
noncompensatory pause
noncompliant plaque
noncompressible appendix
noncontact imaging technology
noncontractile scar tissue
noncontrast phase (NCP)
non-coplanar arc technique
non-coplanar therapy beams
noncoronary cusp
noncoronary sinus
nondecremental
nondelineated nodule
nondependent lung
nondisplaced fracture
nondistensible balloon

nondominant vessel
nonenclosed magnet
nonenhanced CAT scan
nonenhancing nodule
nonenhancing lesion
nonferromagnetic needle
nonfilarial chylocele
nonfilling venous segment
nonforeshortened angiographic view
nonfunctioning thyroid nodule
non-Hodgkin lymphoma
nonhomogeneous consolidation
nonhyperfunctioning adrenal adenoma
nonimmunological fetal hydrops
noninducible tachycardia
noninfarcted segment
noninteger period
noninvasive diagnosis
noninvasive imaging study
nonionic contrast medium
nonionic paramagnetic contrast medium
nonisotropic gradient
nonlethal myocardial ischemic injury
nonlinear excitation profile
nonlingular branches of upper lobe
   bronchus
Nonne-Milroy lymphedema
non-nodular fibrosis
non-nodular silicosis
nonocclusive mesenteric arterial
   insufficiency
nonpeptide angiotensin II antagonist
nonpulsatile mass
nonradiopaque foreign body
nonresonance Raman spectroscopy
nonresponsive to TSH manipulation
nonrheumatic valvular aortic stenosis
nonsegmental areas of opacification
nonselective angiography
non-small cell lung cancer (NSCLC)
nonspecific bowel gas pattern
nonspecific changes

nonspecific esophageal motility
   disorder (NEMD)
nonspecific phenomenon
nonsteroidal antiphlogistics
nonstress test (NST)
nonsubtraction images
nonsyndromic bicoronal synostosis
nonsyndromic unicoronal synostosis
nontrabeculated atrium
nontransmural myocardial infarction
nontransmural match
nontraumatic dislocation
nontraumatic epidural hemorrhage
nontriggered phase-contrast MR
   angiography
nonuniform attenuation
nonuniform rotational defect (NURD)
nonunion of fracture fragments
nonunion, torsion wedge
nonvalved conduit
nonviable scar from myocardial
   infarction
nonvisualization of gallbladder
nonweightbearing view
Noonan syndrome
NoProfile balloon catheter
Norland bone densitometry
Norland pQCT XCT2000 scanner
Norland XR26 bone densitometer
normal
   borderline
   high
   low
normal anatomic variation
normalized average glandular dose
normalized cross-section (NCC)
normal-pressure hydrocephalus
normal-region pixel
normokalemic reperfusion
normotensive
normothermia
normovolemia

normovolemic
normoxia
NOS (not otherwise specified)
nose cone
nosocomial TB (tuberculosis)
   transmission
notch
   acetabular
   anacrotic
   angular
   antegonial
   aortic
   auricular
   cardiac
   cerebellar
   clavicular
   coracoid
   costal
   cotyloid
   craniofacial
   dicrotic
   digastric
   ethmoidal
   fibular
   frontal
   greater sciatic
   interclavicular
   intercondylar
   intercondyloid
   intervertebral
   Kernohan
   lesser sciatic
   radial sigmoid
   scapular
   sciatic
   sigmoid
   spinoglenoid
   sternal
   suprasternal
   trochlear
   ulnar
notched aortic knob

notching of pulmonic valve on echocardiogram
notching, rib
Nothnagel syndrome
Novopaque contrast medium
NOX (number of excitations) on MRI
NP (nephrographic phase)
^{59}NP (iodomethylnorcholesterol)
scintigraphy
NPC (nasopharyngeal cancer)
NPC (nodal premature contraction)
NRH (nodular regenerative
hyperplasia)
NSCLO (non-small cell lung cancer)
nubbin sign
Nuck
canal of
diverticulum of
nuclear bone imaging
nuclear electric quadripole relaxation
nuclear gated blood pool testing
nuclear hepatobiliary imaging
nuclear magnetic resonance (NMR)
(see also *imaging*)
NMR imaging
NMR magnetometer probe
NMR quadrature detection array
NMR scan
NMR spectography
NMR spectrometer
NMR spectroscopy
NMR spectrum
NMR station, MacSpect real-time
NMR tomography of breast

nuclear medicine information system
(NMIS)
nuclear parameters
nuclear perfusion imaging
nuclear relaxation
nuclear renal scintigraphy
nuclear signal
nuclear spin
nuclear spin quantum number
nuclear-tagged red blood cell bleeding
study
nucleonics
nucletron applicator
nucleus (pl. nuclei)
caudate
dentate
Kölliker
lenticular
lentiform
neutron-deficient
residual
nucleus globosus
nucleus pulposus
nuclide analysis
null point
number, clonogen
number of excitations (NEX) on MRI
NURD (nonuniform rotational defect)
nursemaid's elbow
nutation angle measurement
nutcracker esophagus
Nycomed contrast
Nycore angiography catheter

O, o

obstructive hydrocephalus
obstructive hypopnea
obstructive jaundice
obstructive lesion
obstructive pneumonia
obstructive pulmonary disease (OPD)
obstructive pulmonary overinflation
obstructive renal dysplasia
obstructive thrombus
obstructive-type atelectasis
obstructive ventilatory defect
obturating embolus
obturator hernia
obturator internus muscle
obturator nodal chain
obturator node
obturator sign
obtuse marginal (OM) coronary artery
obtuse marginal branch (OMB)
occipital-atlas-axis ligaments
occipital-axis joint
occipital bone
occipital condyle
occipital fissure
occipital fracture
occipital gyrus
occipital lesion
occipital lobe
occipital pole
occipital-temporal sulcus
occipital tip
occipital vessels
occipital view of skull
occipitoanterior
occipitoatlantoaxial fusion
occipitocervical articulation
occipitofrontalis muscle
occipitoposterior
occipitotemporal gyrus
occipitotemporal sulcus
occipitotemporopontine tract

occiput
occlude
occluded graft
occluder
   ameroid
   radiolucent plastic
occluder delivered into left atrium
   under fluoroscopic control
occluding spring emboli
occluding thrombus
occlusal plane
occlusal segment
occlusion
   aqueductal
   arterial
   balloon
   basilar
   bilateral
   complete
   coronary
   deep venous
   ductus arteriosus
   embolic
   fallopian tube
   graft
   intermittent
   intracranial vascular
   late graft
   side branch
   snowplow
   subtotal
   tapering
   total
   traumatogenic
   unilateral
   ureteral
   vascular
   vein graft
   vertebrobasilar
   vessel
occlusion measurement
occlusive arterial thrombus

occlusive cerebrovascular insult
occlusive impedance phlebography
occlusive lesion
occult cerebral vascular malformation (OCVM)
occult fracture
occult lesion
occult, roentgenographically
occult subluxation
OCG (oral cholecystogram)
ochronosis
OCL bowel prep
O'Connor finger dexterity test
OCT (optical coherence tomography)
octagon board
octapolar catheter
OctreoScan radiologic imaging agent
Octreotide scintigraphy
ocular globe topography
ocular pneumoplethysmography (OPG)
oculoauriculovertebral (OAV)
oculomotor apparatus
oculomotor nerve (third cranial nerve)
oculomotor-trochlear nucleus
oculopharyngeal dystrophy
oculoplethysmography (OPG)
oculoplethysmography/carotid phonoangiography (OPG/CPA)
oculopneumoplethysmography
oculosubcutaneous syndrome of Yuge
Oddi, sphincter of
Oden classification of peroneal tendon subluxation
odontogenic fibromyxoma
odontoid bone
odontoid fracture
odontoid process
odontoid view
odontoma
ODQ (opponens digiti quinti) muscle
OEC Series 9600 cardiac system

off-axis dose inhomogeneity
off-axis factor
off-axis point localization
off-center cut
off-center modulation
off-resonance saturation pulse imaging
off-resonance spin-locking
offset, frequency
Ogden classification of epiphyseal fracture
Ogilvie syndrome (pseudo-obstruction of colon)
Ogston line
ohm (pl. ohms)
oil embolism
oil emulsions contrast
oil, peppermint (used with barium enema)
OKT3 monoclonal antibody
OKT4 monoclonal antibody imaging agent
OKT8 monoclonal antibody imaging agent
Okuda transhepatic obliteration of varices
olecranon
olecranon fossa
olecranon process
olecranon tip fracture
oleothorax
Olerud and Molander fracture classification
oligemic lobe
oligoclonal IgG bands in cerebrospinal fluid
oligodactylia
oligodendroglioma tumor
oligodendroma
oligohydramnios
olisthesis
olisthetic vertebra, wedging of
olive ring

Oliver-Cardarelli sign
olivopontocerebellar atrophy
olivopontocerebellar degeneration
Ollier disease
olsalazine
Olympus Gastrocamera GTF-A
Olympus GF-UM3 and CF-UM20
    ultrasonic endoscope
Olympus UM-1W transendoscopic
    ultrasound probe
Olympus VU-M2 and XIF-UM3
    echoendoscope
OM (obtuse marginal) coronary artery
OMB (obtuse marginal branch)
OMB1 (obtuse marginal branch #1)
omental cake
omentum
    colic
    gastric
    gastrocolic
    gastrohepatic
    gastrosplenic
    greater (omentum majus)
    incarcerated
    lesser (omentum minus)
    pancreaticosplenic
    splenogastric
omentum majus
omentum minus
Omniflex balloon catheter
Omnipaque (iohexol) nonionic
    imaging agent
Omnipaque contrast media
Omniscan (gadodiamide) nonionic
    contrast medium
omohyoid muscle
omphalic
omphalocele
omphaloma
on-column preparation
OncoScint breast imaging agent
OncoScint CR/OV (satumomab
    pendetide) contrast medium

OncoScint CR103 (colorectal) and
    OV103 (ovarian) (monoclonal
    antibody B72.3 labeled with
    indium-111)
OncoScint CR372 imaging agent
OncoScint-NSC (non-small cell) lung
    imaging agent
OncoScint PR356 imaging agent
OncoSpect imaging agent
OncoTrac imaging agent
one-part fracture
one-dimensional chemical shift
    imaging (1D-CSI)
one-shot echo planar imaging
onion bulb appearance of myelin
    sheaths
onion bulb changes on biopsy
onion-shaped dilatation of duodenum
onion peel appearance on x-ray
onionskin configuration of collagenous
    fibers
onlay graft
on-line anion exchange purification
on-line portal imaging
opacification
opacified
opacify
opacifying
opacity (pl. opacities)
    diffuse
    ground-glass
    linear
    patchy alveolar
    reticular
opaque media
opaque wire suture
OPD (obstructive pulmonary disease)
OPD4 monoclonal antibody imaging
    agent
open architecture system
open beam
open-break fracture

organ
  accessory
  annulospiral
  circumventricular
  Corti
  critical
  extraperitoneal
  floating
  poles of
  retroperitoneal
  Zuckerkandl
organic brain disease (OBD)
organic granulomatosis
organic liquid scintillator
organification defect
organoaxial
organomegaly
orientation
  coronal
  disk-to-magnetic field
  disturbed
  sagittal
  slice
  spatial
  temporal
  transverse
ORIF (open reduction and internal
  fixation)
orifice
  anal
  aortic
  atrioventricular
  cardiac
  coronary
  coronary sinus
  double coronary
  esophagogastric
  external urethral
  gastroduodenal
  golf-hole ureteral
  hypoplastic tricuspid
  ileocecal

orifice *(cont.)*
  inferior vena cava
  internal urethral
  lingular
  mitral
  narrowed
  pharyngeal
  pulmonary
  pyloric
  rectal
  regurgitant
  segmental
  slitlike
  tricuspid
  ureteral (or ureteric)
  urethral
  vaginal
  valve
orifice-to-annulus ratio
origin
  anomalous
  muscle
origin of artery
origin of vessel
Orion balloon catheter
oroendotracheal tube
orogastric tube
oropharyngeal airway
oropharynx
orotracheal intubation
Orthacor material
orthocephalic
Orthoclone
orthogonal angiographic projection
orthogonal RF coil
orthogonal tag lines
orthogonal view on angiography
orthonormal diameter
orthopantogram
orthoroentgenogram
orthotopic ureter
orthovoltage radiation therapy

Ortner syndrome
os (pl. ossa) (see also *bone*)
   cervical
     coronary sinus
     external cervical
     internal cervical
os acetabuli (acetabulum)
os calcis (calcaneus)
os coxae (hip bone; ilium, ischium, pubis)
os cuboides secondarium (cuboid bone)
os naviculare (navicular bone)
os pubis (pubic bone)
os trigonum (triangular bone of tarsus)
oscillating magnetic field
oscillography
oscilloscope tuning station
Osgood-Schlatter disease
OSI (open systems interconnect)
OSI (optical surface imaging)
Osler disease
Osler-Libman-Sacks syndrome
Osler nodes
Osler sign
Osler triad
Osler-Weber-Rendu telangiectasia
Osm (osmole)
osmotic blood-brain barrier disruption
osmotic demyelination syndrome
osmotic edema
osmotic effect
osseous bridge
osseous destructive process
osseous dysplasia
osseous graft
osseous metastases
osseous outgrowth
osseous remodeling
osseous spiral lamina
osseous structure

osseous survey
osseous union
ossicle, Riolan
ossiferous
ossific nodule
ossific nucleus of navicular
ossification
   abnormal
   enchondral
   endochondral
   heterotopic
   intracartilaginous
   intramembranous
   irregular enchondral
   muscle
   periarticular heterotopic (PHO)
   peripheral
   primary center of
   secondary center of
   soft tissue
ossification center
ossification variant
ossified body
ossifying fibroma of long bone
osteal stenoses
ostealgia
ostemia
ostempyesis
OsteoAnalyzer device
osteoaneurysm
osteoarthritic change
osteoarthritic spur
osteoarthritis (OA)
   degenerative
   erosive
   generalized
   post-traumatic
   traumatic
osteoarticular
osteoblastic bone regeneration
osteoblastic metastasis
osteoblastic tumor

osteocachexia
osteocalcin
osteocartilaginous lesion
osteochondral fracture
osteochondral lesion
osteochondritic loose body
osteochondritic separation of
   epiphyses
osteochondritis dissecans (OD)
osteochondrofibroma
osteochondrolysis
osteochondroma
   epiphyseal
   soft tissue
osteochondromatosis
   multiple
   synovial
osteochondromatous dysplasia,
   epiarticular
osteochondrophyte
osteochondrosarcoma
osteochondrosis deformans juvenilis
osteochondrosis dissecans
osteoclasis
osteoclastic
osteo condensans ilii
osteocystoma
osteocyte
osteodiastasis
osteodystrophy
osteoenchondroma
osteofibrochondrosarcoma
osteofibromatosis
osteogenesis, distraction
osteogenesis imperfecta
osteogenesis imperfecta tarda
osteogenic sarcoma
osteohalisteresis
osteoid osteoma
osteolipochondroma
osteolipoma
osteolysis, scalloping

osteolytic metastases
osteoma
   juxta-articular osteoid
   osteoid
   parosteal
   spongy
   ulcer
osteomalacia
   hematogeneous
   renal tubular
   senile
osteomatosis
osteomesopyknosis
osteomyelitic sinus
osteomyelitis
osteonal bone
osteonecrosis
   dysbaric
   Ficat classification of femoral head
osteopenia
osteopetrosis
osteophyte
   bony
   bridging
   cervical
   fringe of
   horseshoe
   jagged
   marginal
osteophyte formation
   beaklike
   hooklike
   marginal
   nipplelike
osteophytic bone lip
osteophytic lipping
osteophytic proliferation
osteophytosis
osteoporosis
   corticosteroid-induced
   disuse
   juvenile

osteoporosis *(cont.)*
  post-traumatic
  postmenopausal
  senile
osteoporotic bone
osteoradionecrosis
osteosarcoma
  cardiac
  classical
  extraosseous
  fibroblastic
  intracortical
  intraosseous
  juxtacortical
  osteoblastic
  parosteal
  periosteal
  telangiectatic
osteosclerosis
osteosis
osteospongioma
osteothrombosis
OsteoView desktop hand x-ray system
ostia (pl. of ostium)
ostial lesion
ostial stenosis
ostium (pl. ostia)
  aortic
  artery
  atrioventricular
  coronary
  coronary sinus
ostium abdominale tubae uterinae
  (abdominal orifice of uterine tube)
ostium primum defect
ostium secundum defect
Otto pelvis dislocation
out-of-phase GRE images
outcome, clinical
outcomes (radiology outcomes data)
outer table
Outerbridge ridge

Outerbridge scale (articular damage)
outflow
  hypoplastic subpulmonic
  maximum venous (MVO)
  subpulmonic
outflow anastomosis
outflow of ventricle
outflow tract
outgrowth, osseous patellar
outlet
  pelvic
  pyloric
  thoracic
  ventricular
  widened thoracic
outlet chamber, rudimentary
outlet view
outpocketings of mucosa
outpouching
output
  adequate cardiac
  augmented cardiac
  cardiac (CO)
  Dow method for cardiac
  Fick method for cardiac
  Gorlin method for cardiac
  Hetzel forward triangle method
    for cardiac
  inadequate cardiac
  low cardiac
  pulmonic
  reduced systemic cardiac
  stroke
  systemic
  thermodilution cardiac
  ventricular
output amplitude
output point
OV (ovarian)
Ovadia-Beals classification of tibial
  plafond fracture

P, p

P (posterior)
PA (posteroanterior or posterior-anterior)
PA and lateral films
PA and lateral views
PA (pulmonary artery)
Paas disease
PABP (pulmonary artery balloon pump)
pacchionian
pacemaker
pace mapping
Pace Plus System scanner
pack-a-day smoking history
packing
  cubic
  extraction, and calculation technique
  periodic
pack-year smoking history
pack-years of cigarette smoking
PACS (picture archive and communication system)
PACS, PBT Technologies
PACSRO (picture archiving and communications systems in radiation oncology)

pad
  abdominal
  antimesenteric fat
  fat
  fibrocartilaginous
  padding
  UltraEase ultrasound
PADP-PAWP (pulmonary artery diastolic and wedge pressure) gradient
pad sign of aortic insufficiency
PAEDP (pulmonary artery end-diastolic pressure)
Paget abscess
Paget-associated osteogenic sarcoma
Paget disease, "fluffy rarefaction" of
pagetoid bone
Paget osteitis deformans
Paget-Schroetter venous thrombosis of axillary vein
Paget-von Schroetter syndrome
Pais fracture
PALA enhancement
palatal
palate
  bony
  Byzantine arch

panoramic CT scan
panoramic image
panoramic radiography
Panorex x-ray
pansystolic mitral regurgitation
pantalar fusion
pantaloon embolus
pantaloon hernia
Pantopaque contrast medium
Pantopaque myelography
PAP (pulmonary artery pressure)
papilla
   acoustic
   bile
   duodenal
   major duodenal
   minor duodenal
   renal
   Santorini
   urethral
   Vater
papillary epithelial neoplasm
papillary fibroelastoma
papilloma
   choroid plexus
   cockscomb
   Hopmann
   ventricular tumor
PAPVR (partial anomalous pulmonary
  venous return)
para-aortic region
para-articular bone remodeling
para-articular calcification
parabola, metatarsal
paracardiac mass
paracardiac-type total anomalous
  venous return
paracentral lobule
paracervical region
parachute deformity of mitral valve
paracicatricial emphysema
paracoccidioidomycosis

paracolic gutter
paracorporeal
paracostal
paradoxical embolus
paradoxical hyperconcentration of
  contrast medium
paradoxical motion
paradoxical suppression
paraesophageal hernia
paraesophagogastric devascularization
parafascicular nucleus
paraganglioma
paragangliomatosis
parahilar (also perihilar)
parallel analog mapping
parallel and spiral flow patterns
parallel hole image
parallel hole medium sensitivity
  collimator
parallel opposed ports
parallel opposed unmodified ports
parallel-tagged MR images and
  field-fitting analysis
parallel tag planes
Parallel virtual machine
paralysis of diaphragm
paralytic chest
paralytic ileus
paramagnetic artifact
paramagnetic contrast media
paramagnetic Cr-labeled red blood
  cells
paramagnetic relaxation
paramagnetic shift
paramagnetic substances
paramagnetism
paramalleolar arteries
paramedian position
paramedian sagittal plane
paramediastinal glands
parameningeal

parameter
  clinical
  hematologic
  kinetic perfusion
  nuclear
  optimization
  parameters
  physiologic
  scan
  sonographic
  thermal treatment
  ventricular function
paranasal sinus
paraneoplastic cerebellar degeneration
paraneoplastic hypercalcemia
paraneoplastic process
parapatellar plica
parapelvic (also peripelvic)
parapelvic gutter
parapharyngeal abscess
parapharyngeal space
paraprosthetic-enteric fistula
paraprosthetic leakage
pararenal abscess
pararenal aortic aneurysm
pararenal aortic atherosclerosis
parasagittal head region
parasagittal intracranial mass
parasagittal meningioma
parasagittal region
parasellar mass
paraseptal emphysema
paraseptal position
paraspinal abnormality
paraspinal muscles
paraspinal musculature
paraspinal pleural stripe
paraspinal soft tissue mass
paraspinal soft tissue shadowing
paraspinous musculature
parasternal bulge
parasternal long-axis view

parasternal lymph nodes
parasternal motion
parasternal short-axis view
parasternal view of heart
parasternal window
parasympathetic nervous system
paratracheal soft tissues
paratracheal stripe
paratrooper fracture
paravalvar leak
paravalvular
paravertebral gutter
paravertebral musculature
paravertebral nerve plexus
paravertebral region
paravertebral venous plexus
parchment heart syndrome
parchment right ventricle
parenchyma
  cerebral
  liver
  lung
  pulmonary
  spinal cord
parenchymal collaterals
parenchymal consolidation
parenchymal echogenicity
parenchymal fibrous band
parenchymal infarct
parenchymal infiltrates, pulmonary
parenchymal lung disease
parenchymal neurocutaneous
  melanosis
parenchymal tracer accumulation
parenchymal transit
parenchymatous atrophy
parenchymatous cerebellar
  degeneration
parenchymatous hemorrhage
parenchymatous neurosyphilis
parenchymatous phase
parent vein

paresis, hemilingual
parietal band
parietal bone
parietal branches
  paired
  unpaired
parietal cephalohematoma
parietal cortex lesion
parietal cortex, post-rolandic
parietal extension of infundibular
  septum
parietal gyrus
parietal layer
parietal lobe lesion
parietal lobe sign
parietal pericardial calcification
parietal pericardium
parietal pleura
parieto-occipital lesion
parieto-occipital sulcus
parietotemporal area
Paris system
Park Medical Systems scanner
Parks bidirectional Doppler flowmeter
Parks ileal reservoir
Parona space
parosteal chondrosarcoma
parosteal osteogenic sarcoma
parosteal osteosarcoma
parotid gland
parotid pleomorphic adenoma
paroxysmal crisis, hypertensive
parrot-beak meniscus tears
parry fracture
pars interarticularis
Parsons, third intercondylar
  tubercle of
partial anomalous pulmonary venous
  return (PAPVR)
partial-brain radiation therapy
partial collapse of lung
partial dislocation

partial dislodgement
partial K-space sampling
partial liquid ventilation with
  perflubron
partial obliteration of a lateral
  ventricle (on scan)
partial ossicular replacement
  prosthesis (PORP)
partial pericardial absence
partial saturation and spin-echo pulse
  sequence
partial saturation technique
partial-thickness tear
partial volume averaging
partial volume effect, artifact due to
particle (pl. particles)
  beta
  bone
  calcium/oxyanion-containing
  charged
  Ivalon
particle beam
particle debris
particle identification
particle masks
particle size determination
particulate debris
particulates, magnetic
partition
  atrial
  gastric
partition coefficient
parts, fetal small
PAS (pulmonary artery systolic)
  pressure
pascals of force (SI units)
passage of blind catheter
passages, narrowing of bronchiolar
passive clot
passive filling
passively congested lung tissue
passively shimmed superconducting
  magnet

passive pneumonia
passive track detector
passive vascular congestion
passive venous distention
PASTA (polarity-altered spectral-
    selective acquisition) imaging
patch crinkling
patch electrodes placed outside the
    pericardium
patch
    epidural blood
    kinking of
    pericardial
    periosteal
    Peyer
    transannular
    vein
patchy air-space consolidations
patchy alveolar opacities
patchy atelectasis
patchy atrophy of renal cortex
patchy consolidation
patchy distribution of the tracer
patchy infiltrate
patchy migratory infiltrates
patchy zones
patella
    apex of head of
    bipartite
    dislocated
    floating
    high-riding
    lower pole of
    skyline view of
    subluxing
    undersurface of
patella alta (high-riding)
patella baja
patellar button
patellar chondromalacia
patellar contour
patellar dislocation

patellar edge
patellar entrapment
patellar fat pad
patellar fossa
patellar groove
patellar subluxation
patellar tendinosis
patellofemoral articular cartilage
patellofemoral joint space
patellofemoral region
patency
    arterial
    coronary artery
    coronary bypass graft
    ductus arteriosus
    graft
    long-term
    short-term
    vein
patency and valvular reflux of deep
    veins
patency
patency of vein graft
patency of vessel
patency rate
patent bifurcation
patent ductus arteriosus (PDA)
patent foramen ovale
patent trifurcation
patent, widely
Paterson-Parker rules
Pathfinder catheter
pathognomonic sign
pathologic confirmation
pathologic correlation
pathologic diagnosis
pathologic dislocation
pathologic fracture
pathologic reflux
pathology, radiographic
pathophysiologic changes in airways
    obstruction

pathophysiology
pathway
   neural
   optic
   retrovestibular neural
patient motion artifact
pattern
   abdominal wall venous
   A fib (atrial fibrillation)
   air-space filling
   alveolar
   AM (associative memory)
   anhaustral colonic gas
   arterial deficiency
   bigeminal
   blood flow
   bowel
   bowel gas
   branching
   butterfly
   cobblestone
   cobweb
   contractile
   corduroy cloth (on myelogram)
   dP/dt upstroke
   ductal
   early repolarization
   echo
   electron and x-ray diffraction
   enhancement
   extended
   fibrotic cavitating
   filigree
   fine reticular
   fold
   gas
   gastric mucosal
   haustral
   helical
   hemodynamic
   heterogeneous perfusion
   hierarchical scanning

pattern *(cont.)*
   hole
   homogeneous
   honeycomb
   hourglass
   infiltration
   interstitial
   juvenile T wave
   Laue
   left ventricular contraction
   left ventricular strain
   lobular
   M (on right atrial waveform)
   miliary
   macronodular
   marrow edema
   micronodular
   mosaic
   mosaic attenuation
   mosaic duodenal mucosal
   moth-eaten
   movement
   MR enhancement
   M-shaped mitral valve
   mucosal
   nonspecific gas
   parallel
   pin
   P pulmonale
   pseudoinfarct
   pulmonary flow
   pulmonary vascular
   recurrence
   rheologic
   right ventricular strain
   rugal
   sigmoid hair (on spine)
   signet ring
   small bowel mucosal
   SMPTE test
   speckled
   spectral

pattern *(cont.)*
  spiral flow
  star
  stellate
  strain
  sulcal
  surface convexity
  task-rest
  temporal sawtooth
  thermal convection
  tree-in-bud (TIB)
  trigeminal
  ventricular contraction
  vesicular
patulous hiatus
pauciarticular
paucity of bowel gas
pause
  asystolic
  compensatory
  noncompensatory
  pauses
  postextrasystolic
  sinus
Pauwel angle of femoral neck
  fracture
Pauwel fracture classification
Pawlik trigone
PAWP (pulmonary artery wedge
  pressure)
Payr disease
Payr sign
Pb (lead)
Pb-212-labeled monoclonal antibody
  imaging agent
PBF (pulmonary blood flow)
PBPI (penile-brachial pressure index)
  to assess cardiac disease
PBT Technologies PACS
PBVI (pulmonary blood volume
  index)
PC (phase contrast) imaging

PC (posterior commissure)
PCA (posterior cerebral artery)
PCA (posterior communicating artery)
PCL (posterior cruciate ligament)
PCoA (posterior communicating
  artery)
PCP (pulmonary capillary pressure)
PCS (proximal coronary sinus)
PCVD (pulmonary collagen vascular
  disease)
PCWP (pulmonary capillary wedge
  pressure)
Pd (palladium)
PDA (patent ductus arteriosus)
PDA (posterior descending artery)
PDI (power Doppler imaging)
PDR (pulsed brachytherapy)
PE (pericardial effusion)
PE (pulmonary embolism)
peak
  airway pressure
  diffraction
  juxtaphrenic
  main glow
  pressure
  single
peak airway pressure
peak count density
peak dP/dt
peak early diastolic filling velocities
peak enhancement
peak expiratory flow (PEF)
peak expiratory flow rate (PEFR)
peak filling rate (PFR)
peak fitting
peak flow
peak flow variability
peak flow velocity
peak identification
peak-inflation pressures
peak late diastolic filling velocities
peak parenchymal activity

peak profile
peak regurgitant flow velocity
peak regurgitant wave pressure
peak systolic and diastolic ICA/CCA
   ratios
peak systolic pressure
peak systolic velocity (cm/sec)
peak tidal expiratory flow
peak-to-peak pressure gradient
peak velocity of blood flow on
   Doppler echocardiogram
pectoral
pectoralis major muscle
pectoralis major syndrome
pectoralis minor muscle
pectus carinatum
pectus excavatum deformity
pedal artery opacification
pediatric biplane TEE (transesophageal
   echocardiography) probe
pediatric neuroradiology
pedicle
   IMA (internal mammary artery)
   musculofascial
   phrenic
   spinal
   vascular
pedicle bone grafts
pedicle erosion
pedicle of vertebra
pedicle sclerosis
peduncle
   cerebellar
   cerebral
   inferior cerebellar
peduncular segment of superior cerebellar artery
pedunculated myxoma
pedunculated polyp
pedunculated subserous myoma
pedunculated thrombus
pedunculated uterine myoma

pedunculated vesical tumor
pedunculation
PEG (pneumoencephalogram)
Pel-Ebstein disease
Pellegrini-Stieda disease
pellet
   alanine-silicone
   radiopaque
pellet artifact (shotgun pellets)
pellucidum
pelvic abscess
pelvicaliceal changes
pelvicaliceal distention
pelvic bone
pelvic brim
pelvic collateral vessel
pelvic diameter
pelvic floor
pelvic fracture frame
pelvic girdle
pelvic inlet
pelvic node
pelvic notching
pelvic obliquity
pelvic outlet
pelvic rim fracture
pelvic ring fracture
pelvic tilt, bent knee
pelvic traction
pelvic ultrasound
pelvic ultrasound CT scan
pelvic view
pelviectasis
pelvimetry, Mengert index in
pelvis
   android
   anthropoid
   assimilation
   beaked
   bony
   brachypellic
   contracted

pelvis *(cont.)*
  cordate
  cordiform
  Deventer
  dolichopellic
  dwarf
  false
  female
  flat
  frozen
  funnel-shaped
  greater
  gynecoid
  hardened
  heart-shaped
  inverted
  juvenile
  Kilian
  kyphoscoliotic
  kyphotic
  lesser
  longitudinal oval
  lordotic
  male
  masculine
  mesatipellic
  Nägele
  osteomalacic
  Otto
  platypelloid
  portable film of
  Prague
  pseudo-osteomalacic
  rachitic
  reniform
  renal
  Rokitansky
  scoliotic
  small
  spider
  spondylolisthetic
  transverse oval

pelvis *(cont.)*
  true
  ureteral
  ureteric
pelviureteral junction
pelvocaliceal effacement
pencil beam approach
pencil-beam navigator echos
penciling of ribs
Pendred syndrome
pendulous urethra
pendulum movement
penetrating aortic ulceration
penetrating atherosclerotic ulceration
penetrating trauma
penetrating injury
penetrating ulceration
penile urethra
penis
  bulb of
  bulbospongiosus muscle of
  clubbed
  concealed
  corpora cavernosa
  corpus spongiosum
  crura of
  deep fascia of
  dorsal artery of
  dorsal nerve of
  dorsum of
  double
  glans
  ischiospongiosus muscle of
  root of
  suspensory ligament of
  webbed
penoscrotal
PenRad mammography clinical reporting system
Penrose drain
Pentagastrin
pentavalent DMSA

Pentax EUP-EC124 ultrasound
  gastroscope
Pentax-Hitachi FG32UA endosonographic system
pentetreotide indium-111 (^{111}In)
penumbra, dosimetric
penumbra zone
PEP (pre-ejection period)
PE Plus II balloon dilatation catheter
peppermint oil (used with barium
  enema)
peptic ulcer
  acute
  chronic
peptic ulcer disease (PUD)
peptide imaging agent
percentage signal intensity loss (PSIL)
Perception scanner
perceptual linearization
Perchloracap contrast medium
perchlorate washout test
Percor DL balloon catheter
Percor DL-II (dual-lumen) intra-aortic
  balloon catheter
Percor-Stat-DL catheter
percutaneous antegrade biliary
  drainage
percutaneous aortic balloon
  valvuloplasty
percutaneous automated diskectomy
  under fluoroscopy
percutaneous endoluminal placement
  of stent-graft
percutaneous fibrin glue
percutaneous gastrostomy, radiologic
percutaneous insertion via femoral
  vein
percutaneous interventional radiology
percutaneous intracoronary angioscopy
percutaneously cannulated
percutaneous pericardioscopy
percutaneous radiofrequency ablation

percutaneous retrograde transfemoral
  technique
percutaneous transcatheter ductal
  closure (PTDC)
percutaneous transhepatic biliary
  drainage with contrast monitoring
percutaneous transhepatic cholangiogram (PTHC)
percutaneous transhepatic liver biopsy
percutaneous transhepatic portography
  with hemodynamic evaluation
percutaneous transluminal angioplasty
  (PTA)
percutaneous transluminal coronary
  angioplasty (PTCA)
percutaneous transluminal renal
  angioplasty (PTRA)
percutaneous transperineal seed
  implantation
percutaneous transvenous embolization
perflubron contrast
perfluorocarbon F-19 (^{19}F) imaging
  agent
perfluoroctylbromide (PFOB) imaging
  agent
perfluoro-1H,-1H-neopentyl imaging
  agent
perforated diverticulum
perforating aneurysm
perforating arteries
perforating fracture
perforation
  bladder
  cardiac
  transseptal
  ulcer
perforator vessel
perfusate
perfuse
perfusion
  adequate coronary
  antegrade

perfusion *(cont.)*
  coronary
  diminished systemic
  homogeneous
  hypothermic
  intraperitoneal hyperthermic
  (IPHP)
  luxury
  misery
  mosaic
  myocardial
  peripheral
  poor
  pulsatile
  quantitative cardiac
  regional (by mixed venous blood)
  regional cerebral
  renal
  retrograde cardiac
  tissue
perfusion abnormality
perfusion agent
perfusion and ventilation lung scan
perfusion catheter
perfusion defect
perfusion deficit
perfusion gradient
perfusion lung scan
perfusion magnetic resonance imaging
perfusion-metabolism mismatch
perfusion pressure
perfusion scan
perfusion-weighted MRI
perialveolar fibrosis
periampullary diverticulum
periampullary duodenal tumor
periaortic area
periaortic fibrosis
periapical granuloma
periapical lesion
periappendiceal abscess
periaqueductal gray matter

periaqueductal region
periarticular calcification
periarticular fracture
periarticular heterotopic ossification
  (PHO)
peribronchial alveolar spaces
peribronchial connective tissue
peribronchial cuffing
peribronchial distribution
peribronchial fibrosis
peribronchial infiltrate
peribronchial lymph nodes
peribronchial markings
peribronchial thickening
peribronchiolar hemorrhage
pericallosal artery
pericardiacophrenic vein
pericardial absence
  congenital
  partial
pericardial cavity
pericardial constriction, occult
pericardial cyst
pericardial diaphragmatic adhesions
pericardial effusion
pericardial fat pad
pericardial fluid
pericardial fold
pericardial hematoma
pericardial infusion
pericardial reflection
pericardial sac
pericardial sinus
pericardial space
pericardiocentesis, ultrasonic guidance
  for
pericardium
  adherent
  autologous
  bread-and-butter
  calcified
  congenitally absent

pericardium *(cont.)*
   diaphragmatic
   fibrous
   parietal
   serous
   shaggy
   soldier's patches of
   veins of
   visceral
pericardium calcareous deposits
pericardium fibrosum
pericatheter thrombus (pl. thrombi)
pericecal abscess
pericholecystic edema
pericholecystic fluid
pericicatricial emphysema
pericolonic fat
pericystic edema
periductal calcification
periductal fibrosis
peridural fibrosis
perigastric deformity
perigraft hematoma
perihilar (also parahilar)
perihilar density
perihilar edema
perihilar fat
perihilar fibrosis
perihilar infiltrate
perihilar markings
perihilar region
peri-ileal
peri-infarction ischemia
peri-infarctional defect
perilesional bone
perilunate carpal dislocation
perilunate fracture dislocation (PLFD)
perimalleolar pain
perimedullary
perimembranous ventricular septal
   defect
perimuscular plexus

perimylolysis
perinatal respiratory distress syndrome
perineal descent
perineogram
perineoplastic edema
perinephric abscess
perinephric fat
perinephric space
perineural invasion
perineural tumor
perineural fibroblastoma tumor
period
   diastolic filling
   noninteger
   raster
   rapid filling (RFP)
   reduced ventricular filling
periodic packing
periodontal ligament
periorbital Doppler study
periosteal bone formation
periosteal creep
periosteal fibroma
periosteal new bone formation
periosteal osteosarcoma
periosteal reaction
periosteal sarcoma
peripancreatic arteries
peripancreatic fluid collection
peripelvic (also parapelvic)
peripelvic collateral vessel
peripheral air-space disease
peripheral arterial cannula
peripheral blood flow
peripheral circulatory vasoconstriction
peripheral consolidation
peripheral cutaneous vasoconstriction
peripheral embolus
peripheral fracture
peripheral gating technique
peripheral infiltrate

peripheral laser angioplasty (PLA)
peripheral lesion
peripheral loading
peripheral lung disease
peripherally inserted central catheter
    (PICC)
peripheral nerve
peripheral nodule
peripheral ossification
peripheral parenchymal atelectasis
peripheral pulmonary artery stenosis
peripheral pulmonic stenosis
peripheral quantitative computed
    tomography technology (pQCT)
peripheral resistance
peripheral small airways study
peripheral vascular disease,
    arteriosclerotic
peripheral vascular resistance,
    decreased
peripheral veins, absent
peripheral vessels
peripheral washout sign
periphery, echogenic
periportal area
periportal tracking of blood
periprosthetic bone resorption
periprosthetic leak (leakage)
periradicular nerve
periradicular sheath
perirectal abscess
perirenal fat
perirenal hematoma
perirenal hemorrhage
perirenal mass
perirenal septum
perirenal space
perirolandic cortex
perisigmoid colon
perisinusoidal space
peristalsing bowel

peristalsis
    absent
    accelerated
    decreased
    increased
    reversed
    visible
peristaltic contraction
peristaltic rush
peristaltic wave
peristriate cortex
peritoneal cavity
    greater sac of
    lesser sac of
peritoneal catheter
peritoneal enhancement
peritoneal effusion
peritoneal mouse
peritoneal-venous shunt patency test
peritoneogram
peritoneography, CT
peritoneovenous shunt (PVS)
peritoneum
    parietal
    pelvic
    visceral
periureteral fibrosis
perivalvular dehiscence
perivalvular disruption
perivalvular leak
perivascular canal
perivascular distribution
perivascular edema
perivascular fibrosis
perivascular plane
perivascular space of Virchow-Robin
periventricular density
periventricular gray (PVG) matter
periventricular halo
periventricular leukomalacia (PVL)
periventricular white matter
perivenular nodularity

perivesical
permanent brachytherapy
permeability
   capillary
   membrane
   tumor capillary
permeability-type pulmonary edema
permeative lesion
peroneal area
peroneal artery
peroneal muscles
peroneal obliterative thrombus
peroneal-tibial trunk
peroneal vein
peroneus tertius
Persantine thallium stress test
persistent common atrioventricular
   canal
persistent fetal circulation
persistent truncus arteriosus
perspective volume rendering (PVR)
Pertechnegas
pertechnetate sodium (technetium)
Perthes-Bankart lesion
Perthes disease
Perthes epiphysis
pertrochanteric fracture
pertubation, radiation dose
perusal
pervenous catheter
pes abductus
pes adductus
pes anserinus
pes arcuatus
pes calcaneocavus
pes calcaneovalgus
pes calcaneus
pes cavovalgus
pes cavovarus
pes cavus
pes contortus
pes equinovalgus

pes equinovarus
pes equinus
pes excavatus
pes malleus valgus
pes planovalgus
pes plantigrade planus
pes planus
pes pronation
pes pronatus
pes supinatus
pes valgus
pes varus
pessary
PET (positron emission tomography)
   PET balloon, USCI
   PET balloon with window and
      extended collection chamber
   PET metabolic imaging
   PET myocardial fatty acid imaging
   PET perfusion imaging
   PET radioligands
   PET radiopharmaceuticals
   PET target material
petal-fugal flow on angiography
Petit disease
petroclinoid ligament
petroclival region
petromastoid
petro-occipital synchondrosis
petrosal bone
petrosal nerve
petrosal sinus
petrosphenoid
petrosquamosal
petrous bone
petrous carotid canal stenosis
petrous pyramid
petrous ridge
petrous segment of carotid artery
Peutz-Jeghers gastrointestinal
   polyposis
Peyer patch

Pezzer catheter
PF-PACS system
Pfeiffer-Comberg method
Pfeiffer syndrome
PFFD (proximal focal femoral
    deficiency)
PFOB imaging agent
P53-mediated radioresistance
PFR (peak filling rate)
PFWT (pain-free walking time) on
    treadmill
PGK (Panos G. Koutrouvelis, M.D.)
    stereotactic device
phagedenic ulcer
phagocytosis, MR imaging of
phakomatoses
phalangeal bones
phalangeal glenoidal ligament of hand
phalangeal herniation
phalanx (pl. phalanges)
    base of
    waist of
Phalen position
pharmacologic intervention
pharmacologic stress dual-isotope
    myocardial perfusion SPECT
pharmacologic stress echocardiography
pharmacoradiologic disimpaction of
    esophageal foreign body
pharyngeal area
pharyngoesophageal diverticulum
pharyngoesophageal function
pharynx
    laryngeal part of
    nasal part of
    oral part of
phase (see also *period*)
    corticomedullary (CP)
    delayed
    diastolic depolarization
    equilibrium
    expiratory

phase *(cont.)*
    hepatic arterial (HAP)
    inspiratory
    late
    NCP (noncontrast)
    NP (nephrographic)
    parenchymatous
    plateau (in cardiac action
        potentials)
    portal venous (PVP)
    prolonged expiratory
    prolonged inspiratory
    PVP (portal venous)
    rapid filling
    vascular
    ventilation
    wash-in
    washout
phase analysis
phase angle
phase cycling
phase-contrast angiography
phase-contrast imaging
phased-array surface coil
phased array, symmetrical
phase delay
phase difference
phase-encoded motion artifact
phase-encode pulse
phase encode time reduced acquisition
    sequence
phase identification
phase image (imaging)
phase relation
phase sensitive detector
phase shift
phase shifting interferometry
phase-shift velocity mapping
phase-unwrapping method
phase-velocity image
phasic contractions
phenomenological effective surface
    potential

phenomenon (pl. phenomena)
   A
   aliasing
   anniversary
   Aschner
   Ashman
   Austin Flint
   baked brain
   Bancaud
   Bell
   booster
   Bowditch staircase
   combined-flexion
   coronary steal
   crus
   Cushing
   dip
   dip and plateau
   Doppler
   embolic
   extinction
   flare
   flip-flop
   freezing
   Friedreich
   Gaertner (Gärtner)
   Gallavardin
   gap conduction
   Gibbs
   Goldblatt
   Gordon knee
   Gowers
   Hering
   Jod-Basedow
   Kasabach-Merritt
   Katz-Wachtle
   Kernohan notch
   kindling
   Litten diaphragm
   Marin-Amat
   no-reflow
   nonspecific

phenomenon *(cont.)*
   on-off
   Piltz-Westphal
   Robin Hood (steal syndrome)
   R-on-T
   Schellong-Strisower
   Schiff-Sherrington
   Schramm
   staircase
   steal
   steal syndrome
   stone heart
   treppe
   Uhthoff
   unilateral Raynaud
   V
   vacuum joint
   vertebral steal
   Wenckebach
   zone
phentetiothalein contrast medium
pheochromocytoma
Philips CT scanner
Philips DVI 1 system
Philips Gyroscan ACS scanner
Philips Gyroscan NT; NT5; NT15
   scanner
Philips Gyroscan S5 scanner
Philips Gyroscan T5 scanner
Philips linear accelerator (LINAC)
Philips 1.5T NT MR scanner
Philips scanner
Philips Tomoscan 350 CT scanner
Philips Tomoscan SR 6000 CT scanner
Philips ultrasound machine
phlebogram (phlebography), MR
   ascending
   ascending contrast
   direct puncture
   impedance
phlebolith

phleborheography (PRG)
phlebosclerosis
phlebostasis
phlebostenosis
phlebothrombosis
phlegmon
   Holz
   pancreatic
   periurethral
phlegmonous
phoenix abscess
phosphoric acid imaging agent
phosphorus metabolites
phosphorus nuclear magnetic
   resonance spectroscopy (P-MRS)
phosphorus-32 intracavitary irradiation
phosphorus-32 sodium phosphate
photo-plotter film
photoacoustic ultrasonography
photocell plethysmography
photodeficient region
photodetectors, CCD
photodiode
photodisruption
photoelasticity
photographic technique
   Debye-Scherrer
   Laue
photography, CT bone window
photolabel, long wavelength
photon attenuation measurement
photon deficiency
photon deficient lesion
photon densitometry
photon interaction depth
photon-neutron mixed-beam
   radiotherapy
photon, soft
photon therapy beam line
photonic medicine
photopeak
photopenia

photopenic area on film or scan
photopenic defect
photopenic region
photoplethysmographic digit
photoplethysmographic monitoring
photoplethysmography (PPG)
photoreceptor fractional velocity error
photoreceptor motion
photostimulable luminescence intensity
photostimulable phosphor dental
   radiography (PSP)
phrenic artery
phrenic pedicle
phrenoesophageal ligament
phrenogastric gastric
phrenovertebral junction
phrygian cap deformity
phthinoid chest
phthisis, aneurysmal
PHTN (pulmonary hypertension)
Phylax implantable cardioverter-
   defibrillator (Biotronik)
phyllodes tumor
physeal bar
physeal cartilage
physeal closure
physeal damage
physeal distraction
physeal fracture
physeal injury
physeal plate fracture
physicochemical speciation
physiologic flow
physiologic regurgitation
physiologic shunt flow
physis (pl. physes)
   distal tibial
   fibular
   fused
   medial
   unfused
phytobezoar

PI (pulmonic insufficiency)
pia arachnoid
pia mater
pial vessels
PIBC (percutaneous intra-aortic balloon counterpulsation)
pica artifact
PICA (posterior inferior communicating artery)
Pick body
Pick bundle
Pick disease
Picker camera
Picker CT scanner
Picker Magnascanner
Picker MR scanner
Picker PQ 5000 helical CT scanner
Picker PQ-2000 spiral CT scanner
Picker SPECT attenuation correction
Picket Fence fiducial localization stereotactic system
picture archive and communication system (PACs) for imaging
picture archiving and communications systems in radiation oncology (PACSRO)
picture element (pixel)
picture frame pattern of vertebral bodies
PIE (pulmonary interstitial emphysema)
piece, chin-occiput
Piedmont fracture
pigeon-breeder's lung
pigeon chest
pigeon-fancier's lung
Pigg-O-Stat x-ray chair for child
piggybacking
pigtail catheter
Pillar view
pillion fracture
pillow fracture

pilonidal cyst
pilonidal sinus
pin pattern
PIN (posterior interosseous nerve) entrapment
pinchcock mechanism at esophago-gastric junction
pinched nerve
pincushion distortion, radiographic
pineal apoplexy
pineal body, calcified
pineal calcification displaced from midline
pineal gland, calcified
pineal gland tumor
pinealoma tumor
pineal region
pineoblastoma
pineocytoma
ping-pong fracture
pinhole, bone
pinhole collimator
pinhole image
Pinnacle 3 radiation therapy planning system
PION (posterior interosseous nerve)
PIP (proximal interphalangeal)
    PIP articulation
    PIP joint
pipestem arteries
pipe-stemming of ankle-brachial index
PIPIDA (P-isopropylacetanilide-iminodiacetic acid)
    ^{99m}TcPIPIDA hepatobiliary scan
PIPJ (proximal interphalangeal joint)
Pipkin classification of femoral fracture
Pirie bone
piriform muscle
pisiform bone of wrist
pisotriquetral joint
pistoning

piston sign
pit
  anal
  articular
  auditory
  central
  colonic
  costal
  cutaneous
  gastric
  postanal
pitch
  scan
  spiral CT
pitch ratio
pituitary fossa
pituitary gland
pituitary microadenoma
pituitary stalk distortion (PSD)
pituitary tumor
pivoting table
pixel (picture element)
  edge-region
  normal-region
pixel-block, 8 x 8
pixel noise
pixel-oriented algorithms
Pixsys FlashPoint camera
placement
  annular
  catheter
  intracoronary stent
  intrapericardial patch lead
  percutaneous endoluminal
  radiotherapy field
  shent
  shim
  subannular
  subject
placement of radiation therapy fields,
  ultrasonic guidance for

placenta
  abnormal adherence of
  accessory
  adherent
  annular
  battledore
  bilobate
  chorioallantoic
  chorioamniotic
  cirsoid
  deciduate
  Duncan
  fetal
  first-trimester
  fundal
  horseshoe
  incarcerated
  kidney-shaped
  marginal
  maternal
  nondeciduate
  panduriform
  retained
  Schultze
  second-trimester
  third-trimester
  velamentous
  villous
placenta previa
  central
  complete
  incomplete
  lateral
  marginal
  partial
  total
placental abruption (abruptio placentae)
placental localization
placental polyp
placental souffle
placentography

plane of cleavage of tumor
planigram
planigraphy
planimeter
planimetry
planogram
planography
planovalgus foot deformity
plantar aponeurosis
plantar axial view
plantar calcaneal spur
plantar compartment
plantar flexion-inversion deformity
plantar hyperplasia
plantar spur
plantar vault
plantaris muscle
plantaris rupture
plantarward
plaque (also plaquing)
   arterial
   arteriosclerotic
   atheromatous
   atherosclerotic
   calcific
   calcified
   concentric atherosclerotic
   coral reef
   disrupted
   eccentric
   eccentric atherosclerotic
   echogenic
   echolucent
   endocardial
   fatty
   fibrofatty
   fibrotic
   fibrous
   fissured atheromatous
   gastrointestinal
   Hollenhorst

plaque *(cont.)*
   Hutchinson
   iliac
   infiltrating
   intraluminal
   Lichtheim
   lipid-laden
   luminal
   multiple sclerosis (MS)
   neuritic senile
   noncompliant
   obstructive
   pleural
   pulverized
   Randall
   residual
   sclerotic
   senile
   sessile
   stenotic
   talc
   ulcerated
   uncalcified
plaque cleaving
plaque compression
plaque-containing artery
plaque constituents
plaque erosion
plaque fracture (or fracturing)
plaquelike linear defect
plaque regression
plaque remodeling
plaque rupture
plaque splitting
plaque tearing
plaque vaporization
plaquing (see *plaque*)
plasma radioiron disappearance rate
plasma radioiron turnover rate
plasma volume
plastic clot

plate
    acetabular reconstruction
    alar
    anal
    auditory
    axial
    basal
    bone
    bone flap fixation
    bony
    budding
    cap-and-anchor
    cardiogenic
    cartilaginous growth
    chorionic
    clinoid
    cloacal
    cloverleaf
    coaptation
    compression
    condylar
    connecting
    cortical
    cranial bone fixation
    cribriform
    dorsal
    dual
    dynamic compression (DCP)
    end
    epiphyseal cartilage
    ethmovomerine
    femoral
    fibrocartilaginous
    flat
    flexor palmar
    foot
    frontal
    fusion
    growth
    hilar
    interfragmentary
    intertrochanteric

plate *(cont.)*
    localization-compression grid
    meningioma of cribriform
    microfixation
    nail
    neutralization
    occipitocervical
    orbital
    orthotic
    overlay
    palmar
    pedicle
    planar
    plantar
    pterygoid
    skull
    stabilization
    stainless steel
    stem base
    subchondral bone
    supracondylar
    tarsal
    tectal
    tendon
    3-D or 3D (three-dimensional)
    titanium
    vertebral body
    volar
plate and screw system, MRI-compat-
    ible
plateau
    multiple sclerosis
    tibial
plateau fracture
platelet-activating factor inhibitor
platelet-rich thrombus
platelet survival study
platelike atelectasis
platform, Cemax PACS
platinum coil
platybasia
platycephaly

platypellic pelvis
platypelloid pelvis
platypodia
platyspondylosis
platyspondyly
PLC (posterolateral corner) of knee
pleating of ligamentum flavum
pleating of small bowel
pleomorphic xanthoastrocytoma
pleomorphism, nuclear
plesiography (brachytherapy)
plethora of findings
plethoric
plethysmogram
plethysmography
  air
  body box
  digital
  Doppler ultrasonic velocity
    detector segmental
  exercise strain gauge venous
  impedance (IPG)
  Medsonic
  photocell
  strain-gauge
  venous
pleura (pl. pleurae)
  cervical
  congested
  costal
  costodiaphragmatic recess of
  diaphragmatic
  edematous
  mediastinal
  parietal
  pericardiac
  pulmonary
  silicotic visceral
  visceral
  wrinkled
pleural adhesions, fibrous
pleural apical hematoma cap

pleural-based area of increased
  opacity
pleural cap
pleural cavity
pleural cupula (pl. cupulae)
pleural effusion
  ipsilateral
  liquid
  loculated
pleural empyema
pleural exudate
pleural fibrosis, asbestos-induced
pleural fistula
pleural flap
pleural fluid
pleural implants, malignant
pleural line
pleural margins
pleural plaque
pleural reflection
  costal
  mediastinodiaphragmatic
  sternal
  vertebral
pleural rind
pleural sac
pleural space
pleural thickening
pleurisy
  acute
  blocked
  chronic
  circumscribed
  costal
  diaphragmatic
  diffuse
  double
  dry
  encysted
  exudative
  fibrinous
  hemorrhagic

pleurisy *(cont.)*
  ichorous
  indurative
  interlobular
  latent
  mediastinal
  metapneumonic
  plastic
  primary
  proliferating
  pulmonary
  pulsating
  purulent
  sacculated
  secondary
  serofibrous
  serous
  single
  suppurative
  typhoid
  visceral
pleurocutaneous fistula
pleuroparenchymal plaque
pleuroperitoneal canal
pleuropulmonary adhesion
plexiform
plexus
  abdominal aortic
  anterior coronary
  anterior pulmonary
  aortic
  Auerbach mesenteric
  autonomic
  axillary
  basilar
  Batson
  biliary
  brachial
  calcification of choroid
  cardiac
  carotid
  cavernous

plexus *(cont.)*
  celiac
  cervical
  choroid
  ciliary ganglionic
  coccygeal
  colic
  colonic myenteric
  common carotid
  coronary
  cystic
  deep cardiac
  deferential
  enteric
  esophageal
  Exner
  extradural vertebral
  facial
  femoral
  gastric
  gastroesophageal variceal
  great cardiac
  hemorrhoidal
  hepatic nerve
  hypogastric
  ileocolic
  inferior mesenteric
  intermesenteric
  lumbar
  lumbosacral
  lymph
  Meissner
  myenteric
  nerve
  pampiniform
  paravertebral nerve
  paravertebral venous
  pelvic
  perimuscular
  pharyngeal
  presacral
  prostatic venous

plexus *(cont.)*
   pulmonary
   rectal
   right coronary
   sacral
   sciatic
   solar
   spinal nerve
   submucosal venous
   superficial
   superior hypogastric
   superior mesenteric
   uterovaginal
   vaginal
   vascular
   venous
   vertebral
   vertebral venous
   vesical
   vesical venous
plexus injury
plica (pl. plicae)
   medial
   parapatellar
   suprapatellar
   synovial
plication defect
P-LINK software
PLL (posterior longitudinal ligament)
ploidy, DNA
P loop (on vectorcardiography)
plots, cluster
PLSA (posterolateral spinal artery)
plug
   meconium
   mucus
Plummer disease
Plummer-Vinson syndrome
plump vessel
plurality of slices
plutonium, environmental
PM (posterior mitral)

PMD (papillary muscle dysfunction)
PML (posterior mitral leaflet)
pmol (picomole)
P-MRS (phosphorus magnetic resonance spectroscopy)
PMT (pyridoxyl-5-methyl tryptophan) imaging agent
PMT robotic fulcrumless tomographic system
PMV (percutaneous mitral balloon valvuloplasty)
PMV (prolapsed mitral valve)
PMVL (posterior mitral valve leaflet)
PNC (premature nodal contraction)
PNET (primitive neuroectodermal tumor)
pneumatic bone
pneumatization
pneumatocele
pneumencephalography, lumbar
pneumoarthrogram
pneumocele
pneumocephalus
pneumoconiosis
pneumoconstriction
pneumocystic infection
pneumocystis pneumonia (PCP)
pneumocystography
pneumocystotomography
pneumoencephalogram (PEG)
pneumoencephalographic pattern
pneumoencephalography
pneumoencephalomyelogram
pneumoencephalomyelography
pneumogastrography
pneumogram
pneumography
   cerebral
   retroperitoneal
pneumogynogram
pneumohemothorax
pneumointestinalis

pneumolith
pneumomediastinography
pneumomediastinum
  postoperative
  radiolucent
pneumomyelography
pneumonia (see also *pneumonitis*)
  acute
  alcoholic
  allergic
  amebic
  anthrax
  apex
  apical
  aspiration
  asthmatic
  atypical bronchial
  atypical interstitial
  bacterial
  bilious
  bronchial
  Buhl desquamative
  capillary
  caseous
  catarrhal
  central
  cerebral
  cheesy
  chelonian
  chemical
  chronic eosinophilic
  classic interstitial
  consolidative
  contusion
  Corrigan
  deglutition
  delayed resolution of
  desquamative interstitial (DIP)
  diffuse
  double
  Eaton agent
  embolic

pneumonia *(cont.)*
  exogenous lipoid
  eosinophilic
  ephemeral
  exogenous
  fibrinous
  fibrous
  Friedländer
  fungal
  gangrenous
  giant cell
  granulomatous
  gray hepatization stage of
  Hecht
  hypersensitivity
  hypostatic
  incomplete resolution of
  indurative
  infantile
  inhalation
  interstitial plasma cell
  irradiation
  lingular
  lipoid
  lobar
  lobular
  lymphoid interstitial
  massive
  metastatic
  migratory
  mycoplasmal
  necrotizing
  nonbacterial
  nosocomial
  obstructive
  oil-aspiration
  parenchymatous
  passive
  pertussoid eosinophilic
  Pittsburgh
  plague

pneumonia *(cont.)*
  plasma cell
  pleuritic
  pleurogenic
  pneumocystis
  postobstructive
  postoperative
  post-traumatic
  primary atypical
  protozoal
  purulent
  radiation
  red hepatization stage of
  resolving
  respiratory syncytial viral
  rheumatic
  rickettsial
  right-sided
  secondary
  segmental
  septic
  staphylococcal
  streptococcal
  subacute allergic
  superficial
  suppurative
  terminal
  toxic
  toxemic
  traumatic
  tuberculous
  tularemic
  typhoid
  unresolved
  varicella
  viral
  walking
  wandering
  white
  woolsorter's
pneumonic infiltrate

pneumonitis (see also *pneumonia*)
  acid aspiration
  acute interstitial
  aspiration
  bacterial
  chemical
  cholesterol
  chronic
  congenital rubella
  cytomegalovirus
  early
  granulomatous
  hypersensitivity
  interstitial
  lipoid
  lymphocytic interstitial
  malarial
  manganese
  Mycoplasma (mycoplasmal)
  pigeon breeder's
  plasma cell (PCP)
  radiation
  staphylococcal
  trimellitic anhydritic
  uremic
  ventilation
pneumonocirrhosis
pneumopericardium
pneumoperitoneum
pneumopreperitoneum
pneumopyelography
pneumoradiography
pneumoroentgenogram
pneumoscrotum
pneumothorax
  artificial
  basilar
  closed
  congenital
  diagnostic
  extrapleural
  induced

pole *(cont.)*
  germinal
  inferior
  kidney
  lower
  middle
  patellar
  scaphoid
  superior
  temporal
  upper
pole figure texture analysis
Polhemus 3 digitizer
pollex pedis
polyarticular symmetric tophaceous
  joint inflammation
polyclonal IgG
polycystic kidney disease
polydactyly
polygelin colloid contrast medium
polygon mirror
polygyria
polyhydramnios
polymer
  friction-reducing
  PLA (polyactic acid)
polymer-coated drug-eluting stent
polymeric endoluminal paving stent
polynomial step-wise multiple-linear
  regression
polyostotic bone lesion
polyostotic fibrous dysplasia
polyp
  adenomatous
  benign
  bleeding
  broad-based
  bronchial
  cardiac
  cervical
  choanal
  colon

polyp *(cont.)*
  colonic
  colorectal
  cystic
  dental
  duodenal
  endometrial
  fibrinous
  fibroepithelial
  fibrovascular
  gastric
  hamartomatous gastric
  Hopmann
  hydatid
  hyperplastic gastric
  inflammatory fibroid
  juvenile
  laryngeal
  lipomatous
  lymphoid
  malignant
  metaplastic
  metastatic
  mucous
  multiple
  myomatous
  nasal
  neoplastic
  osseous
  pedunculated
  Peutz-Jeghers
  placental
  postinflammatory
  rectal
  regenerative
  retention
  sessile
  sigmoid
  single
  stalk of
  tubular
  tubulovillous

polyp *(cont.)*
    uterine
    vascular
    villous
polypoid calcified irregular mass
polypoid filling defect
polypoid lesion
polypoid lymphoid hyperplasia
polyposis
    adenomatous
    diffuse mucosal
    familial adenomatous (FAP)
    familial colorectal
    familial gastrointestinal
    familial intestinal
    FAP (familial adenomatous)
    filiform
    gastric
    hamartomatous
    intestinal
    juvenile
    multiple
    Peutz-Jeghers gastrointestinal
polyp stalk
polysplenia
Polystan venous return catheter
polystyrene, cross-linked
polytomographic radiology
polytomography
polytrauma
polyurethane foam embolus
polyurethane stent
polyvinyl alcohol particle size
Pompe disease
pond fracture
P1-P4 segments of posterior cerebral
    artery (PCA)
pons (pl. pontes)
    caudal
    infarction of
pons and midbrain, tegmentum of
pontine angle

pontine contusion
pontine glioma tumor
pontine hemorrhage
pontine infarction
pontine-medullary levels
pontocerebellar fibers
pontocerebellar glioma
pontomedullary junction
pontomesencephalic junction
pool
    blood
    focal
    vascular blood
pooling of blood in extremities
pooling, venous
poor shimming of MRI magnet
popcorn calcification
popliteal aneurysm
popliteal artery entrapment syndrome
popliteal artery occlusive disease
popliteal bypass
popliteal fossa
popliteal in situ bypass
popliteal recess
popliteal space
popliteal to distal in situ bypass
popliteal trifurcation
popliteal vein
porcelain gallbladder
porencephalic cyst
porencephalous
porencephaly
porosis, cerebral
porous ingrowth
porous metallic stent
port
    BardPort implantable
    parallel opposed unmodified
    single
    tangential
    treatment
portable C-arm image intensifier
    fluoroscopy

portable x-ray
portable film
Port-A-Cath
portacaval anastomosis, end-to-side
portacaval shunt
portal-systemic shunt (or portosystemic)
portal-to-portal bridging
portal triad
portal vein thrombosis
portal venography
portal venous phase (PVP)
PortalVision radiation oncology
   system
Portnoy ventricular catheter
porto-azygos collaterals
portogram
portography
   arterial
   CT arterial
   double-spiral CT arterial
   percutaneous transhepatic
   splenic
portopulmonary shunt
portosystemic (or portal-systemic)
Posicam HZ PET scanner
POSICAM PET (positron emission
   topography) system
position (see also *projection*; *view*)
   anatomic
   anterior oblique
   antero-oblique
   barber chair
   bayonet fracture
   beach chair
   Bertel
   catheter tip
   decubitus
   dorsal
   dorsosacral
   erect
   Fowler

position *(cont.)*
   frogleg
   full lateral
   horizontal
   infragenicular
   infrapulmonary
   LAO (left anterior oblique)
   lateral
   left anterior oblique (LAO)
   left-side-down decubitus
   lordotic
   lotus
   LPO (left posterior oblique)
   near anatomic
   neutral hip
   normal anatomic
   park bench
   Phalen
   prone
   pulmonary capillary wedge
   RAO (right anterior oblique)
   rectus
   recumbent
   reverse Trendelenburg
   right anterior oblique (RAO)
   right posterior oblique (RPO)
   right-side-down decubitus
   side-lying
   steep Trendelenburg
   supine
   swimmer's
   three-quarters prone
   Trendelenburg
   upright
position confirmed by fluoroscopy
   with aid of radiopaque marking
positioning error
position of joint, near anatomic
positive GI contrast agent
positive predictive value
positive-pressure pneumothorax
positive tilt test

Positrol II catheter
positron emission computed
    tomography (PET) scan
positron emitters
positron imaging
positron scanning (see *PET scan*)
postablation
postangioplasty aortogram
postangioplasty mural thrombosis
postangioplasty stenosis
post beat filtration
postcapillary venules
postcardiotomy lymphocytic
    splenomegaly
postcentral (sensory) gyrus
postcentral sulcus
postcontrast MR imaging
postcricoid area
postcubital
postdilatation arteriogram
postdrainage cystogram
postdrainage projection
postductal type of coarctation
posterior-anterior (PA)
posterior-aorta transposition of great
    arteries
posterior apical segment
posterior axillary line
posterior cervical triangle
posterior circulation
posterior colliculus
posterior column deficits (of spine)
posterior commissure
posterior communicating artery (PCA)
posterior compartment lesion
posterior coronary plexus (of heart)
posterior cusp
posterior descending artery (PDA)
posterior fossa
posterior fracture-dislocation
posterior free wall
posterior gray column of cord

posterior gray horns of the spinal
    canal
posterior inferior cerebellar artery
    (PICA)
posterior inferior communicating
    artery (PICA)
posterior intercostal artery
posterior interventricular groove
posterior interventricular vein
posterior joint syndrome
posterior-lateral (posterolateral)
posterior lip
posterior lumbar interbody fusion
    (PLIF)
posterior mediastinum
posterior neck surface coil
posterior olive in brain
posterior papillary muscle
posterior pulmonary plexus
posterior root entry zone (PREZ)
posterior root ganglia
posterior segment
posterior skull view
posterior spine fusion (PSF)
posterior spinocerebellar tract
posterior tibial artery
posterior tibiofibular ligament
posterior tibiotalar ligament
posterior wall myocardial infarction
posterior wall thickness
posteroanterior (PA)
posterobasal wall myocardial
    infarction
posterolateral aspect
posterolateral spinal artery (PLSA)
posterolateral wall myocardial
    infarction
posteromedial
postevacuation film
postganglionic gray fibers
postglomerular arteriolar constriction
post-glucose loading exam

postictal cerebral blood flow scan
postinfarction ventricular aneurysm
postinfarction ventriculoseptal defect
postinflammatory pulmonary fibrosis
post-injection image
postirradiation vascular insufficiency
postischemic recovery
postlymphangiography
postmastectomy lymphedema
   syndrome
postmetrizamide CT scan
postmyocardiotomy infarction
postobstructive pneumonia
postoperative bronchopneumonia
postoperative chylothorax
postorchiectomy para-aortic
   radiotherapy
postpartum pituitary apoplexy
postperfusion lung syndrome
postphlebitic incompetence
postprimary tuberculosis
postprocedure nephrostogram
post-PTCA residual stenosis
post-pyelonephritis cortical scarring
postradiation fibrosis
postreduction x-ray
postsphenoidal bone
poststenotic dilatation
poststress ankle/arm Doppler index
poststress images
postsurgical
post-thrombolytic coronary
   reocclusion
post-tourniquet occlusion angiography
post-transplant acute renal failure
   (ARF)
post-transplant coronary artery disease
post-traumatic or posttraumatic
post-traumatic angulation
post-traumatic cavus
post-traumatic fibrosis
post-traumatic neuroma

post-traumatic osteoporosis
post-ulnar bone
postvenography phlebitis
postvoid residual (PVR)
postvoid residual urine volume
postvoid(ing) film
potassium perchlorate contrast medium
potassium-43 imaging agent
   (myocardial perfusion imaging)
potassium-perchlorate
potential
   electrostatic
   phenomenological effective surface
   sorption
potentiometer
Pott fracture
Pott puffy tumor
potter's asthma
pouce flottant (floating thumb)
pouch
   antral
   apophyseal
   blind
   blind upper esophageal
   branchial
   Broca pudendal
   celomic
   deep perineal
   Douglas rectouterine
   dural root
   endodermal
   gastric
   Hartmann
   haustral
   Heidenhain
   hepatorenal
   hypophysial
   ileoanal
   ileocecal
   jejunal
   Kock
   Morison

preferential shunting
preformed clot
preformed guide wire
prefrontal bone of von Bardeleben
pregnancy
   abdominal
   ampullar
   bigeminal
   broad ligament
   cervical
   combined
   compound
   cornual
   ectopic
   extrauterine
   fallopian
   false
   heterotopic
   hydatid
   gemellary
   heterotopic
   interstitial
   intraligamentary
   intraperitoneal
   intrauterine
   membranous
   mesenteric
   molar
   multiple
   mural
   ovarian
   ovarioabdominal
   oviductal
   parietal
   phantom
   plural
   post-term
   prolonged
   pseudointraligamentary
   sarcofetal
   sarcohysteric
   spurious

pregnancy *(cont.)*
   stump
   toxemia of
   tubal
   tuboabdominal
   tuboligamentary
   tubo-ovarian
   tubouterine
   twin
   uteroabdominal
   uterotubal
Preiser disease
preliminary film
premature atherosclerosis
premature closure of ductus arteriosus
premature mid-diastolic closure of
   mitral valve
premature rupture of membranes
premature valve closure
premedullary arteriovenous fistula
preoperative renal angiography
preoperative resting MUGA scan
prep (preparation)
   bowel
   kit
   on-column
   touch
prepared and draped (prepped and
   draped)
prepatellar bursa
prepectorally
preponderance
preponderant
prepontine cistern
prepped and draped
prepulse, spin-lock
prepyloric antrum
prepyloric atresia
prepyloric fold
prereduction x-ray
prerenal
presacral mass

presaturation
  fat-selective
  projection
  spatial
presbyesophagus
presbyophrenia
prescan, MRI
prescapula
presentation of fetus
  breech
  brow
  cephalic
  compound
  face
  footling
  frank breech
  parietal
  shoulder
  transverse
  vertex
presenting part
pre-slip changes on x-ray
presphenoidal bone
PRESS sequence
PRESS spectroscopy
pressure
  A wave (left or right atrial
    catheterization)
  alveolar
  ankle-arm
  ankle systolic
  AO or Ao (aorta)
  aortic
  aortic root
  arterial (ART or Art.)
  arterial peak systolic
  atmospheres of
  bile duct
  blood (BP)
  brachial artery
  brachial artery cuff
  brachial artery end-diastolic

pressure *(cont.)*
  brachial artery peak systolic
  C wave (right atrial catheterization)
  capillary
  capillary wedge
  cardiac filling
  central aortic
  central venous (CVP)
  coronary artery perfusion (CPP)
  coronary wedge
  cuff blood
  diastolic blood (DBP)
  diastolic filling (DFP)
  diastolic perfusion
  diastolic pulmonary artery
  distal coronary perfusion
  Doppler ankle systolic
  Doppler blood
  Doppler calf systolic
  Doppler thigh systolic
  elevated
  end-diastolic
  end-systolic (ESP)
  endocardial
  equalized diastolic
  esophageal peristaltic
  extravascular
  femoral artery (FAP)
  filling
  hepatic wedge
  high filling
  high interstitial
  high wedge
  in vivo balloon
  interstitial fluid hydrostatic
  intraluminal esophageal
  jugular venous
  LA (left atrium)
  left atrial (LAP)
  left atrial end-diastolic
  left subclavian central venous
    (LSCVP)

pressure *(cont.)*
  left ventricular (LV)
  left ventricular cavity
  left ventricular end-diastolic
    (LVEDP)
  left ventricular filling
  left ventricular peak systolic
  left ventricular systolic (LVS)
  left-sided heart
  LES (lower esophageal sphincter)
  maximum inflation
  mean
  mean aortic
  mean arterial (MAP)
  mean atrial
  mean blood
  mean brachial artery
  mean circulatory filling
  mean left atrial
  mean pulmonary artery (MPAP)
  mean pulmonary artery wedge
  mean right atrial
  minimum blood
  PA (pulmonary artery) systolic
  PAD (pulmonary artery diastolic)
  PAS (pulmonary artery systolic)
  passage
  peak
  peak regurgitant wave
  peak systolic
  peak systolic aortic (PSAP)
  peak-inflation
  perfusion
  phasic
  portal venous (PVP)
  pulmonary arterial wedge (PAWP)
  pulmonary artery (PAP)
  pulmonary artery diastolic (PAD)
  pulmonary artery end-diastolic
    (PAEDP)
  pulmonary artery mean (PAM)
  pulmonary artery peak systolic

pressure *(cont.)*
  pulmonary artery/pulmonary
    capillary wedge
  pulmonary artery systolic (PAS)
  pulmonary artery wedge (PAWP)
  pulmonary capillary (PCP)
  pulmonary capillary wedge
    (PCWP)
  pulmonary venous capillary (PVC)
  pulmonary venous wedge
  pulmonary wedge
  pulse
  PV (pulmonary vein)
  PVC (pulmonary venous capillary)
  RA (right atrial)
  recoil
  regional cerebral perfusion (rCPP)
  right atrial (RAP)
  right-sided heart
  right subclavian central venous
    (RSCVP)
  right ventricular (RVP)
  right ventricular diastolic (RVD)
  right ventricular end-diastolic
  right ventricular peak systolic
  right ventricular systolic (RVS)
  right ventricular volume
  RV (right ventricular)
  RVD (right ventricular diastolic)
  RVS (right ventricular systolic)
  segmental lower extremity Doppler
  stump
  subatmospheric
  supersystemic pulmonary artery
  SVC (superior vena cava)
  systemic
  systolic
  systolic blood (SBP)
  toe systolic
  transmyocardial perfusion
  transpulmonary (PTP)

pressure *(cont.)*
   V wave (left or right atrial
      catheterization)
   venous
   ventricular
   wedge
   wedged hepatic venous (WHVP)
   withdrawal
   X' (prime) wave (right atrial
      catheterization)
   Y wave
   Z point
pressure catheter
pressure cuff
pressure difference, aortic-left
pressure equalization
pressure flow gradient
pressure fracture
pressure gradient on pullback
pressure injector
pressure measurement
pressure overload
pressure perfusion study
pressure pneumothorax
pressure pullback
pressure readings
pressure study
pressure waveform
Pressurometer
pretectal lesion
pretectal nucleus (region of midbrain)
pretectal region
pretendinous bands (of hand)
pretendinous cord
pretherapy imaging
pretibial region
prevertebral fascia
prevertebral soft tissue
PREZ (posterior root entry zone)
PRG (phleborheography)
primarily pulmonary hypertension
  (PPH)

primary bronchi, right and left
primary, cancer of unknown (CUP)
primary complex
primary megaloureter
primary motor strip
primary neoplasm
primary pulmonary hypertension
primary pulmonary plasmacytoma
primary rhabdomyosarcoma
primary sarcoma
primary thrombus
primary tuberculosis
primary vesical calculus (pl. calculi)
primary visual cortex
primitive dislocation
primitive neuroectodermal tumor
  (PNET)
principal bronchus
principal eigenvector
principle, uncertainty
print reflectance modulation
printer
   Codonics color
   raster scanning
   Winprint laser
Priodax contrast medium
prism interpolation
prism method for ventricular volume
Pro-Flo XT catheter
probability
   absolute emission
   emission
probe
   AngeLase combined mapping-laser
   Chandler V-pacing
   Doppler flow
   echocardiographic
   electromagnetic flow
   gamma
   hand-held
   hand-held exploring electrode
   hand-held mapping

probe *(cont.)*
  high-frequency miniature
  laparoscopic Doppler
  magnetometer
  Medrad Mrinnervu endorectal
    colon
  NRM magnetometer
  nuclear
  oligonucleotide
  pediatric biplane TEE
  sapphire contact
  side-hole cannulated
  Siemens-Elema AB pulse transducer
  system, USCI
  Teflon
  truncated NMR
  ultrasound
Probe balloon-on-a-wire dilatation
probehead, MRI
PROBE-SV spectrometer
probing catheter, USCI
procedure (see *imaging*)
process (pl. processes)
  accessory
  acromial
  alar
  alveolar consolidative
  apical
  articular
  ascending
  auditory
  basilar
  bony
  calcaneal
  caudate
  clinoid
  cochleariform
  condyloid
  conoid
  consolidative
  coracoid
  coronoid

process *(cont.)*
  costal
  energy transfer
  ensiform
  ethmoidal
  falciform
  fibroplastic
  frontal
  frontonasal
  frontosphenoidal
  glenoid
  inflammatory
  jugular
  knobby
  left ventricular posterior superior
  lumbar transverse
  neoplastic
  odontoid
  olecranon
  osseous destructive
  pterygoid
  sacral
  spinous
  styloid
  transverse
  trochlear
  uncinate
  vermiform
  vertebrospinous (or vertebral
    spinous)
  vertebral
  xiphoid
  zygomatic
processor, sequence
proctogram
  balloon
  video
proctographic features
proctosigmoidoscopy
procurvature deformity
product cipher
product, daughter

prolapsed tumor through mitral valve
  orifice
prolapsing scallop
proliferation
  angiofibroblastic
  bile duct
  bony
  fibroplastic
  glandular
  myointimal
  nodular
  osteophytic
  papillary
  synovial
  villous
prolonged interval
prolonged left ventricular impulse
prominence
  aortic
  bony (spur)
  hilar
  mediastinal
  tibial tubercle
prominent rim of radiolucency
  surrounding ulcer
prominent septal lymphatics
prominent xiphoid process
promontory, sacral
prompt-gamma neutron activation
pronation
pronator quadratus
prone lateral view
prone position
prone view
properitoneal flank stripe
property (pl. properties)
  CTA dosimetric
  ferromagnetic
  ionic
proportional counter
propria
  lamina

propria *(cont.)*
  substania
  tunica
propulsive mechanism
propyliodone contrast medium
prospective analysis
ProSpeed CT scanner
ProstaScint diagnostic imaging agent
ProstaScint monoclonal antibody
  imaging agent
prostate
  apex of
  carcinoma of
  inferolateral surfaces of
  lateral lobe of
  lymph vessels of
  median lobe of
  posterior surface of
prostate implant
prostate seeding
prostatic urethra
prosthesis (pl. prostheses)
  acetabular
  aortic valve
  aortofemoral
  ball-and-cage valve
  ball-cage
  ball valve
  bifurcated aortofemoral
  bileaflet valve
  bilioduodenal
  closure
  collar
  convexo-concave valve
  disk valve
  esophageal
  femoral
  femorofemoral crossover
  intraluminal sutureless
  intravascular
  iridium
  monostrut cardiac valve

prosthesis *(cont.)*
   outflow tract
   tilting-disk aortic valve
   total hip replacement
   total knee replacement
prosthesis cup
prosthesis dehiscence
prosthetic femorodistal graft
prosthetic heart valve
protection
   myocardial
   radiation
protein kinase C localization (brain)
protein synthesis rate
protocol
   MNP10
   MPRAGE
   neon particle
   RTOG
   2D GRE dynamic
   UCLA imaging
   urokinase
protodensity MRI image
protodiastolic reversal of blood flow
proton density
proton density images (MRI)
proton density-weighted images
proton irradiation
proton magnetic resonance
   spectroscopy
proton MR spectroscopy
protons
   methyl
   91-41 MeV
   precessing
protrude
protruding atheroma
protrusion
   disk
   spicular
   spoonlike (of leaflets)
   vascular

protrusion of navicular
protuberance, occipital
proximal anastomosis
proximal and distal portion of vessel
proximal anterior tibial artery
proximal articular set angle (PASA)
proximal carpal row
proximal circumflex artery
proximal coil
proximal focal femoral deficiency
   (PFFD)
proximal interphalangeal (PIP) joint
proximal popliteal artery
proximal segment
proximally
Pruitt-Inahara balloon-tipped perfusion
   catheter
pruned appearance of pulmonary
   vasculature
PS (pulmonary sequestration)
PS (pulmonic stenosis)
PSA (power spectral analysis)
psammoma body
psammoma, Virchow
psammomatous meningiomas
pseudarthrosis
pseudoaneurysm
pseudoangiomatous stromal
   hyperplasia
pseudocapsule
pseudocirrhosis, cholangiodysplastic
pseudocoarctation of aorta
pseudocolor B-mode display
pseudocyst
   adrenal
   mature pancreatic
   pancreatic
   pulmonary
pseudodextrocardia
pseudodislocation
pseudodiverticulum

pseudodynamic MR imaging of the
temporomandibular joints
pseudoepiphysis
pseudoextrophy
pseudofracture artifact
pseudogestational sac
pseudohaustration
pseudojoints
pseudoluxation
pseudolymphoma, gastric
pseudomembrane
pseudomeningocele
pseudomitral leaflet
pseudoneuroma
pseudo-obstruction
   bowel
   chronic idiopathic intestinal (CIIP)
   colonic
   familial intestinal
   idiopathic intestinal
   nonfamilial intestinal
pseudo-orbital tumor
pseudopolyp
pseudopolyposis
pseudopregnancy
pseudosac
pseudosacculation
pseudosclerosis, spastic
pseudosheath
pseudostone
pseudothrombosis
pseudotumor
   fibrosing inflammatory
   orbital
pseudotumor cerebri (PTC)
PSF (posterior spine fusion)
PSG (peak systolic gradient)
PSIL (percentage signal intensity loss)
P623-Gd imaging agent
psoas abscess
psoas muscle shadow, obliteration of
PSP (photostimulable phosphor dental
radiography)

P, substance
pSV-b-Gal plasmid imaging agent
pT3 tumor
pT4 tumor
PTA (percutaneous transluminal
angioplasty)
pTa-T2 tumor
PTBD (percutaneous transhepatic
biliary drainage) catheter
PTBD (percutaneous transluminal
balloon dilatation)
PTC (percutaneous transhepatic
cholangiography)
PTC (pseudotumor cerebri)
PTCA (percutaneous transluminal
coronary angioplasty)
PTCA catheterization
PTCA coronary angiogram
PTD (percutaneous transhepatic
drainage)
PTDC (percutaneous transcatheter
ductal closure)
pterion
pterygoid bone
pterygoid chest
pterygoideus hamulus
PTF (posterior talofibular) ligament
PTHC (percutaneous transhepatic
cholangiogram)
P-31 MR spectroscopy
PTL (posterior tricuspid leaflet)
ptosis
ptotic
PTRA (percutaneous transluminal
renal angioplasty)
PTT (pulmonary transit time)
PTV (posterior terminal vein)
pubic bone
pubic ramus (pl. rami)
   inferior
   superior
pubic symphysis

pulmonary cavitation
pulmonary cavity
pulmonary circulation
pulmonary cirrhosis
pulmonary compliance, reduced
pulmonary compression by pleural
   fluid or gas
pulmonary confluence
pulmonary congestion
pulmonary consolidation
pulmonary contusion
pulmonary cyanosis
pulmonary cystic lymphangiectasis
pulmonary edema
   acute
   cardiogenic
   frank
   fulminant
   high-altitude
   interstitial
   negative image
   neurogenic
   noncardiac
   noncardiogenic
   permeability-type
   postoperative
   reexpansion
pulmonary embolism (embolus, pl.
   emboli) (PE)
pulmonary emphysema
pulmonary eosinophilic infiltrates
pulmonary failure
pulmonary fibrosis (see *fibrosis*)
pulmonary fistula, congenital
pulmonary flotation catheter
pulmonary gangrene
pulmonary gas exchange
pulmonary hemorrhage
pulmonary hilus
pulmonary histoplasmosis
pulmonary incompetence
pulmonary infarction

pulmonary infiltrate
pulmonary insufficiency
pulmonary interstitial emphysema
   (PIE)
pulmonary interstitial idiopathic
   fibrosis
pulmonary interstitium
pulmonary ligament
pulmonary microcirculation
pulmonary microvasculature
pulmonary nodule enhancement
pulmonary orifice
pulmonary outflow tract
pulmonary overdistention
pulmonary parenchymal changes
pulmonary parenchymal infiltrates
pulmonary parenchymal window
pulmonary perfusion and ventilation
pulmonary perfusion imaging
pulmonary pleura
pulmonary plexus
pulmonary quantitative differential
   function study
pulmonary regurgitation
pulmonary sarcoidosis
pulmonary scars
pulmonary scintigraphy
pulmonary sequestration (PS)
pulmonary stenosis
pulmonary/systemic flow ratio
pulmonary TB (tuberculosis)
pulmonary thromboembolism (PTE)
pulmonary thrombosis
pulmonary time activity curve
pulmonary trunk idiopathic dilatation
pulmonary tuberculosis (TB)
pulmonary valve annulus
pulmonary valve atresia
pulmonary valve deformity
pulmonary valve insufficiency
pulmonary valve stenosis
pulmonary vascular bed impedance

pulmonary vascular congestion
pulmonary vascular markings
pulmonary vascular obstruction
pulmonary vascular pattern
pulmonary vascular redistribution
pulmonary vascular reserve
pulmonary vascular resistance (PVR)
pulmonary vascular resistance index
  (PVRI)
pulmonary vasculature
pulmonary vasoconstriction, hypoxic
pulmonary vein apoplexy
pulmonary vein atresia
pulmonary vein, congenital stenosis of
pulmonary vein fibrosis
pulmonary vein stenosis
pulmonary vein wedge angiography
pulmonary veno-occlusive disease
pulmonary venous anomalous
  drainage
pulmonary venous anomalous
  drainage to right atrium
pulmonary venous congestion
pulmonary venous drainage
pulmonary venous hypertension
pulmonary venous obstruction
pulmonary venous system
pulmonary venous-systemic air emboli
pulmonary venous wedge pressure
pulmonary ventilation imaging
pulmonary vesicles
pulmonary vessels
pulmonary wedge angiography
pulmonary wedge pressure (PWP)
pulmonic atresia with intact
  ventricular septum
pulmonic infiltrate
pulmonic regurgitation
pulmonic stenosis-ventricular septal
  defect
pulmonic valve stenosis

pulposus, nucleus
pulsate
pulsatile flow, dampened
pulsatile perfusion
pulsatile tinnitus
pulsatility index (PI)
pulsation balloon
pulse (pl. pulses)
  adiabatic slice-selective rf (RF)
    (radiofrequency)
  DANTE-selective
  fat suppression
  narrow-band spectral-selective
    90 RF
  navigator
  phase-encode
  radiofrequency (rf or RF)
  section-select
  spatially selective inversion
  2D spatially selective RF
pulsed brachytherapy (PDR)
pulsed Doppler transesophageal
  echocardiography
pulsed Doppler ultrasound
pulse deficit
pulsed electron paramagnetic NMR
pulsed gradient
pulsed infrared laser
pulsed L-band ESR spectrometer
pulse Doppler interrogation
pulsed magnetization transfer contrast
  MRI
pulsed ultrasound
pulse duration
pulsed-wave Doppler echocardiography
pulse height spectral analysis
pulse indicator, xylol
pulse length
pulse reappearance time
pulse sequence, single-shot adiabatic
  localization

pulse sequencing
PulseSpray injector
PulseSpray pulsed infusion system
pulse voltage
pulse volume recording (PVR)
pulse volume waveforms
pulse wave
pulse width
pulsion
pulverized plaque particulate matter
pulvinar region
pump
   angle port
   balloon
   cardiac balloon
   intra-aortic balloon (IABP)
   ion
   pulmonary artery balloon (PABP)
punctate area
puncture
   fine-needle
   stereotactic
   venous
puncture fracture
puncture wound (types I-IV)
purification, one-line anion exchange
purified water contrast
purity, radionuclide
putamen
putaminal hemorrhage, nondominant
PV (pulmonic valve)
PVD (peripheral vascular disease)
PVG (periventricular gray) matter
PVL (periventricular leukomalacia)
PVP (portal venous pressure)
PVR (peripheral vascular resistance)
PVR (perspective volume rendering)
PVR (postvoiding residual)
PVR (pulmonary vascular resistance)
PVR (pulse volume recorder)
PVR fly-through viewing

PVRI (pulmonary vascular resistance
   index)
PW (posterior wall)
PW (pulse width)
PWT (posterior wall thickness)
pyelectasia
pyelectasis
pyelocaliceal
pyelocaliectasis
pyelocaliceal
pyelofluoroscopy
pyelogram
   antegrade
   excretory intravenous
   intravenous (IVP)
   retrograde
pyelographic appearance time
pyelography
pyelostogram
pyelotubular backflow
pyemia
   cryptogenic
   portal
pyknomorphous
pyloric channel
pyloric hypertrophy
pyloric insufficiency
pyloric outlet obstruction
pyloric ring
pyloric stenosis
pyloric string sign
pyloric ulcer
pyloric valve
pyloroduodenal junction
pylorospasm, persistent
pylorus, hypertrophic
pyocephalus
pyogenic granuloma
pyonephrosis
pyopneumothorax
pyothorax

Q, q

Q (cardiac output)
Q (quotient, as in V/Q, ventilation perfusion scan)
QCA (quantitative coronary arteriography)
Q-cath catheterization recording system
Q space
QCT (quantitative computed tomography) test for bone loss
QDR-1500 or QDR-2000 bone densitometer
QHS (quantitative hepatobiliary scintigraphy)
QM (quantization matrix)
QO_2 (oxygen consumption)
QPD (quadrature phase detector)
QR pattern
QRS interval
QRS loop, counterclockwise superiorly oriented frontal
QRS score
QRS synchronized shock
QRS vector
QRS vertical axis
QRS-T angle, wide
quad resonance NMR probe circuit

Quad-Lumen drain with radiopaque stripe
quadrangle cartilage
quadrangulation of Frouin
quadrant
   left lower (LLQ)
   left upper (LUQ)
   left upper outer
   right lower (RLQ)
   right upper (RUQ)
   right upper outer
quadrant of death (anterosuperior quadrant of hip)
quadrate lobe of liver
quadrature phase detector (QPD) artifact
quadrature RF receiver coil
quadrature setting
quadrature surface coil system
quadrature T/L surface coil
quadratus femoris muscle
quadratus, pronator
quadriceps muscle
quadrigeminal plate
quadrigeminy
quadrilateral brim
quadripolar catheter

Quain fatty degeneration of the heart
qualitative study
quality factor
quantification
  automated
  flow
quantify
quantitative analysis
quantitative cardiac perfusion
quantitative computed tomography
  (QCT)
quantitative coronary arteriography
  (QCA)
quantitative CT during expiration
quantitative Doppler assessment
quantitative electroencephalography
  (QEEG)
quantitative exercise thallium-201
  variables
quantitative fluorescence imaging
quantitative gated SPECT (QGS)
quantitative hepatobiliary scintigraphy
  (QHS)
quantitative magnetization transfer
quantitative regional myocardial flow
  measurement
quantitative scan
quantitative spirometrically controlled
  CT
quantity, spectrophotometric
quantization
    sequent scalar (SSQ)
    wavelet scalar (WSQ)
quantization matrix (QM) scaling
quantizer-design algorithms
quantum number
quench
quenching
Quénu-Muret sign
Quervain fracture
quiescence
Quik-Prep, Quinton
Quincke angioedema disease
Quinton PermCath
Quinton Quik-Prep
Quinton vascular access port
quotient, Rayleigh
QW 3600 contrast agent

R, r

R (roentgen)
RA (right atrial) pressure
RA (right atrium) oxygen saturation
RA (rheumatoid arthritis) factor
Raaf Cath (vascular catheter)
RAAPI (resting ankle-arm pressure
    index)
RAB (remote afterloading brachy-
    therapy)
RACAT (rapid acquisition computed
    axial tomography)
rachioscoliosis
rachitic rosary sign
Racobalamin-57 radioactive agent
rad (radiation absorbed dose)
radiability
radial artery catheter
radial artery to cephalic vein fistula
radial bone
radial collateral ligament
radial deviation
radial drift
radial epiphyseal displacement
radial facing of metacarpal heads
radial forearm flap
radial fossa
radial head fracture

radial head subluxation (RHS)
radial ray defect
radial styloid process fracture
radial tuberosity
radial vascular thermal injury
radialized
radiate ligament
radiation (see also *radiation therapy*)
    adjuvant
    Cerenkov
    diagnostic
    external beam
    ionizing
    monochromatic
    synchrotron
    therapeutic
    ultraviolet
radiation-absorbed dose (rad)
radiation changes
radiation dosages
radiation dose pertubation
radiation dosimetry calculation
radiation fibrosis
radiation fistula
radiation-induced ulceration
radiation-induced up-regulation
radiation intensity

radiation interrogation
radiation monitor
radiation necrosis
radiation osteonecrosis
radiation pericardial disease
radiation port
radiation protection
radiation scatter
radiation source
   intracavitary
   intrastitial
radiation therapy (also radiotherapy)
   accelerated hyperfractionated
   combined-modality
   concomitant boost
   conformal
   conformal neutron and photon
   conventionally fractionated
     stereotactic
   craniospinal axis
   dynamic
   external beam (EBRT)
   eye-view 3D-CRT
   fractionated external beam
   fractionated stereotaxic
   hyperfractionated
   hypofractionated
   I-B1 radiolabeled antibody
     injection
   ICRU 50
   interstitial
   intracavitary
   intraoperative (IORT)
   large-field
   megavoltage
   neuroaxis
   orthovoltage
   palliative
   partial-brain
   photon-neutron mixed-beam
   postorchiectomy para-aortic
   rotational

radiation therapy *(cont.)*
   short-distance (brachytherapy)
   split-course accelerated
   split hyperfractionated accelerated
   stereotactic or stereotaxic
   three-dimensional conformal
   3D-CRT
   upper mantle
   whole-brain
radiation therapy planning (RTP)
   system
radiation toxicity syndrome
radical mastectomy
radicle, biliary
radicular arteries
radicular compression
radicular cyst
radicular vessels to spinal cord
radiculomedullary artery
radiculospinal artery
radioactive aerosol
radioactive bolus
radioactive cancer-specific targeting
   agent
radioactive cobalt
radioactive emissions from heart
radioactive fibrinogen scan
radioactive iodinated serum albumin
   (RISA) imaging agent
radioactive iodine uptake test (RAIU)
radioactive isotope (see *imaging*
   agent)
radioactive label (labeling)
radioactively tagged
radioactive marker
radioactive material
radioactive source
radioactive string markers
radioactive thallium
radioactive tracer
radioactive xenon clearance
radioactive xenon gas inhalation

radioaerosol clearance
radioaerosol imaging studies
radioallergosorbent test (RAST)
radioccipital
radiobiological
radiobiology
radiocalcium
radiocapitellar joint
radiocarcinogenesis
radiocardiogram
radiocardiography
radiocarpal angle
radiocarpal dislocation
radiocarpal joint
radiocarpal portal
radiochemical study
radiochemistry
radiochromic film
radiocurable
radiode
radiodiagnosis
radiodiagnostics
radiodigital
radioelement application
   interstitial
   intracavitary
   surface
radioelement solution
radiofluorinated
Radiofocus Glidewire for angiography
radiofrequency (RF)
   RF ablation (RFA) therapy
   RF catheter ablation (RFCA)
   RF coil
   RF energy
   RF field
   RF-generated thermal balloon
     catheter
   RF hypertheramia
   RF magnetic shield
   RF overflow artifact
   RF period

radiofrequency *(cont.)*
   RF pulse
   RF saturation bands
   RF screen
   RF modification transcatheter
   RF spatial distribution problem
   RF spatial distribution problem
     reconstruction artifact
   RF transmitter
radiogenic leukopenia
radiogold
radiogram (radiograph) (see *imaging*)
radiographic control
radiographic hallmark
radiographic imaging system,
   intensified (IRIS)
radiographically firm synostosis
radiography (see *imaging*)
radiohumeral articulation
radioimmunity
radioimmunoassay (RIA)
radioimmunoassay, scintillation
   proximity
radioimmunodetection (RAID)
radioimmunodiffusion
radioimmunoelectrophoresis
radioimmunoimaging
radioimmunoscintigraphy
radioimmunoscintimetry
radioimmunosorbent
radioimmunotherapy
radioiodinated serum albumin (RISA)
radioiodination
   direct
   electrophilic
radioiodine
radioiron oral absorption
radioiron red cell utilization
radioisotope (isotope) (see *imaging
   agent)*
radioisotope assay, thyroxine (T_4RIA)
radioisotope cisternography

radioisotope clearance assay
radioisotope-labeled antibody
radioisotope-labeled antigen
radioisotope labeling
radioisotope lung scan
radioisotope (static) scanning
radioisotope stent
radioisotope uptake
radioisotope voiding cystography
radiolabeled antifibrin antibody
radiolabeled compound
radiolabeled estrogen analog F-18 (^{18}F)
   estradiol (FES)
radiolabeled fibrinogen
radiolabeled MoAb
radiolabeled peptide alpha-M2
   imaging agent
radiolabeled platelets
radiolabeled water study
radiolabeled WBCs
radiolesion
radioligand
radiologic-anatomic correlation
radiologic gastrostomy
radiologic guidance
radiologic-histopathologic study
radiologic-pathologic correlation
radiologic percutaneous gastrostomy
radiologic protection
radiologist
radiology
   computed (CR)
   diagnostic
   interventional
   neurointerventional
   percutaneous interventional
   polytomographic
   skeletal
   storage phosphor
   therapeutic
radiology outcomes data
radiolucency, soap-bubble

radiolucent area
radiolucent center
radiolucent cleft
radiolucent focus (pl. foci)
radiolucent pneumomediastinum
radiolucent spine frame
radiolucent stone
radiolunotriquetral ligament
radiolymphoscintigraphy,
   intraoperative
radiomuscular
radionecrosis, cerebral
Radionics CRW stereotactic head
   frame
radionitrogen
radionuclear venography
radionuclide (see *imaging agent*)
   absorption of
   concentration of
   inhalation of
   inhaled
   injection of
   uptake of
radionuclide angiocardiogram
radionuclide angiogram (RNA)
radionuclide blood flow (dynamic)
   studies
radionuclide carrier system
radionuclide cineangiography
radionuclide cisternography
radionuclide cystography
radionuclide flow scan
radionuclide gated blood pool
   scanning
radionuclide injection
radionuclide label (labeling)
radionuclide liver scan
radionuclide mammography
radionuclide milk scan
radionuclide purity
radionuclide scan (scanning)
radionuclide shuntogram

radionuclide signals
radionuclide study, blood pool
radionuclide testicular scintigraphy
radionuclide ventriculogram
radionuclide voiding study
radiopacity
radiopaque calculus
radiopaque contrast medium
radiopaque density
radiopaque distal tip for location on
   fluoroscopy
radiopaque fluid, extravasation of
radiopaque marker
radiopaque medium
radiopaque nanoparticulate
radiopaque pellet
radiopaque suture
radiopaque urine
radiopaque vesical calculi
radiopaque wire of counteroccluder
   buttonhole
radiopaque xenon gas
radiopathology
radiopharmaceutical (see *imaging*
   agent)
radiopharmaceutical ablation
radiopharmaceutical dacryocystography
radiopharmaceutical localization
radiopharmaceutical therapy
radiopharmaceutical voiding
   cystogram
radiopharmaceutical volume-dilution
   technique
radiophobia
radiophotography
radiophylaxis
radiopotassium
radiopulmonography
radioreaction
radioresistance
radioscaphocapitate ligament
radioscaphoid joint

radioscaphoid ligament
radioscapholunate ligament
radioscintigraphy
radioscopically tagged antihuman
   antibody
radiosensibility
radiosensitive
radiosensitivity, fibroblast
radiosensitizer
   carbogen
   halogenated thymidine analogue
   nicotinamide
radiostereoscopy
radiostyloid process
radiosulfur
radiosurgery
   Bragg-peak
   charged-particle
   dynamic stereotactic
   gamma knife
   heavy-charged particle Bragg peak
   image-guided
   interstitial
   LINAC or Linac (linear accelerator)
   multiarc LINAC
   stereotactic or stereotaxic
radiosurgically
radiotherapeutic agent
radiotherapist
radiotherapy (see *radiation therapy*)
radiotherapy with hyperthermia
radiotherapy without hyperthermia
radiotherapy field placement
radiotoxemia
radiotoxicity
radiotracer activity
radiotracer foil method
radiotracer foil method for sorption
   studies
radiotracer technique
radiotracer uptake
radiotransparency

radiotropic
radioulnar joint
radioulnar subluxation
radioulnar surface
radium radioactive source
radius
RadNet radiology information system
radon seeds radioactive source
RADstation radiology workstation
radwaste radioactivity detection
RAE (right atrial enlargement)
Raeder-Arbitz syndrome
Raeder paratrigeminal syndrome
ragpicker's disease
RAID (radioimmunodetection)
railroad track pattern on x-ray in
    Sturge-Weber syndrome
railroad track sign
Raimiste sign
Raimondi ventricular catheter
raised intracranial pressure
RAIU (radioactive iodine uptake test)
rake retractor
rake ulcer
Raman spectroscopy
Ramesh and Pramod algorithms
rami (see *ramus*)
ramp, folded step
Ramsay Hunt cerebellar myoclonic
    dyssynergia
ramus (pl. rami)
    dorsal
    dorsal primary
    inferior
    inferior pubic
    ischiopubic
    pubic
    superior
    ventral
    ventral primary
ramus intermedius artery branch

ramus medialis artery branch
R&F camera
Rand microballoon
random field, Gibbs
randomly distributed cortical perfusion
    defects
Ranfac LAP-013 cholangiographic
    catheter
Ranfac ORC-B cholangiographic
    catheter
Ranfac XL-11 cholangiographic
    catheter
range
    absorbed dose
    grayscale
    normal
    reference
    therapeutic
range-gated Doppler spectral flow
    analysis
Ranke angle
Ranke complex
Ranvier groove
Ranvier node
RAO (right anterior oblique)
    RAO position for cardiac
        catheterization
    RAO projection
    RAO view
RAP (right atrial pressure)
raphe
    abdominal
    amniotic
    anococcygeal
    anogenital
    longitudinal
    median
    palpebral
    penile
    pterygomandibular
    scrotal
    tendinous

rapid acquisition with relaxation
   enhancement (RARE)
rapid axial MRI
rapid deceleration injury
rapid dephasing
rapid early repolarization phase
rapid filling phase
rapid filling wave
rapid image transfer
rapid inspiratory flow rates
rapid oscillatory motion
rapid repolarization phase
rapid sequence intravenous pyelogram
   (IVP)
rapid sequential CT scan
rapid thoracic compression technique
rapid ventricular filling phase
rapid ventricular rate
rapid ventricular response
Rappaport classification of gastric
   lymphoma
Rappaport disability rating scale
raptus of attention
RARE (rapid acquisition with
    relaxation enhancement) MRI
RARE-derived pulse sequence
rarefaction of cortex
rarefied area
Rashkind double umbrella device
Rashkind septostomy balloon catheter
Rasmussen mycotic aneurysm
Rastelli atrioventricular canal defect
   (type A, B, or C)
raster frequency
raster lines
raster period
raster scanning printer
raster spacing error
rate
   complication
   deposition
   instantaneous enhancement

rate *(cont.)*
   patency
   protein synthesis
   shear
   slew
   transverse relaxation
   valley-to-peak
rate meter
Rathke pouch
Rathke duct
Rathke pouch (in the brain)
rating scale
ratio
   AH:HA
   ankle-brachial pressure
   AO:AC (aortic valve opening to
     aortic valve closing)
   aortic root
   artery/aortic velocity
   brain-to-background
   C/N (contrast to noise)
   cardiothoracic (CT, CTR)
   CBV/CBF
   cerebral blood volume/cerebral
     blood flow
   chemical-shift
   CK:AST
   compression
   conduction (number of P waves to
     number of QRS)
   contrast-to-noise (C/N)
   E:A (on echocardiography)
   escape-peak
   ESP-ESV
   ESWI-ESVI (end-systolic wall
     stress index to end-systolic
     volume)
   FL/AC (femur length to abdominal
     circumference)
   gray to white matter activity (also
     gray/white matter activity)
   gray to white matter utilization

ratio *(cont.)*
- gyromagnetic
- HC/AC (head circumference to abdominal circumference)
- heart-to-background
- heart-to-lung
- Holdaway
- inferior-anterior (I-A) count
- Insall (in patella alta)
- Insall-Salvati
- inverse inspiratory–expiratory time
- isotopic
- I–E (inspiration to expiration, or inspiratory to expiratory)
- kidney-to-background
- LA–AR (left atrium/aortic root)
- L/A (liver/aorta) peak
- L/B
- L/LP (liver/liver peak)
- left ventricular systolic time interval
- lesion-to-background
- lesion-to-muscle
- lesion to non-lesion count
- liver/aorta (L/A) peak
- liver/liver peak (L/LP)
- magnetogyric
- maximum diameter to minimum diameter
- metatarsal length
- nasal-to-plasma radioactivity
- orifice-to-annulus
- P:A (peroneal to anterior compartment)
- PASP–SASP (pulmonary to systemic arterial systolic pressure)
- patellar ligament-patellar
- peak systolic and diastolic
- pitch
- Poisson
- P:QRS

ratio *(cont.)*
- P–S flow (pulmonic–systemic)
- pulmonary–systemic blood flow
- pulmonary to systemic flow
- R/S amplitude
- R/S wave
- risk–benefit
- RVP–LVP (right ventricular to left ventricular systolic pressure)
- RV6:RV5 voltage
- scatter-to-primary
- septal to free wall
- serum glucose:CSF glucose
- SI joint to sacrum
- signal-to-clutter
- signal-to-noise (S/N)
- spleen-to-liver
- stroke volume
- target-to-background
- thallium-to-scalp
- TME (trapezium-metacarpal eburnation)
- tumor-to-normal brain
- T–D (thickness to diameter of ventricle)
- VLDL-TG to HDL-C

Ratliff classification of avascular necrosis

rat-tail appearance on pancreatogram

Rau, apophysis of

Rauchfuss triangle

rauwolfia derivative

RAW (airway resistance)

ray (pl. rays)
- central
- digital
- grenz
- hypermobile first
- keV gamma
- long axis
- pollicized

ray amputation

ray-casting method
Rayleigh quotient
Rayleigh scattering law
Raymond-Cestan syndrome
Raynaud phenomenon
ray-sum projection
ray-sum views
Ray-Tec x-ray detectable surgical
   sponge
Ray TFC (threaded fusion cage)
Ray ventricular cannula
Rb (rubidium)
   ^{82}Rb-based cardiac imaging
RBBB (right bundle branch block)
RBC (red blood cell)
   labeled
   technetium-99m-labeled
RBG (red, blue, green)
RCA (retained cortical activity)
RCA (right coronary artery)
RCA (rotational coronary
   atherectomy)
rCBF (regional cerebral blood flow)
   PET scan
rCBV (regional cerebral blood
   volume) PET scan
rCMRO$_2$ (regional cerebral metabolic
   rate for oxygen)
rCPP (regional cerebral perfusion
   pressure)
RCT (retinocortical time)
rd (rutherford) radioactive unit
RDG (retrograde duodenogastroscopy)
RDW (red cell diameter width)
RE (reflux esophagitis)
RE (rehabilitation engineering)
Re (rhenium)
reabsorption, bony
reaccumulation
reaction
   endoergic
   exoergic

reaction (cont.)
   hilar
   hypersensitivity
   lamellar
   periosteal
   pleural
   sarcoid-like
reactivation tuberculosis
reactive airways disease (RAD)
reactive airways dysfunction syndrome
reactive arterioles
reactive disease of smooth muscle
reactive hyperemia
reactivity, bronchial
Reader paratrigeminal syndrome
reading
   batch-
   wet x-ray
readout wavelength
reagent, Wittig
real-time assessment
real-time biplanar needle tracking
real-time chirp Z transformer
real-time color flow Doppler
   imaging of blood flow
real-time CT fluoroscopy
real-time DAP (dose area product)
   real-time equipment
real-time display
real-time edge enhancement
real-time format converter
real-time images
real-time MR imaging tracking
real-time respiratory feedback
real-time scan ultrasound
real-time sonogram (sonography)
real-time two-dimensional (2D) blood
   flow imaging
real-time ultrasound (ultrasonography)
real-time volume rendering
realign
realignment, patellofemoral

reapproximating
reapproximation
rebleeding of aneurysm
rebreathing ventilation scan
re-bypass
recalcitrant
recanalization technique
   angiographic
   argon laser
   laser
   percutaneous transluminal coronary
   peripheral laser (PLR)
recanalized artery
recanalized ductus
recanalizing
receiver coil
receiver operating characteristics
   (ROC)
receptor (pl. receptors)
   baro-
   benzodiazepine
   dopamine
   D2
   GABA
   serotonin
   S2
   transferrin
receptor antagonist
receptor binding
recess
   attic
   cecal
   cerebellopontine
   cochlear
   costodiaphragmatic
   costomediastinal
   duodenojejunal
   epitympanic
   hepatorenal
   ileocecal
   inferior duodenal
   infraglenoid

recess *(cont.)*
   intersigmoid
   optic
   popliteal
   paraduodenal
   peritoneal
   pleural
   prestyloid
   retrocecal
   retroduodenal
   sacciform
   splenorenal
   sublabral
   subphrenic
   subscapularis
   superior duodenal
recession, nasion
recheck
reciprocal changes
reciprocating conduction
recirculation peak
Recklinghausen disease of bone
recoarctation of aorta
recognition, high-order curve
recoil
   arterial
   catheter
recoil pressure
recombinant human granulocyte
   colony stimulating factor
   (r-metHuG-CSF)
recon pitch
reconstituted via collaterals
reconstitution of blood flow in artery
reconstitution via profunda artery
reconstitution via collaterals
reconstructed with a 1:1 pitch at
   1 mm increments
reconstruction
   aortic
   Dor
   external gamma dose

redistribution study
Redi-Vu teleradiology system
red Robinson catheter
red rubber catheter
reduced cardiac output
reduced circulation
reduced compliance of chamber
reduced plasma volume
reduced prominence of pulmonary vessels
reduced pulmonary compliance
reduced signal intensity
reduced stroke volume
reducible hernia
reduction
  afterload
  anatomic
  blood viscosity
  closed
  concentric
  congruent
  electrolytic
  fracture
  manual
  manual fracture
  open
  stable
  surgical
  thoracic volume
  trial
redundancy of interposed colon segment
redundant aortic valve leaflets
redundant carotid artery
redundant mitral valve leaflets
redundant scallop of posterior annulus
reefing, capsular
reefing of medial retinaculum of knee
re-entry point
reexpansion of lung
reexpansion pulmonary edema
reexploration

reference coordinate system
reference line
reference site
reference standards, Wilmad
reference, sternospinal
referred pain
REFI (regional ejection fraction image)
refill, capillary
reflectant
reflected edge of Poupart ligament
reflection
  costopleural
  epicardial
  hepatoduodenal
  hepatoduodenoperitoneal
  mediastinal
  mediastinodiaphragmatic pleural
  pericardial
  peritoneal
  sternal pleural
  vertebral pleural
reflectivity, high
reflectometer tuning unit
reflex (pl. reflexes)
reflux
  abdominojugular
  acid
  bile
  duodenobiliary
  duodenogastric (DGR)
  duodenopancreatic
  free
  gastric
  gastroesophageal (GE, GER)
  hepatojugular (HJ)
  intra-renal
  nasopharyngeal
  nocturnal gastric
  vesicoureteral
reflux atrophy
reflux esophagitis

reflux gastritis
reflux grades I through V
refluxing spastic neurogenic bladder
reflux of activity
reflux regurgitation
reformation, multiplanar
reformatted planar "Christmas tree"
  MR appearance of endolymphatic
  sac
reformatting, multiplanar
refractoriness, ventricular
refractory congestive heart failure
refractory hypertension
refractory hypoxemia
refractory period of myocardium (see
  period)
refractory to treatment
refracture
region
  anesthesic
  Broca
  dark
  insular
  interseptal
  midfrontal
  periaqueductal
  photodeficient
  photopenic
  septal
  subfrontal
  task-activated brain
  temporal
  Wernicke
regional cerebral blood flow (rCBF)
  PET tomography
regional cerebral blood volume
  (rCBV) PET scan
regional cerebral metabolic rate for
  oxygen (rCMRO$_2$)
regional cerebral oxygen saturation
regional cerebral perfusion pressure
  (rCPP)

regional ejection fraction image
  (REFI)
regional left ventricular function
regional lymph nodes
regional myocardial uptake of thallium
regional oxygen extraction fraction
  (rOEF)
regional perfusion by mixed venous
  blood
regional pulmonary perfusion
regional tracer uptake
regional ventilation
regional ventricular function
regional wall motion abnormality, left
  ventricular
regional washout measurements
region of interest (ROI)
region-of-interest fluoroscopy
region-of-interest imaging technique
registration
  landmark
  robust
  spatial
  surface
  two-dimensional portal image
registration and alignment of 3D
  images
registry, STAR
Regnauld degeneration of MTP joint
regress
regression
  plaque
  polynomial step-wise multiple-
    linear
  spontaneous
  stepwise
regrowth delay
regular wedge
regulation, defective volume
regurgitant flow
regurgitant jet
regurgitant lesion

regurgitant pandiastolic flow
regurgitant pocket
regurgitant stream
regurgitant velocity
regurgitant volume
regurgitation
   aortic (AR)
   aortic valve
   congenital
   congenital aortic
   congenital mitral (CMR)
   Dexter-Grossman classification of
      mitral
   Grossman scale for
   ischemically mediated mitral
   massive aortic
   mitral
   mitral valve
   pansystolic mitral
   paravalvular
   physiologic
   pulmonary
   pulmonic (PR)
   pulmonic valve
   silent
   sour fluid
   transient tricuspid (of infancy)
   tricuspid (TR)
   tricuspid orifice
   tricuspid valve
   trivial mitral
   valvular (VR)
regurgitation index
rehabilitation (rehab), cardiac
rehydrated
Reichek method of calculating end-
   systolic wall stress
Reichert flexible sigmoidoscope
Reichert-Mundinger-Fischer
   stereotactic frame
Reid baseline
Reil, island of

reimplantation technique
reinfarction
reinjection thallium stress exam
reinnervation, motor
reinsertion
reintimalization
reintubation
re-irradiation
re-irrigation
Reiter disease
rejection
   accelerated acute
   acute
   acute renal
   allograft
   borderline severe
   chronic
   chronic humoral
   end-stage
   first-set
   focal moderate
   hyperacute
   low moderate
   resolved
   resolving
   second-set
   severe acute
   transplant
   vasculitic
rejection crisis
relapsing course
relation
   end-diastolic pressure-volume
   end-systolic pressure-volume
   force-frequency
   force-length
   force-velocity
   Frank-Starling (of heart)
relationship
   dentoskeletal
   dose-volume
   globe-orbit

relative hypoxia
relative refractory period (RRP)
relative shunt flow
relativistic mass
relaxation
   ferromagnetic
   longitudinal
   multispin
   nuclear
   nuclear electric quadrupole
   paramagnetic
   reciprocal agonist-antagonist
   spin-spin
   spin-lattice
   spin-spin
   T2 star
   tissue-based T2
   transverse
relaxation atelectasis
relaxation rate
relaxation techniques
relaxation time
   T1
   T2
relaxivity
relaxometer
   Bruker PC-10
   IBM Field-Cycling Research
Reliance urinary control stent
relief, mucosal
relief pattern
reloading, anode tube
remineralization
remitting course
remnant
   ductal
   heart
remodeling
   bone
   craniofacial
   para-articular bone
   regressive
   thrombus

remote afterloader
remote afterloading brachytherapy
   (RAB)
remote afterloading high intensity
   brachytherapy
remote control afterloading high-dose-
   rate intracavitary brachytherapy
remote control afterloading machines
remote-controlled implantation of
   radioactive source
remote-controlled production
remote diagnosis
remote history
remote lower motor neuron lesion
remyelination
renal agenesis
renal angiogram
renal angiography
renal angiomyolipoma
renal arteriography
renal artery aneurysm
renal artery occlusion
renal artery stenosis
renal atrophy
renal axis
renal calculus
renal capsule
   fatty
   fibrous
renal cocktail
renal cortex, patchy atrophy of
renal cortical isotope scanning agent
renal cortical necrosis
renal cross-fused ectopia
renal cyst study
renal duplex scan
renal dysplasia
renal failure
renal flow curve
renal function impairment
renal hemangiopericytoma
renal hypertension

renal impression on liver
renal injury
renal isthmus
renal lithiasis (renolithiasis)
renal mass lesion
renal osteodystrophy
renal parenchymal disease
renal pelvic urothelial carcinoma
renal pelvis
renal perfusion
renal pyramids
renal resistive index
renal scan, diuretic
renal scarring
renal sclerosis
renal shadow
renal shutdown
renal sinus echo
renal sinus fat
renal transplant
renal trauma
renal tubules
renal ultrasound
renal vascular damage
renal vascular hypertension (RVH)
renal vein
renal vein thrombosis
rendering
    perspective volume
    surface projection
    3D
    transparent
    volume
    voxel gradient
Rendu-Osler-Weber disease or syn-
    drome (also Weber-Osler-Rendu)
reniform contour
renin-angiotensin dependent outer
    cortex
renin-angiotensin mechanism
renin-secreting tumor
Renkin model

Renografin contrast medium
Renografin 60
renogram curve
renography, DTPA
renolithiasis (renal lithiasis)
Reno-M contrast medium
Reno-M-Dip contrast medium
Reno-M-30 contrast medium
Reno-M-60 contrast medium
renovascular hypertension
renovascular reconstruction
renovascular stent
Renovist II contrast medium
Renovue-Dip contrast medium
Renshaw cell
rent (tear or rupture)
Rentrop infusion catheter
reocclusion, post-thrombolytic
    coronary
reoxygenation
repeatability
repeated FID (free induction decay)
repeated microtraumas
reperfuse
reperfusion
    acute myocardial infarction
    controlled aortic root
    coronary
    normokalemic
reperfusion injury of postischemic
    lungs
reperfusion therapy
repetition time (TR)
repetitive seizures
repetitive strain (or stress) injury
    (RSI)
rephasing gradient
replacement
    aortic root
    aortic valve (AVR)
    ascending aneurysm
    bone

residual urine
residual urine accumulation
residual volume (RV)
residual volume/total lung capacity
　　(RV/TLC)
residue, fecal
residuum morphology
resilient artery
resistance
　　airway (RAW)
　　arteriolar
　　calculated
　　coronary vascular
　　decreased peripheral vascular
　　decreased systemic
　　expiratory
　　fixed pulmonary valvular
　　increased airways
　　increased cerebral vascular
　　increased outflow
　　increased peripheral
　　increased pulmonary vascular
　　index of runoff
　　nasal airway
　　peripheral vascular (PVR)
　　pulmonary arteriolar
　　pulmonary vascular (PVR)
　　systemic vascular (SVR)
　　total peripheral (TPR)
　　total pulmonary (TPR)
　　vascular
　　vascular systemic
　　Wood units index of
resistance blood flow
resistive exercise table
resistive index (RI)
resistive magnet
resolution
　　contrast
　　high temporal
　　interval
　　spatial

resolution stage
resolved (or resolving) rejection
resolving time
resonance
　　bandbox
　　cough
　　cracked-pot
　　nuclear magnetic (NMR)
　　skodaic
　　tympanic
　　vesicular
　　vesiculotympanic
　　vocal
　　whispering
　　wooden
resonance line
resonant frequency
resonant percussion note
resonator
　　bridged loop-gap
　　multicoupled loop-gap
resorbable pin
resorbable plate
resorbable rod
resorbable screw
resorption
　　bone
　　bony
　　dependent edema fluid
　　fluid
　　osteoclastic
resorption phase of healing
respiration gated three-dimensional
　　(3D) reconstruction
respiratory atrium
respiratory compensation
respiratory complications
respiratory compromise
respiratory decompensation
respiratory disturbance of acid base
respiratory embarrassment
respiratory excursions full and equal

respiratory frequency
respiratory gating technique
respiratory insufficiency
respiratory modulation of vascular
    impedance
respiratory motion artifacts
respiratory muscle weakness
respiratory ordered phase encoding
    (ROPE)
respiratory spasm
respiratory status, compromised
respiratory stridor
respiratory tract obstruction,
    mechanical
response
    abnormal ejection fraction
    cardioinhibitory
    controlled ventricular
    hemodynamic
    metabolic
    rapid ventricular
    regional cerebral blood flow
    slow ventricular
    therapeutic
    vagal
    vasoactive
    vasoconstrictor
    vasodepressor
    vasodilatory
    ventricular
responsive to TSH manipulation
responsiveness, airway
re-stenosis after angioplasty
restiform body
resting electrocardiogram
resting end-systolic wall stress
resting heart
resting imaging
resting MUGA scan, preoperative
resting perfusion
resting phase of cardiac action
    potentials

resting pulse
resting-redistribution thallium-201
    scintigraphy
resting regional myocardial blood
    flow
resting regional myocardial
    hypoperfusion
rest injection
rest LV (left ventricular) function
rest-redistribution exam
rest RV (right ventricular) function
rest thallium-201 myocardial imaging
restoration algorithm
restoration of sinus rhythm
restriction, unilateral flow
restrictive abnormality
restrictive bulbo-ventricular foramen
restrictive cardiac syndrome
restrictive defect
restrictive hemodynamic syndrome
restrictive lung disease
restrictive myocardial disease
restrictive-obstructive lung disease,
    mixed
restrictive pattern
restrictive ventilatory defect
result (pl. results)
    concordant
    false-positive
    false-negative
    suboptimal
resurrection bone
retained cortical activity (RCA)
retained foreign body
retained secretions
retained urine
retard premature rewarming
rete (pl. retia)
rete pegs
rete ridges
retention of barium
retention of stool

reticular activating formation (RAF)
reticular activating substance
reticular activating system (RAS)
reticular formation of brain stem
reticular infiltrate
reticular opacity
reticulation artifact
reticulocortical pathway
reticuloendothelial contrast agent
reticuloendothelial system
reticulogranular appearance
reticulogranular pattern
reticulonodular infiltrate
reticulospinal tract
reticulum
   hematopoietic (of marrow)
   arcoplasmic
reticulum cell sarcoma
retina, angiomatosis of
retinacular disruption
retinacular ligaments
retinaculum
   avulsed
   extensor
   flexor
   patellar
   superior peroneal (SPR)
retinal exudate
retinoblastoma
retraction (pl. retractions)
   chest-wall
   clot
   costal
   inspiratory
   intercostal
   late systolic
   leaflet
   midsystolic
   mild subcostal
   nipple
   postrheumatic cusp
   sternocleidomastoid

retraction *(cont.)*
   sternum
   substernal
   suprasternal
   systolic
re-treating
retrieval
   microvascular
   transvaginal oocyte
retroappendiceal fossa
retroareolar dysplasia
retrobulbar hemorrhage
retrocalcaneal bursa
retrocalcaneal exostosis
retrocalcaneal spur
retrocardiac density
retrocardiac infiltrate
retrocardiac space
retrocecal appendix
retroclavicular
retrocrural lymph nodes
retroesophageal subclavian artery
retroflexed scope
retroflexed view
retroflexion
retrograde aortogram
retrograde arterial catheterization
retrograde atherectomy
retrograde atrial activation mapping
retrograde blood flow across valve
retrograde blood velocity
retrograde conduction
retrograde coronary sinus infusion
retrograde duodenogastroscopy (RDG)
retrograde femoral arterial approach
retrograde flow on barium enema
retrograde imaging
retrograde injection
retrograde percutaneous femoral
   artery approach for cardiac
   catheterization
retrograde perfusion

retrograde peristalsis
retrograde pyelogram
retrograde pyelography
retrograde refractory period
retrograde transfemoral aortography
retrograde ureterogram
retrograde ureterography
retrograde ureteropyelogram
retrograde urethrogram
retrograde ventriculoatrial conduction
retrohepatic vena cava
retroileal appendix
retrolisthesis
retromammary space view in mammography
retromedullary arteriovenous
  malformation
retronuchal muscle
retroorbital space
retropancreatic preaortic space
retropancreatic tunnel
retropectoral mammary implant
retroperfusion
  coronary sinus
  synchronized
retroperitoneal actinomycosis
retroperitoneal approach
retroperitoneal area
retroperitoneal fibrosis
retroperitoneal hematoma
retroperitoneal region
retroperitoneal space
retroperitoneal tumor
retroperitoneal tunnel
retroperitoneally
retroperitoneum
retropharyngeal abscess
retropulsion of bone fragment into
  spinal canal
retrosellar region
retrosomatic cleft
retrosternal chest pain

retrosternal thyroid
retrotorsion, femoral
retroversion, femoral
retrovestibular neural pathway
retrusion, midface
return
  anomalous
  anomalous pulmonary venous
  central arterial
  infracardiac-type total anomalous
    venous
  paracardiac-type total anomalous
    venous
  pulmonary venous
  supracardiac-type total anomalous
    venous
  systemic venous
  total anomalous pulmonary venous
  total anomalous venous
  venous
return to baseline
Retzius
  ligament of
  line of
  space of
  system of
  vein of
REU (rectal endoscopic ultrasonography)
revascularization
  cerebral
  coronary
  coronary ostial
  endosteal
  foot
  graft
  heart
  infrainguinal
  myocardial
  percutaneous
  surgical
revascularized tissue

reverberation echos
reversal of blood flow
reversal of cervical lordosis
reversal, shunt
reversal sign
reverse Barton fracture
reverse Colles fracture
reverse distribution
reverse immunoassay
reverse redistribution
reverse transport
reversed coarctation
reversed differential cyanosis
reversed greater saphenous vein
reversed Mercedes-Benz sign
reversed peristalsis
reversed 3 sign
reversible (or resolving) ischemic
    neurologic deficit (RIND)
reversible airways disease (RAD)
reversible atrial pacing
reversible defect
reversible ischemia
reversible obstructive airway disease
    (ROAD)
reversible organic brain syndrome
reversible perfusion defects
revolving Ge-68 pins as transmission
    sources
Reye syndrome
Reynolds number
REZ (root exit zone)
RF (rapid filling)
RFA (radiofrequency ablation)
RFCA (radiofrequency catheter
    ablation)
RFP (rapid filling period)
RFW (rapid filling wave)
Rh (rhodium) isoimmunization
rhabdoid suture
rhabdoid tumor
rhabdomyolysis

rhabdomyoma of heart
rhabdomyosarcoma
    alveolar
    cardiac
    childhood
    primary
rhebosis
Rhees views of orbits
rhenium (Re)
    ^{186}Re hydroxyethylidene diphos-
        phate (HEDP)
    ^{188}Re-labeled antibodies
rheologic pattern
rheumatic adherent pericardium
rheumatic aortic insufficiency
rheumatic aortic stenosis
rheumatic chorea
rheumatic fever (RF)
rheumatic heart disease (RHD)
rheumatic lesion
rheumatic mitral stenosis
rheumatic nodule
rheumatic pneumonia
rheumatic valvular disease
rheumatoid arthritis (RA) factor
rheumatoid arthritis-associated
    interstitial lung disease
rheumatoid nodule
rheumatoid spondylitis
rheumatologist
rhinocerebral mucormycosis
rhodium (Rh)
rhomboid fossa
rhomboid ligament
rhomboid major muscle
rhomboideus muscle
rhonchus (pl. rhonchi)
RHS (radial head subluxation)
RHV (right hepatic vein)
rhythmic segmentation
RI (resistive index) angiography
RIA (radioimmunoassay) test

ridge *(cont.)*
Outerbridge
palatine
pectoral
petrous
radial
ridging
sagittal
semicircular
septal
sphenoid
supra-aortic
supracondylar
supracoronary
supraorbital
tentorial
transverse
triangular
ulnar
urethral
vastus lateralis
wolffian
riding embolus
Ridley sinus
Ridley syndrome
Riedel lobe
Riedel struma
Rieux hernia
RIF-1 tumor
right and left atrial phasic volumetric
function
right and retrograde left heart
catheterization
right-angle chest tube
right-angled telescopic lens
right anterior oblique (RAO) position
right aortic arch with mirror image
branching
right atrial enlargement
right atrial extension of uterine
leiomyosarcoma
right atrial patch positioned over the

right atrioventricular sulcus
right atrial pressure (RAP)
right atrium
right border of heart
right bundle branch block (RBBB)
right bundle branch block with left
anterior (or posterior) hemiblock
right coronary artery, dominant
right heart catheter
right heart failure
right heart pressure
right inferior epigastric artery
right internal iliac artery
right internal jugular artery
right internal mammary anastomosis
right Judkins catheter
right lateral decubitus view
right-left disorientation
right lower lobe (RLL) of lung
right main stem bronchus
right middle lobe (RML) of lung
right middle lobe lingula
right posterior oblique (RPO) position
right side down decubitus position
right-sided empyema
right-sided heart failure
right-sided pneumonia
right subclavian artery, retroesophageal
right-to-left shift
right-to-left shunt with pulmonic
stenosis
right-to-left shunting
right to left shunt of blood
right upper lobe (RUL) consolidation
right upper quadrant (RUQ)
right ventricle
augmented filling of
double-outlet
parchment
right ventricle adherent to posterior
table of sternum

right ventricle outflow tract
right ventricle-pulmonary artery
  conduit
right ventricular assist device (RVAD)
right ventricular coil
right ventricular conduction defect
right ventricular ejection fraction
  (RVEF)
right ventricular end-diastolic volume
  (RVEDV)
right ventricular end-systolic volume
  (RVESV)
right ventricular failure
right ventricular hypertrophy (RVH)
right ventricular impulse,
  hyperdynamic
right ventricular obstruction,
  intraventricular
right ventricular outflow obstruction
right ventricular outflow tract
right ventricular overload
right ventricular pressure (RVP)
right ventricular stroke volume
right ventricular stroke work (RVSW)
right ventricular stroke work index
  (RVSWI)
right ventricular systolic time interval
rigid ureter
Rigiflex TTS balloon catheter
Rigler sign
RIGScan CR49
rim
  dark signal intensity
  glenoid
  high-density
  low-density
  sclerotic
  signal intensity
rimlike calcium distribution
rim sign
RIND (reversible or resolving
  ischemic neurologic deficit)

Rindfleisch, fold of
ring (pl. rings)
  abdominal
  Ace-Colles half
  amnion
  annular
  anorectal
  aortic subvalvular
  apex of external
  arc
  atrial
  atrioventricular
  Bickel
  Cannon
  Carpentier
  cartilaginous
  CBI stereotactic
  centering
  Charnley centering
  choroidal
  ciliary
  common tendinous
  congenital (of aortic arch)
  constriction
  Crawford suture
  crural
  distal esophageal
  double-flanged valve sewing
  doughnut
  drop-lock
  esophageal A
  esophageal B
  esophageal contractile
  esophageal mucosal
  esophageal muscular
  external
  external inguinal
  femoral
  fibrocartilaginous
  fibrous
  Fischer
  fracture

R/O (rule out)
ROA (regurgitant orifice area)
ROAD (reversible obstructive airway disease)
road-mapping for interventional radiography
road-mapping mode
Robengatope radioactive agent
Robertson sign
Robicsek vascular probe (RVP)
Robin Hood phenomenon (steal syndrome)
Robinson catheter, red rubber
Robinson-Chung-Farahvar clavicular morcellation
robotics-controlled stereotactic frame
robust registration technique
ROC (receiver operating characteristics)
rocking curve measurement
rocking precordial motion
Rockwood classification of acromioclavicular injury
rod, TLD (thermoluminescent dosimeter)
RODEO (rotating delivery of excitation off-resonance), 3D
Rodriguez-Alvarez catheter
Roederer obliquity
rOEF (regional oxygen extraction fraction)
roentgen (R)
roentgen knife
roentgen stereophotogrammetric analysis (RSA)
roentgenkymography
roentgenogram
roentgenographic control
roentgenographic silhouette
roentgenography
roentgenologist
roentogenographically occult

Rogan teleradiology system
Roger syndrome
Roger ventricular septal defect
ROI (region of interest)
Rokitanski-Aschoff sinus
Rokitansky-Cushing ulcer
Rokitansky diverticulum
Rokitansky pelvis
Rolando angle
Rolando area
Rolando fissure
Rolando fracture
Rolando line
Rolando point
Rolando tubercle
roll, radiolucent
Rolleston rule for systolic blood pressure
Romano-Ward syndrome
Romberg-Wood syndrome
Romhilt-Estes score for left ventricular hypertrophy
ROMI (rule out myocardial infarction)
ROMIed
roof
    acetabular
    intercondylar
root
    anatomical
    cochlear
    coronary sinus
    cranial
    dental
    dilated aortic
    facial
    insula
    lingual
    lung
    motor
    nerve
    palatine

root *(cont.)*
  retained
  sensory
  spinal
  ventral
  ventricle
rootlets of nerve
root-mean-squared gradient measure
ROPE (respiratory ordered phase encoding)
rope-like cord (in thrombophlebitis)
ropy
Roques syndrome
Rosch catheter
rose bengal sodium ^{131}I radioactive biliary agent
Rosenbach syndrome
Rosen-Castleman-Liebow syndrome
Rosenmüller, fossa of
Rosenthal, basal vein of (BVR)
rosette appearance of anus
rostral brain stem ischemia
rostral cervical nerve
rostral connection
rostral hypothalamus
rostral medulla
rostral pons
rostral spinal cord
rostral terminus
rostrally
rostrum of corpus callosum
rostrum sphenoidale
rotary instability
rotary scoliosis
rotary subluxation
rotary thoracolumbar scoliosis
rotatable pigtail catheter
rotating bur (or burr)
rotating delivery of excitation off-resonance), 3D (RODEO)
rotating frame imaging
rotating frame of reference

rotating gamma camera
rotating tomographic projection
rotating tourniquets for pulmonary edema
rotation
  360°
  tube position
rotation therapy
rotational alignment
rotational atherectomy system (RAS)
rotational coronary atherectory (RCA)
rotational flaps
rotational force
rotational radiotherapy
rotator cuff tear
rotatory loads on spine
Rotch sign in pericardial effusion
Roubin-Gianturco flexible coil stent
rough zone
roughened state of pericardium
roughened surface
rouleaux formation
round cell tumors
round pronator (pronator radii teres)
rounded border of lung
rounded convex borders
routine magnfication view
routine view
Rouviere, ligament of
Roux-en-Y anastomosis
Roux-en-Y limb
row, carpal
row mode sinogram images
Rowe calcaneal fracture classification
Rowe-Lowell fracture-dislocation classification system
Royal Flush angiographic flush catheter
Royer-Wilson syndrome
RPA (right pulmonary artery)
rpm (rotations per minute)
RPO (right posterior oblique) position

RPT (rapid pull-through) technique
RPV (right pulmonary vein)
RSA (roentgen stereophotogrammetric
    analysis)
Rsch-Uchida transjugular liver access
    needle-catheter
RSCVP (right subclavian central
    venous pressure)
RSI (repetitive stress injury)
RT (repetition time)
RT 3200 Advantage ultrasound
    scanner
RT 6800 ultrasound scanner
RTL cassette
RTOG protocol
RTP (radiation therapy planning)
    system
RTV cassette
rubidium (Rb)
    ^{82}Rb-based cardiac imaging
Rubin test
Rubratope-57 radioactive agent
rubrospinal tract
rubrous
rudimentary bone
rudimentary ribs
rudimentary sinus
rudimentary ventricular chamber
RUE (right upper extremity)
Ruedi-Allgower tibial plafond fracture
    classification
ruga (pl. rugae)
rugal fold
rugal pattern
rugger jersey spine
RUL (right upper lobe) of lung
rule-based scheme
rule out (R/O)
rule out myocardial infarction (ROMI)
rules, Paterson-Parker
Rumel catheter

runoff
    absent
    aortic
    aortofemoral
    arterial
    digital
    distal
    inadequate
    peripheral
    single-vessel
    suboptimal
    three-vessel
    two-vessel
    vessel
runoff arteriogram
runoff resistance, index of
runoff vessel
runoff views, aortofemoral
    arteriography with
rupture
    abdominal aortic aneurysm
    aneurysma
    appendix
    Achilles tendon
    arch
    arterial
    buttonhole
    cardiac
    chordae tendineae
    chordal
    complete Achilles tendon
    contained aneurysmal
    forniceal
    interventricular septal
    myocardial
    nodal
    papillary muscle
    plantaris (tennis leg)
    plaque
    silicone implant
    ventricular free wall

rupture *(cont.)*
   ventricular septal
   vessel
rupture of membranes (ROM)
ruptured capillaries
ruptured chordae tendineae
ruptured disk
ruptured emphysematous bleb
ruptured intracranial aneurysm
ruptured thoracic duct
RUQ (right upper quadrant)
Russell-Rubinstein classification of cerebrovascular malformation
Russell-Silver syndrome
rutherford (rd) radioactive unit
Ruysch disease
RV (residual volume)
RV (right ventricle) pressure
RVA (right ventricular apical) electrogram
RVBF (reversed vertebral blood flow)
RVD (right ventricular diastolic) pressure
RVD (right ventricular dimension)
RVE (right ventricular enlargement)
RVFW (right ventricular free wall)
RVH (renal vasular hypertension)
RVH (right ventricular hypertrophy)
RVID (right ventricular internal diameter)
RVM (right ventricular mass)
RVOT (right ventricular outflow tract)
RVP (right ventricular pressure)
RVP–LVP (right ventricular to left ventricular systolic pressure) ratio
RVS (right ventricular systolic) pressure
RVSTI (right ventricular systolic time interval)
RVSW (right ventricular stroke work)
RVSWI (right ventricular stroke work index)
RV/TLC (residual volume/total lung capacity)

S, s

SAA protein
SAB (sinoatrial block)
Sabathie sign
saber shin
sac
   abdominal
   abnormal gestational
   air
   alveolar
   amniotic
   aneurysmal
   aortic
   bursal
   chorionic
   common dural
   cystic
   decidual
   dental
   double decidual
   dural
   effacement of dural
   embryonic
   endolymphatic
   enterocele
   false
   fluid-filled
   gestational

sac *(cont.)*
   greater peritoneal
   heart
   hernia
   indirect hernia
   intrauterine
   lesser peritoneal
   narrowing of thecal
   pericardial
   peritoneal
   pleural
   spinal
   terminal air
   thecal
   tight dural
   wide-mouth
   wrapped aneurysmal
   yolk
sacciform recess
saccular aneurysm
saccular appearance, lobulated
saccular bronchiectasis
saccular collection
saccular mass
sacculated pleurisy
sacculation
saccule

sacculus ventricularis
Sack-Barabas syndrome
saclike spaces
sacral ala
sacral cyst
sacral dermatomes
sacral gutter
sacral insufficiency fracture (SIF)
sacralization of vertebrae
sacralized transverse process
sacral plexus
sacral promontory
sacroabdominoperineal pull-through
sacrococcygeal chordoma
sacrococcygeal joint
sacrococcygeal remnant tumor
sacrococcygeal teratoma
sacrococcyx
sacroiliac (SI)
sacroiliac articulation
sacroiliac disease
sacroiliac joint
sacroiliac sprain
sacroiliac subluxation
sacropubic diameter
sacrosciatic foramen
sacrosciatic notch
sacrospinalis muscle
sacrotuberous ligament
sacrouterine
sacrovertebral angle
sacrum (sacral spine)
    alae of
    assimilation
    cornua of
    promontory of
    scimitar
    tilted
SACT (sinoatrial conduction time)
saddle-area anesthesia
saddle coil
saddle embolism or embolus

saddle joint
saddle points
SADIA (small angle double incidence angiograms)
Sadowsky breast marking system
SaECG (signal-averaged electro-cardiogram)
SAFHS (sonic-accelerated fracture-healing system)
Sage-Salvatore classification of acromioclavicular joint injury
sagittal gradient echo image
sagittal groove
sagittal image
sagittal oblique images
sagittal orientation
sagittal plane
sagittal plane faults
sagittal plane loop
sagittal roll spondylolisthesis
sagittal section
sagittal sinus
sagittal slice
sagittal suture
sagittal T-1 image
sagittal tomogram
sagittal transabdominal image
sagittal ultrasound
SAH (subarachnoid hemorrhage)
sail sign (of fat pad in elbow joint)
Sakellarides classification of calcaneal fracture
saline
    heparinized
    hypertonic
    sterile
saline-enhanced MR arthrography
saline-enhanced RF tissue ablation
saline loading
saline solution
saline torch
salivary gland function study

Salkowski test
salpingitis
  chronic interstitial
  follicular
  gonococcal
  hemorrhagic
  interstitial
  pseudofollicular
  purulent
  tuberculous
salpingogram
salpingography, selective osteal
salpinx (pl. salpinges)
Salpix contrast medium
salt and pepper duodenal erosion
salt wasting, cerebral
Salter-Harris classification of fracture
  (I through VI, or 1-6)
Salter-Harris-Rang classification of
  fracture
salvage, interventional limb
salvage of myocardium
salvage surgery
salvage therapy
salvo of echoes
salvo of premature ventricular
  complexes
SAM (scanning acoustic microscope)
SAM (systolic anterior motion) on
  2-D echocardiogram
samarium (Sm)
  ^{153}Sm ethylene diamine tetramethy-
    lene phosporic acid imaging
    agent
same-day microsurgical arthroscopic
  lateral-approach laser-assisted
  (SMALL) fluoroscopic diskectomy
sample points
sampling
  adrenal vein
  tissue
  zonal

SAN (sinoatrial node)
Sanchez-Perez automatic film changer
sandbag hazard
sandbagging fracture of long bones
Sandhoff disease
Sandrock test for thrombosis
sandwich patch closure, anterior
Sanfilippo syndrome
SA (sinoatrial)
SA nodal reentry tachycardia
SA node (also called sinus)
Sansom sign in pericardial effusion
Santiani-Stone classification of
  pancreatitis
Santorini
  duct of
  papilla of
saphenofemoral junction
saphenous varices
saphenous vein
  greater
  reversed greater
saphenous vein bypass graft
saphenous vein graft (SVG)
saphenous vein incompetence
sarcoid-like reaction
sarcoid of Boeck
sarcoidosis
  hepatic
  spinal cord
sarcoma (see also *carcinoma*, *tumor*)
  Abernethy
  alveolar soft part
  ameloblastic
  angiolithic
  botryoid
  cardiac
  clear cell
  endobronchial Kaposi
  endometrial stromal
  epithelioid
  Ewing

sarcoma *(cont.)*
   gastric Kaposi
   giant cell monstrocellular
   granulocytic
   hemangioendothelial
   high-grade surface osteogenic
   immunoblastic
   intracolonic Kaposi
   intracortical osteogenic
   intrathoracic Kaposi
   Ito cell
   Jensen
   juxtacortical osteogenic
   Kaposi epicardial
   Kupffer cell
   leukocytic
   lipoblastic
   low-grade central osteogenic
   lymphatic
   malignant myeloid
   medullary
   mixed cell
   multicentric osteogenic
   multiple idiopathic hemorrhagic
   myelogenic
   myeloid
   myocardial infiltration by Kaposi
   neurogenic
   osteogenic
   Paget associated osteogenic
   parosteal osteogenic
   periosteal
   postirradiation osteogenic
   primary
   pulmonary Kaposi
   reticulum cell
   right atrial
   small cell osteogenic
   spindle cell
   synovial
   telangiectatic osteogenic
   vasoablative endothelial (VABES)

Sarns wire-reinforced catheter
SAS (supravalvular aortic stenosis)
Sassone score of appearance in
   transvaginal ultrasound
satellite lesion
satellite nodule
satumomab pentetide (OncoScint
   CR/OV) imaging agent
saturation
   jugular venous oxygen
   oxygen
   regional cerebral oxygen
saturation inversion projection (SIP)
saturation recovery sequence
saturation recovery technique
saturation stripe
saturation transfer
saucer-shaped excavation
saucerization of vertebra
sausage finger, in syringomyelia
sausaging of vein
sawtooth (also saw-toothed)
   appearance
sawtooth irregularity of bowel contour
SBDX (scanning-beam digital x-ray)
SBF (systemic blood flow)
SBFT (small bowel follow-through)
SBO (small bowel obstruction)
SBO (spina bifida occulta)
SBP (systolic blood pressure)
SBSP (simultaneous bilateral
   spontaneous pneumothorax)
SCA (superior cerebellar artery)
SCAD (spontaneous coronary artery
   dissection)
SCA-EX ShortCutter catheter with
   rotating blades
scalar quantization, wavelet (WSQ)
scale
   false color
   fish
   gray

scalene fat pad
scalene musculature
scalenus anterior muscle
scalenus anticus muscle hypertrophy
scalenus anticus syndrome
scalenus minimus
scallop of posterior annulus,
    redundant
scallop, prolapsing
scalloped bowel lumen
scalloped commissure
scalloped luminal configuration
scalloping of margin of vertebral body
scan (scintiscan) (see *imaging; scanner*)
scan decrement
scan defect
Scanditronix PET scanner
Scanmaster DX scanner
Scanmaster DX x-ray film digitizer
scanned-slot detector system
scanner (also digitizer)
   Acoma
   Acuson 128EP
   Acuson ultrasound
   Advanced NMR systems
   Agfa Medical
   All-Tronics
   Aloka ultrasound linear
   Aloka ultrasound sector
   American Shared-CuraCare
   ANMR Insta-scan MR
   Artoscan MRI
   ATL Mark 600 real-time sector
   ATL real-time Neurosector
   Aurora MR breast imaging system
   Biospec MR imaging system
   Bruel-Kjaer ultrasound
   Bruker
   Canon
   Cemax/Icon
   Cencit surface
   charge-coupled device

scanner *(cont.)*
   cine CT (computed tomography)
   Compuscan Hittman computerized
     electrocardioscanner
   CT Max 640
   CT9000
   CTI 933/04 ECAT
   CTI PET
   Delarnette
   Diasonics ultrasound
   Dornier
   DuPont
   Dynamic Spatial Reconstructor
     (DSR)
   Eastman Kodak
   electron beam CT
   Elscint CT
   Elscint MR
   Elscint Twin CT
   EMED
   EMI CT
   Fonar
   4096 Plus PET
   Galen Scan
   Gammex RMI
   GE (General Electric)
   GE Advance PET
   GE CT Max
   GE 9800 CT
   GE 8800 CT/T
   GE Genesis CT
   GE GN 500 MHz
   GE HiSpeed Advantage helical CT
   GE Max MR
   GE 9800 high-resolution CT
   GE Omega 500 MHz
   GE 1.5 Tesla Signa
   GE Pace CT
   GE QE 300 MHz
   GE Signa 1.5 Tesla
   GE Signa 4.7 MRI
   GE Signa 5.2 with SR-230 3-axis
     EPI gradient upgrade

scanner *(cont.)*
  GE single axis SR-230 echo-planar
  GE Vectra MR
  Gyroscan S15
  helical CT
  Hewlett-Packard
  high field open MRI
  high field strength
  Hilight Advantage System
  Hispeed CT
  Hitachi CT
  Hitachi MR
  Hitachi 0.3T unit
  Hitachi Open MRI System
  Hologic 2000
  Howtek Scanmaster DX
  IDSI
  Imatron C-100 ultrafast CT
  Imatron C-100XL CT
  Imatron C-150L EBCT
  Imatron Fastrac C-100 cine x-ray
    CT
  Imatron Ultrafast CT
  Innervision MR
  InstaScan
  Integris 3000
  intensified radiographic imaging
    system (IRIS)
  Irex Exemplar ultrasound
  Konica
  large bore 0.6T imaging system
  large bore 1.5T imaging system
  Lumiscan
  Lunar
  LymphoScan nuclear imaging
    system
  Magna-SL
  Magnetom 1.5 T
  Magnetom SP63
  Magnes 2500 WH (whole blood)
  Magnex MR
  Mallinckrodt

scanner *(cont.)*
  Max Plus MR
  MedImage
  Medison
  Medspec MR imaging system
  midget MRI
  modified electron-beam CT
  MR catheter imaging and
    spectroscopy system
  multiple jointed digitizer
  multisensor structured light range
    digitizer
  NeuroSector
  Nishimoto Sangyo
  Norlan pQCT XCT2000
  Olympus endoscopic ultrasound
  Oxford 2T large bore imaging
    system
  Pace Plus System
  Park Medical Systems
  Perception
  PETite
  Philips CT
  Philips 1.5T NT MR
  Philips 4.7 T small bore system
  Philips Gyroscan ACS
  Philips Gyroscan NT; NT5; NT15
  Philips Gyroscan S5
  Philips Gyroscan T5
  Philips tomoscan 350 CT
  Picker CT
  Picker MR
  Picker PQ 5000 helical CT
  Picker PQ-2000 spiral CT
  Polhemus 3 digitizer
  Posicam HZ PET
  PQCT micro-scanner
  ProSpeed CT
  Quad MRI
  Quick CT9800
  rectilinear
  RT 3200 Advantage ultrasound

scanner *(cont.)*
    RT 6800 ultrasound
    Scanditronix PET
    Scanmaster DX x-ray film digitizer
    scintillation (scintiscanner)
    sector
    Shimadzu CT
    Shimadzu MR
    Siemens CT
    Siemens DRH CT
    Siemens Magnetom GBS II
    Siemens Magnetom Impact
    Siemens Magnetom 1.5 T
    Siemans Magnetom SP 4000
    Siemens Magnetom Vision
    Siemens One Tesla
    Siemens Somaform 512 CT
    Siemens Somatom DR2 whole-
       body; also DR3
    Siemens Somatom PLUS-S
    Siemens Sonoline Elegra ultra-
    sound
    Siemens SP 4000
    SieScape ultrasound
    Signa 1.5T
    Signa Horizon
    Signa I.S.T. MRI
    single-field hyperthermia combined
       with radiation therapy and ultra
       sound
    Smart Prep
    Somatom DR CT
    Somatom Plus-S CT
    spiral CT
    spiral XCT
    Swissray
    TCT900S helical CT
    Tecmag Libra-S16 system
    3D surface digitizer
    3M
    Toshiba CT
    Toshiba helical CT

scanner *(cont.)*
    Toshiba MR
    Toshiba 900S helical CT
    Toshiba 900S/XII
    Toshiba TCT-80 CT
    Toshiba Xpress SX helical CT
    Trionix
    ultrafast computed tomography
    Ultramark
    UM 4 real-time sector
    Vidar
    Vision MRI
    Vision Ten V-scan
    whole-body 1.5T Siemens Vision
    whole-body 3T MRI system
    Xpress/SX helical CT
scanning (see *imaging*)
scanning acoustic microscope (SAM)
scanning-beam digital x-ray (SBDX)
scanning laser ophthalmoscopy
scanning locus
scanogram (see *imaging*)
scanography (see *imaging*)
scan pacing
scan parameters
scan pitch
scan time
scan volume Scan-O-Grams of lower
    extremies
scan with contrast enhancement
scan without contrast enhancement
scaphocapitate joint
scaphocephalic head shape
scaphocephaly
scaphoid abdomen
scaphoid bone (navicular)
    pole of
    waist of
scapholunate (SL)
scapholunate arthritic collapse (SLAC)
    wrist
scapholunate dissociation

Schmidt optics system
Schmitt disease
Schmorl disease
Schmorl node
Schneider PTCA instruments
Schneider-Shiley catheter
Schneider Wallstent
Schonander film changer
Schönlein purpura
Schoonmaker multipurpose catheter
Schüller view
Schwann tumor
schwannoma
   facial
   orbital
   vestibular
Schwarten balloon dilatation catheter
Schwartz test for patency of deep
   saphenous veins
SCI (spinal cord injury)
sciatic artery, persistent
sciatic endometriosis
sciatic foramen
   greater
   lesser
sciatic nerve irritation
sciatic notch
   greater
   lesser
sciatic plexus
sciatica
Sci-Med or SciMed
Sci-Med Express Monorail balloon
Sci-Med SSC "Skinny" catheter
scimitar deformity
scimitar-shaped flap
scimitar-shaped shadow
scimitar sign on chest radiograph
scimitar vein
Scinticore multicrystal scintillation
   camera
scintigram

scintigraphic imaging
scintigraphic study
scintigraphy
   ACE inhibition
   AMA-Fab (antimyosin monoclonal
     antibody with Fab fragment)
   antifibrin
   bone
   bone marrow
   brain perfusion
   cortical
   dipyridamole thallium-201
   dual intracoronary
   exercise stress-redistribution
   exercise thallium
   gallium
   gated blood pool
   hepatobiliary
   indium (In)
     ^{111}In-WBC (indium with white
      blood cells)
   infarct-avid hot-spot
   iodine (I)
     ^{131}I-19-iodocholesterol
     ^{131}I MIBG
   isotope
   labeled FFA (free fatty acid)
   MIBG (metaiodobenzylguanidine)
   microsphere perfusion
   myocardial cold-spot perfusion
   NEFA (non-esterified fatty acid)
   NP-59
   planar thallium
   pulmonary
   pyrophosphate
   quantitative hepatobiliary (QHS)
   radioistope
   resting-redistribution thallium-201
   single photon planar (SPPS)
   SPECT brain perfusion
   SPECT thallium
   technetium ^{99m}Tc-PYP (pyrophos-
     phate)

scintigraphy *(cont.)*
  thallium
  thallium perfusion
  thallium-201 myocardial
  three-phase bone (TPBS)
  vesicoureteral
  white blood cell (WBCS) with
    indium-111 (^{111}In)
scintillating scotoma (pl. scotomata)
scintillation camera
scintillation counter
scintillation crystal
scintillation detector
scintillation, migrainous-like
scintillation proximity radioimmunoassay
scintillation scan
scintillation spectrometry
scintillator
  aqueous
  benzene
  CeI
  cyclohexane
  organic liquid
  toluene
scintimammography (SMM)
scintiphotograph
scintirenography
scintiscan (see *imaging*)
scintiscanner (see *scanner*)
scintiscanning
Scintiview nuclear computer system
Scintron IV nuclear computer system
scirrhous carcinoma
scirrhous lesion
scissor gait
scissoring of legs
SCL (sinus cycle length)
SCLC (small-cell lung cancer)
scleroderma of esophagus
sclerosing nonsuppurative osteomyelitis

sclerosis
  Ammon horn (mesial temporal)
  aortic
  arterial
  arteriocapillary
  arteriolar
  Baló
  calcified
  congenital hippocampal
  coronary
  diffuse
  disseminated
  endocardial
  esophageal variceal
  familial amyotrophic lateral
  gastric
  hepatic
  hepatoportal
  hippocampal
  incisural
  Krabbe diffuse
  laser
  lobar
  medial calcific
  mesenteric
  mesial temporal
  Mönckeberg
  multiple (MS)
  pedicle
  posterolateral (of the spinal cord)
  progressive systemic
  pulmonary and cardiac
  renal
  segmental vein
  subchondral
  subendocardial
  tuberous
  valvular
  variceal
  vascular
  venous
sclerotic area

sclerotic coronary arteries
sclerotic degeneration
sclerotic plaque (plaquing)
sclerotic rims in gout
scoliosis
   adolescent idiopathic (AIS)
   Aussies-Isseis unstable
   Cobb measurement of
   dextrorotary
   dextro-
   Dwyer correction of
   Fergusson method for measuring
   fixation of a
   functional
   idiopathic
   King classification of thoracic
   King-Moe
   levorotary
   levo-
   lumbar
   lumbar component of
   Moe and Kettleson distribution of
     curves in
   rotary
   S-shaped
   thoracic
   thoracolumbar
   uncompensated rotary
   Winter-King-Moe
scoliotic spine
SCOOP 1 transtracheal oxygen
  catheter
SCOOP 2 catheter with distal and
  side openings
score
   late effects toxicity
   LENT (late effects of normal
     tissues)
   mean wall motion
   thallium SPECT
   wall motion
scorings on bone on x-ray

scotoma (pl. scotomata)
   absolute
   bilateral
   cecocentral
   central
   dense
   fortification
   homonymous scintillating
   paracentral
   relative
   scintillating
scotometry
scotomization
scout film
scout image
scout negative film
ScoutView targeting
scrambled image
screen
   guilt
   Lanex Medium
   RF (radiofrequency)
screen craze artifact
screen-film mammogram
screening-detected abnormality
screening mammography
screw
   cancellous
   metallic
   transfixing
screw and plate (screw-plate)
screw fixation
screw-in ceramic acetabular cup
scrotal hernia
SCT (star-cancellation test)
SCTA (spiral CT angiography)
scybalum (pl. scybala)
scyphoid
SDBP (systemic diastolic blood
  pressure)
SDH (subdural hemorrhage)
S distortion

SDRI (small, deep, recent infarct)
SE (spin-echo) image
SE 1500/40 MR images
SE 300/17 MR images
SEA (spinal epidural abscess)
seal and suction
seat belt fracture
seat belt injury
seat belt sign
sebaceum, adenoma (in tuberous
   sclerosis)
second cranial nerve (optic)
second portion of duodenum
secondary cartilaginous joint
secondary electron production
secondary extravasation of
   intravascular contents
secondary fracture
secondary hypertension
secondary sonographic findings
secondary venous insufficiency
secretin
secretion-filled medium-sized bronchi
secretory capacity of the ACTH
   dependent inner adrenal cortex
section
   axial
   cesarean
   Compton scattering cross-
   coronal
   cross-
   elastic cross-
   flood
   sagittal
   serial
   serpiginous
   step
   transverse
section-select flow compensation
section-select pulse
section-sensitivity profiles

sector
   lower field visual
   Sommer (of the hippocampus)
sector echocardiography
sector probe, biplane
sector scan echocardiography
sector scanning
secundum atrial septal defect (ASD)
Seddon classification of nerve injuries
seeding
   intracranial
   metastatic
   prostate
   radioactive
   TheraSeed (palladium-103) active
     isotope in titanium capsule
   tumor
seed points
seed voxel
segment
   akinetic
   angulated
   anterior
   anterior basal
   anterobasal
   anterolateral
   apex
   apical
   apicoposterior
   arterial
   bronchopulmonary
   cardiac
   coarcted
   contiguous
   diaphragmatic
   distal
   endarterectomized
   expansile aortic
   hypokinetic
   infarcted lung
   inferior

segment *(cont.)*
   inferior basal
   inferoapical
   inferoposterior
   interleaved inversion-readout
   liver
   meatal
   nonfilling venous
   noninfarcted
   posterior
   posterior apical
   posterobasal
   posterolateral
   proximal
   pulmonary
   septal wall
   septum
   superior
   Ta
   vaterian
   venous
segment distraction
segmental atelectasis
segmental bone loss
segmental bowel infarction
segmental branch of artery
segmental bronchus (pl. bronchi)
   cardiac
   lateral
   lateral basal
   medial
   medial basal
   posterior
   posterior basal
   superior
segmental consolidation
segmental defect
segmental distribution of
   syringomyelia
segmental fracture
segmental ischemia

segmental lesion
segmental limb pressure
segmental lower extremity Doppler
   pressures
segmental narrowing
segmental orifice
segmental perfusion abnormality
segmental plethysmography
segmental pneumonia
segmental renal artery waveform
segmental sign
segmental symptoms
segmental wall motion abnormality
   akinetic
   dyskinetic
   hyperkinetic
   hypokinetic
segmentation
   automatic lumen edge
   Cannon
   lung
   MR imaging
   rhythmic
   vascular
segmentation method for real-time
   display
segmented k-space cardiac tagging
segmented k-space time-of-flight MR
   angiography
segmented k-space turbo gradient
   echo breath-hold sequence
segmenting dual echo MR head scan
Segond fracture
SEH (spinal epidural hemorrhage)
SeHCAT (selenium-labeled homo-
   cholic acid conjugated with
   taurine) test
SEI (subendocardial infarction)
Seikosha video printer for scans
Seinsheimer classification of femoral
   fracture

senile dementia, Alzheimer type (SDAT)
senile emphysema
senile nevus
senile osteoporosis
senile subcapital fracture
Senographe 500 T mammography
sensing coil
sensitive plane projection reconstruction imaging
sensitive point scanning
sensitive volume
sensitivity
   line-shape
   percussion
   uniform
sensitize
sensitization
sentinel fold
sentinel loop
sentinel node
sentinel pile (hemorrhoid)
sentinel transoral hemorrhage
separation
   AC (acromioclavicular)
   aortic cusp
   atlantoaxial
   atlanto-occipital
   carrier-free
   chromatographic
   costochondral junction
   fracture fragment
   leaflet
   selective
   shoulder
sepsis, intra-abdominal (IAS)
septal accessory pathway
septal amplitude
septal arcade
septal area
septal band
septal cardiac defect

septal collateral
septal cusp of valve
septal defect
   atrial
   atrioventricular
   interventricular
septal dip
septal hypertrophy, asymmetric
septal hypokinesis
septal hypoperfusion on thallium scan
septal infarction
septal leaflet
septal necrosis
septal papillary muscle
septal pathway
septal perforation
septal perforator branch
septal perforators
septal region
septal ridge
septal separation
septal thickness
septal wall thickness
septation
septic embolus (pl. emboli)
septic lung syndrome
septic necrosis
septic pleurisy
septic pulmonary emboli
septic pulmonary infarction
septic shock
septic thrombosis
septicemia
septomarginal trabecula
septum (pl. septa)
   alveolar
   anal intermuscular
   anteroapical trabecular
   aortic
   aortopulmonary
   asymmetric hypertrophy of
   atrial

septum *(cont.)*
  atrioventricular
  bronchial
  bulbar
  canal
  cartilaginous
  conal
  conus
  crural
  distal bulbar
  dyskinetic
  femoral
  gingival
  infundibular
  intact ventricular
  interatrial (IAS)
  interhaustral
  interlobar
  interlobular
  intermuscular
  internal intermuscular
  interventricular (IVS)
  mediastinal
  membranous
  muscular atrioventricular
  nasal
  perirenal
  posterior median (of cord)
  rectovaginal
  rectovesical
  sinus
  thickened
  ventricular
sequela (pl. sequelae)
  clinical
  late normal tissue
  neuroendocrinological
  significant
sequence (pl. sequences)
  breath-hold GRE
  Carr-Purcell
  Carr-Purcell-Meiboom-Gill

sequence *(cont.)*
  conventional pulse
  CPMG
  DANTE
  diffusion pulse
  diffusion-weighted pulse
  dual echo
  dual GRE pulse
  echo-planar
  echo-planar pulse sequence
  FFE
  FLAIR
  FISP
  FLASH 3D
  flow-compensated gradient-echo
  FMPSRGR
  gradient echo
  gradient-echo imaging
  gradient-echo pulse
  GRASS pulse
  in-phase
  interleaved GRE
  inversion recovery
  Klippel-Feil
  magnetization-prepared rapid
    acqusition gradient-echo
  MP-RAGE (magnetization
    prepared 3D gradient-echo)
  multi-slice spin echo
  multiecho
  opposed-phase
  partial saturation
  PRESS
  pulsed
  saturation recovery
  short T1 inversion recovery (STIR)
  single-shot adiabatic localization
    pulse
  SPAMM
  spin echo
  spin-echo pulse
  spin-echo imaging

sequence *(cont.)*
  spiral pulse
  susceptibility-sensitive
  3DFT-CISS
  3D GRE (gradient-recalled echo)
  3D-PSIF
  3D spoiled GRE
  TONE (tilted optimized nonsaturating excitation)
  Turbo-FLASH
  voiding
  three-dimensional time-of-flight MR angiographic
  turbo SE
sequence processor
sequence time
sequential balloon inflation
sequential bypass graft
sequential dilatations
sequential extraction-radiotracer technique
sequential graft
sequential image acquisition
sequential in situ bypass
sequential monophasic shocks
sequential obstruction
sequential pacing
sequential plane imaging
sequential point imaging
sequential quantitative MR imaging
sequential scalar quantization (SSQ)
sequential compression device, Kendall
sequestered lobe of lung
sequestration
  fluid
  third space
sequestrum (pl. sequestra)
  associated
  bony
  necrotic
  primary

sequestrum *(cont.)*
  secondary
  tertiary
SER-IV (supination, external rotation-type IV) fracture
serendipity view
serial changes
serial contrast MR
serial cut film technique
serial duplex scan
serial images
serial lesions
serialography
serial splinting
serial static image
series
  abdominal
  acute abdominal
  dynamic
  sinus
  small bowel
  upper GI (gastrointestinal)
Series-II humeral head
seriography
seromuscular layer
serosa
serosal surface
serosanguineous fluid
serotonin (5-HIAA)
serotonin (S2) receptors
serous cystadenoma
serous membrane
serous pericardium
serous pleurisy
serpiginous ulceration
serrated catheter
serration, marginal
serratus anterior muscle
Sertoli-Leydig cell tumor
sesamoid bones of foot
  accessory
  bipartite

shag, aortic
shagging of cardiac borders
shaggy aorta syndrome
shagreen patches in tuberous sclerosis
Shames model
shape (shaped)
  barrel-
  boat
  brachycephalic head
  dumbbell-
  half-moon
  head
  horseshoe
  hourglass
  mesocephalic head
  oval
  ovoid-
  S-
  scaphocephalic head
  scaphoid
  sickle
  spherical
  spheroid-
Shape Maker system
shape recovery
sharp border of lung
sharp carina
sharp dissection
sharp lateral margin
Sharp-Purser test
shaver catheter
shaving
  femoral condylar
  patellar
shavings, residual metal fragment
Shaw catheter
SHC (sclerosing hepatic carcinoma)
shear fracture
shearing forces (on sacroiliac joints in
  runners)
shearing of white matter (in head
  injury)

shearing stress
shear rate
shear stress
sheath
  angioplasty
  anterior rectus
  arterial
  carotid
  catheter
  caudal
  check-valve
  common synovial flexor
  Cordis
  crural
  dentinal
  dural
  extensor carpi ulnaris
  fascial
  femoral artery
  fenestrated
  fibrous
  flexor tendon
  ganglionic cyst in synovial tendon
  guiding
  Henle
  intratendon
  introducer
  muscle
  myelin
  nerve
  nerve root
  neural
  peel-away
  periradicular
  pilar
  plicated dural
  posterior rectus
  rectus
  Schwann cell of myelin
  self-expanding tulip
  synovial
  tearaway

shock-monitoring method
Shone anomaly
short-arm Grollman catheter
short axis acquisition
short axis images
short axis parasternal view
short axis plane on echocardiography
short axis slice
short bone
short-distance radiotherapy (brachytherapy)
short echo time
short echo time proton spectroscopy
short half-life
short head of biceps
short inversion time inversion
   recovery (STIR) (MRI)
short pulse
short rib-polydactyly syndrome
short T1 inversion recovery (STIR)
   sequence
short T1 relaxation time
short TE, long TR
short TR/TE (repetition time/echo
   time) (T1-weighted image)
shortening
   Achilles tendon
   fractional myocardial
   leg
   mean rate of circumferential
   phalangeal
   skeleton
   suboccipital
   tendon
   T2 (second thoracic vertebra)
shotty lymph node
shoulder
   baseball
   drop
   flail
   frozen
   knocked-down

shoulder *(cont.)*
   Little Leaguer
   loose
   Neviaser classification of frozen
   ring man (in gymnasts)
   sprained
   swimmer's
   tennis
shoulder compression test
shoulder depression test
shoulder-hand-finger syndrome
shoulder immobilizer
shoulder of heart
shoulder pointer
shoulder prosthesis
shoulder rock test
shoulder separation
shoulder-upper extremity-thoracic
   outlet syndrome
shower of echoes
shrinkage, graft
shrinkage of ganglion cells
shrugging sign
shrunken gallbladder
SHU 454 (Echovist) imaging agent
SHU 508A (Levovist) imaging agent
shudder of carotid arterial pulse
shunt (also shunting)
   aorta to pulmonary artery
   aorticopulmonary
   aortopulmonary
   apicoaortic
   arteriovenous (A-V)
   ascending aorta to pulmonary
     artery
   atrial right-to-left
   barium-sulfate impregnated
   bidirectional
   biliopancreatic
   Blalock
   Blalock-Taussig
   Buselmeier

shunt *(cont.)*
   cardiac
   cardiovascular
   central aortopulmonary
   Cordis-Hakim
   CSF (cerebrospinal fluid)
   cysto-atrial
   Davidson
   Denver hydrocephalus
   Denver peritoneal venous
   descending aorta-pulmonary artery
   descending thoracic aorta to
      pulmonary artery
   dialysis
   distal splenorenal (DSR)
   DVP flush
   end-to-side portacaval
   esophageal
   extracardiac right-to-left
   gastric venacaval
   Glenn
   Gore-Tex
   Gott
   Hakim-Cortis ventriculoperitoneal
   hermetic external
   Heyer-Schulte neurosurgical
   high-pressure
   Holter
   Hyde
   infant
   intracardiac right-to-left
   intrapericardial aorticopulmonary
   intrapulmonary
   ISCI
   Javid endarterectomy
   left-to-right
   LeVeen peritoneal
   Linton
   low-pressure
   lumbar arachnoid peritoneal
   lumboperitoneal (LP)
   medium-pressure

shunt *(cont.)*
   mesocaval H-graft
   mesocaval interposition
   migration of
   modified Blalock-Taussig
   net
   Ommaya ventriculoperitoneal
   one-piece
   peritoneal-atrial
   peritoneocaval
   peritoneovenous (PVS)
   portacaval
   portopulmonary
   portosystemic vascular
   posterior fossa-atrial
   Potts
   preferential
   proximal splenorenal
   Pruitt-Inahara carotid
   Pudenz
   Quinton-Scribner
   reversed (right-to-left)
   right-to-left (reversed)
   side-to-side portacaval
   small-bowel
   Spetzler lumboperitoneal
   splenorenal
   subclavian artery to pulmonary
      artery
   subclavian-pulmonary
   subdural to peritoneal
   Sundt loop
   supracardiac
   systemic-pulmonary artery
   T-tube
   thecoperitoneal
   transjugular intrahepatic
      portosystemic
   UNI-SHUNT hydrocephalus
   vena cava to pulmonary artery
   venoarterial
   ventriculoatrial (VA)

shunt *(cont.)*
   ventriculojugular (VJ)
   ventriculoperitoneal (VP)
   ventriculopleural
   ventriculovenous
   Wakabaushi
   Warren splenorenal
   Waterston
   Waterston-Cooley
shunted blood
shunted tracer
shunt flow
   anatomic
   physiologic
   relative
shunt function, cerebrospinal fluid
shunting of blood
   left-to-right
   marked
   right-to-left
shuntogram
shunt quantification
shunt reservoir
shunt reversal
shunt syndrome, lumbar thecoperitoneal
shunt valve
shutdown, renal
SI (sacroiliac) joint
   SI joint to sacrum ratio
SI (saturation index) of bile
SI (signal intensity)
SI (sinus irregularity)
SI (stroke index)
Si(Li) x-ray detector
sialography CT
sialography MRI
Sibson fascia
sick sinus node
sick sinus syndrome (SSS)
   extrinsic
   intrinsic

sickle cell disease
sickle-shaped fold
SICOR (computer-assisted cardiac
   catheter recording system)
side branch occlusion
side-by-side transposition of great
   arteries
side-hole catheter
side-to-side anastomosis
siderosis
siderotic splenomegaly
sideswipe elbow fracture
sidewall, pelvic
sidewinder catheter
Siemens AG system
Siemens DRH CT scanners
Siemens gamma camera
Siemens LINAC (linear accelerator)
Siemans Magnetom 1.5 T
Siemans Magnetom SP 4000 scanner
Siemens Mevatron 74 linear
   accelerator
Siemens One Tesla scanner
Siemens Satellite CT Evaluation
   Console
Siemens Somaform 512 CT scanner
Siemens Somatom DR2 whole-body
   scanner (also DR3)
Siemens Somatom PLUS-S imager
   (scanner)
Siemens SP 4000 scanner
sigmoid cavity of radius
sigmoid cavity of ulna
sigmoid colon volvulus
sigmoid curve
sigmoid notch
sigmoid omentum
sigmoid sinus
sigmoid valve
sign
   Aaron
   Abrahams

sign *(cont.)*

    ace of spades (on angiogram)
    Achilles bulge
    Adson
    Allen
    Allis
    Amoss
    amputation
    angel wing
    Anghelescu
    antecedent
    anterior tibial
    antler
    anvil
    aortic arch aneurysm
    aortic nipple
    apical cap
    Apley
    applesauce
    Ashhurst
    Auenbrugger
    Babinski
    Baccelli (of pleural effusion)
    bagpipe
    ball-bearing eye
    Ballance
    Bamberger
    banana
    Bancroft
    barber pole
    Barlow
    Battle
    bayonet
    beading
    Becker
    Beevor
    Bethea
    beveled edge
    Biermer
    bilateral pyramidal
    Biot
    Bird

sign *(cont.)*

    Blumberg
    Bouillaud
    bow-tie
    bowler hat
    bowstring
    Boyce
    Bozzolo
    Bragard
    brain stem
    Branham arteriovenous fistula
    Braunwald
    brim
    Broadbent inverted
    Brockenbrough-Braunwald
    Brudzinski
    Bryant
    Burton
    buttock
    camelback
    Cantelli
    Cardarelli
    cardinal
    cardiorespiratory
    Carnett
    carotid string
    Carvallo
    Castellino
    Cegka
    cerebral
    Chaddock
    chain of lakes
    Chilaiditi
    choppy sea
    Christmas tree
    Chvostek-Weiss
    Claybrook
    Cleeman
    clockwise whirlpool
    cobblestoning
    Codman
    Cogan lid twitch

sign *(cont.)*

   cogwheel
   Cole
   Collier
   colon cut-off
   commemorative
   Comolli
   contralateral
   Coopernail
   cord
   Corrigan
   cortical
   corticospinal tract
   coughing
   Courvoisier
   cranial nerve
   crescent
   crescent-in-doughnut (for
      intussusception)
   cross-chest impingement
   crossed sciatica
   Cruveilhier
   cuff
   Cullen
   D'Amato
   Dance
   Dawbarn
   Dejerine
   de la Camp
   de Musset (aortic aneurysm)
   de Mussey (pleurisy)
   Delbet
   Delmege
   delta
   Demianoff
   dense sigmoid sinus
   dense vein
   Desault
   Deyerle
   displaced fat pad
   doll's eye
   doorbell

sign *(cont.)*

   Dorendorf
   dorsal column
   double bubble
   double-bubble duodenal
   double camelback
   Drummond
   Duchenne
   Dupuytren
   dural trail
   Duroziez
   d'Espine
   E
   Ebstein
   Egawa
   Ellis
   empty delta
   Erb
   Erichsen
   Ewart
   extrapyramidal tract
   Fajersztajn crossed sciatic
   false localizing
   fan
   fat pad
   Federici
   figure 3
   fingertip
   Finkelstein
   Fischer
   fissure
   flapping tremor
   Fleck
   Fleischner
   focal neurologic
   Forestier bowstring
   Frank
   Fränkel
   Franz
   Friedreich
   Froment paper
   frontal lobe

sign *(cont.)*
    Fürbringer
    Gaenslen
    Gage
    Galant
    Galeazzi
    Gerhardt
    Gilbert
    Glasgow
    gloved finger
    Goldthwait
    gooseneck
    Gordon
    Gowers
    Grancher
    Green-Joynt
    Greene
    Grey Turner
    Griesinger
    Grocco
    Grossman
    guarding
    Guilland
    Gunn crossing
    Hall
    halo
    Hamman pneumopericardium
    harlequin eye
    Hart
    Heim-Kreysig
    Helbing
    Henning
    Hill
    Hirschberg
    Hoffmann
    Homans
    Honda
    Hoover
    Hope
    Horn
    hot-cross-bun skull
    hot nose

sign *(cont.)*
    Howship-Romberg
    Huchard
    Hueter fracture
    Huntington
    hyperdense middle cerebral artery
    hyperintensive ring
    iliopsoas
    inverted V
    J
    Jaccoud
    Jackson
    Jenet
    jugular
    jump
    Jürgensen
    Kanavel
    Kantor
    Kaplan
    Karplus
    Katz-Wachtel
    Keen
    Kehr
    Kellgren
    Kellock
    Kernig
    Kerr
    Klemm
    knuckle
    Kocher-Cushing
    Korányi-Grocco
    Kussmaul venous
    Lachman
    Laënnec
    Lancisi
    Landolfi
    Langoria
    Lasègue
    lateralizing
    Laugier
    Lazarus
    Leichtenstern

sign *(cont.)*
- lemon
- Lennhoff
- Leri
- Leser-Trelat
- Levine
- Lhermitte
- Linder
- linguine (in breast)
- liver flap
- liver-jugular
- Livierato abdominocardiac
- localizing neurological
- lollipop tree
- long-tract
- Lorenz
- Lowenberg
- lower motor neuron
- Ludloff
- Macewen
- Mahler
- Maisonneuve
- Mannkopf
- Marie-Foix
- McBurney
- McCort
- McGinn-White
- McMurray
- Meltzer
- Mendel-Bekhterev
- meningoencephalitic
- meniscus
- Mennell
- Mercedes-Benz
- Minor
- Morquio
- Morton-Horwitz nerve cross-over
- Moschcowitz (of arterial occlusive disease)
- motor
- moulage
- movie

sign *(cont.)*
- Mulder
- Müller (Mueller) aortic regurgitation
- Murphy
- Musset (de Musset)
- mute toe
- Myerson
- Naffziger
- Neer impingement
- negative delta (on CT)
- Negro
- Nelson
- Neri bowing
- neurologic soft
- Nicaladoni-Branham
- nubbin
- obturator
- oculomotor
- Oliver-Cardarelli
- ominous
- Oppenheim
- orbicularis
- organic (of brain damage)
- Ortolani
- Osler
- pad
- panda
- parietal lobe
- Parrot
- patent bronchus
- pathognomonic
- pathologic lid retraction
- Paul
- Payr
- percussion
- Perez
- peripheral washout
- peritoneal
- peroneal
- Pfuhl-Jaffé
- Phalen

sign *(cont.)*
  phonatory
  piano key
  pillow
  Pins
  Piotrowski
  piston
  pivot-shift
  plane
  plumb-line
  Plummer
  positive bottle
  postural motor
  Potain
  Pott
  Pottenger
  precursor
  premonitory
  Prevel
  Prévost
  pronation
  pronator
  pruning
  Prussian helmet
  pseudo-Babinski
  pseudobulbar
  pseudo-Foster-Kennedy
  pseudo-Romberg
  psoas
  puddle
  pupillary
  pyloric string
  pyramidal
  Queckenstedt
  Quénu-Muret
  Quincke
  rabbit ear
  raccoon eyes
  rachitic rosary
  radialis
  railroad track
  Raimiste

sign *(cont.)*
  rat-tail
  rebound
  Renee creak
  reversal
  reversed 3
  reversed Mercedes Benz
  Rigler
  rim
  ring of cribriform plate fracture
  Riordan
  Risser
  Rivero-Carvallo
  Riviere
  Robertson
  Romberg
  Rosenbach
  Rotch
  Rothschild
  Rovighi
  Rovsing
  Rust
  Sabathie
  sail
  Sanders
  Sansom
  Sarbo
  sawtooth appearance
  Schepelmann
  Schick
  Schlesinger
  Schoeber
  scimitar
  seat belt
  segmental
  Seguin
  Seitz
  setting-sun
  Shapiro
  Shibley
  shrugging
  Sister Mary Joseph

sign *(cont.)*

    Skoda

    Smith

    soft neurologic

    somatic

    sonographic Murphy

    Soto-Hall

    Spalding

    Speed

    spinal

    spread suture

    Spurling

    square-root

    stairs

    steeple

    Steinberg thumb

    Steinmann

    Sterles

    Sterling-Okuniewski

    Sternberg

    Stewart-Holmes

    Stierlin

    Strauss

    string

    string of pearls

    stripe

    Strümpell (Struempell)

    Strunsky

    Sumner

    tandem Romberg

    target

    Terry fingernail

    Terry-Thomas

    tethered-bowel

    theater

    Thomas

    thorn

    thumbprinting

    Thurston-Holland

    tibialis (of Strümpell)

    Tinel percussion

    toe spread

sign *(cont.)*

    trapezius ridge

    Traube aortic regurgitation

    Trimadeau

    tripod

    Troisier

    Trömner (Troemner)

    Trousseau

    Turner

    Turyn

    Uhthoff

    unilateral Babinski

    upper motor neuron

    VAD (voluntary anterior drawer)

    Vanzetti

    vein

    versive motor

    vital

    voluntary posterior drawer (VPD)

    Voshell

    VPD (voluntary posterior drawer)

    Waddell

    Walter-Murdoch wrist

    Wartenberg

    Weill

    Weiss

    Westermark

    wet leather

    whirlpool

    white cerebellum

    white matter

    Williams

    Williamson

    Wilson

    wind sock (echocardiogram)

    windshield wiper

    winking owl spinal

    Wintrich

    Yergason

Signa GEMS MR imaging system

Signa Horizon scanner

Signa I.S.T. MRI scanner

Signa 1.5T scanner
signal
  color Doppler
  D
  differential
  disk water
  Doppler flow
  flow
  hyperintense
  hypointense
  lipid
  magnetic resonance
  mosaic-jet
  NAA metabolite
  stimulus-correlated
  water
signal acquisitions
signal blooming
signal dephasing
signal fallout
signal intensity (SI)
signal intensity curve
signal intensity time curves
signal loss
signal magnification
signal mass
signal time-course
signal-to-clutter ratio
signal-to-noise ratio (SNR or S/N
  ratio)
signal void
signature, echo
signet ring appearance
signet ring carcinoma
signet ring pattern
significant axis deviation
significant, clinically
significant residual deficit
significant sequelae
Silastic catheter
Silastic stent
silence, electrocerebral (ECS)

silent areas of brain
silent gallstone
silent ischemia
silent mitral stenosis
silent myocardial infarction
silent myocardial ischemia
silent patent ductus arteriosus
silent regurgitation
silhouette
  cardiac (large thymus shadow
    obscuring)
  cardiovascular
  enlarged cardiac
  luminal
  roentgenographic
  widened cardiac
silhouette image
Silicon Graphics Reality Engine
  system
silicone implant rupture (seen on MRI)
Silicore catheter
silicosis
silicotic fibrosis of lung
silicotic nodule with central necrosis
silicotic visceral pleura
silicotuberculosis
silver-fork deformity
silver-fork fracture
SIM (small intestine mesentery)
Simmons 1, 2, and 3 catheter
Simmons-type sidewinder catheter
Simon nitinol percutaneous IVC filter
simple dislocation
simple fracture, complex
simple shift
simplex, xanthoma tuberosum
Simplus PE/t dilatation catheter
Simpson atherectomy catheter
Simpson atherectomy device, PET balloon
Simpson Coronary AtheroCath (SCA)
  system

sinus venous defect
sinuvertebral nerve (of Luschka)
SIP (saturation inversion projection)
siphon, carotid
SIR angiogram
Sister Mary Joseph node
site
    de-airing
    fracture
    ipsilateral antegrade
    reference
site of arterial puncture
site of maximal intensity
site-specific labeling
sitting-up view
situs ambiguus of atria
situs
    atrial
    D-loop ventricular
    L-loop ventricular situs
situs atrialis solitus
situs concordance
situs inversus
situs inversus totalis
situs inversus viscerum
situs perversus
situs solitus
    atrial
    visceral
situs transversus
situs viscerum inversus
6-[^{18}F] fluoro-DOPA
sixth compartment
sixth cranial nerve (abducens nerve)
sixth intercostal space
60° left anterior oblique projection
60 MHz Fourier Transform NMR
    spectrometer
60 MHz Rapid Scan spectrometer
64 x 64 byte mode
size and caliber
size and configuration

size estimation error
size, particle
sizer, prosthetic valve
sizing, balloon
sizing ring
Sjögren syndrome
SJS (Schwartz-Jampel syndrome)
skeletal amyloidosis
skeletal bed
skeletal disruption
skeletal emphysema
skeletal hyperostosis
skeletal hypoplasia
skeletally immature
skeletally mature
skeletal metastases
skeletal radiology
skeletal survey, isotopic
skeletal traction
skeleton
    appendicular
    articulated
    axial
    bony
    cardiac
    fibrous
    gill arch
    spidering
    spiky
    sulcal
    visceral
skeleton shortening
skeletonizing
skier's fracture
skier's thumb
Skillern fracture
skin bridge
skin crease artifact
skin depth
skin fold artifact
skin lesion artifact
skin lines

Skinny over-the-wire balloon catheter
skin-rolling scapular tenderness
skin thickening
Skiodan contrast medium
skip lesions of Crohn disease
Skoda sign
skull
   beaten silver appearance of
   cloverleaf
   foramen magnum of
   hammer-marked, secondary to
     thinning
   hot-cross-bun
   lytic lesion of the
   molding of
   sonolucent
skull asymmetry
skull base
skullcap
skull defect, postoperative
skull films
skull fracture
   basilar
   compound
   depressed
   depressed and compound
   linear
   simple
   stellate
   undepressed
skull hyperostosis
skull plate
skyline view of patella
SL (scapholunate) joint
slab (pl. slabs)
   coronal
   interleaved axial
SLAC (scapholunate arthritic collapse)
   wrist
slant hole collimator
SLAP (superior labrum anterior
   posterior) lesion

slate-gray cyanosis
SLE (systemic lupus erythematosus)
slew rate
slice
   angled
   apical short-axis
   axial
   basal short-axis
   contiguous
   coronal
   digitized CT
   horizontal long-axis
   intermediate CT
   long axis
   mid-ventricular short-axis
   plurality of
   sagittal
   serial CT
   short-axis
   texture
   tissue
   tomographic
   transaxial
   transverse
   vertical long-axis
slice format
slice fracture
slice orientation
slice-overlap artifact
slice sensitivity profile (SSP)
slice thickness
slice volume
slicing planes
sliding-type hiatal hernia
Slinky catheter
slip angle
slip-in connection
slippage, film
slipped capital femoral epiphysis
slipped disk
slipped tendon
slipped upper femoral epiphysis
   (SUFE)

slipping rib syndrome
slip-ring camera
slip-ring CT
slip-ring technology
SLJD (Sinding-Larsen-Johansson
   disease)
slope
   closing (on echo)
   D to E (of mitral valve)
   decreased E to F (E-F)
   disappearance
   E to F (of mitral valve)
   flat diastolic
   flattened E to F
   opening (on echo)
   ST/HR (ST segment/heart rate)
   valve opening
slot blot analysis
sloughed mucosa
sloughed papilla
sloughed urethra syndrome
slow-channel blocking drugs
slow filling wave
slow-flow lesions
slow-flow vascular anomaly
slow-flow vascular malformation
slow neutron
sludge
   biliary
   blood
   gallbladder
sluggishly flowing blood
Sm (samarium)
SMA (smooth muscle antibody)
SMA (superior mesenteric artery)
SMALL (same-day microsurgical
   arthroscopic lateral-approach laser-
   assisted) fluoroscopic diskectomy
small airway dysfunction
small angle multiple scattering
small aorta syndrome
small bowel contents

small bowel follow-through (SBFT)
small bowel infarct
small bowel series
small bowel transit time
small cardiac vein
small cell carcinoma of the lung
small cell lung cancer (SCLC)
small cuff syndrome
small feminine aorta
small field-of-view (FOV) MR
   imaging
small-lunged emphysema
small saphenous vein
small vessel stroke
small water-hammer pulse
Smart Prep imaging agent
Smart Prep scanner
SmartSpot high resolution digital
   imaging system
SMAS (superior mesenteric artery
   syndrome)
smear fragment
Smec balloon catheter
SMIS console
Smith fracture
SMM (scintimammography)
smokelike echoes
smooth hyperplasia
smooth muscle tumor
SMPTE (Society of Motion Picture
   and Television Engineers) test
   pattern (teleradiology)
SMV (superior mesenteric vein)
S/N (signal-to-noise) ratio
snake graft
snapping hip syndrome
snapshot, contrast-enhanced dynamic
Sneppen fracture of talus
snowman appearance of heart
snowman deformity
snowplow occlusion
snowstorm shadow on chest x-ray

SNR (signal-to-noise ratio)
SNRT (sinus node recovery time)
snuffbox, anatomic
snufftaker's pituitary disease
soap bubble appearance of exudate
soap bubble radiolucency
soapsuds enema (SSE)
socket/residuum interface
socket-stump interface
sodium diatrizoate contrast medium
sodium iodide contrast medium
sodium iodide ring
sodium iodipamide contrast medium
sodium iodohippurate contrast
    medium
sodium iodomethamate contrast
    medium
sodium iothalamate contrast medium
sodium ipodate contrast medium
sodium methiodal contrast medium
sodium pertechnetate ^{99m}Tc
sodium thorium tartrate contrast
    medium
sodium tyropanoate contrast medium
soft-copy computed radiography
soft disk herniation
soft neurologic sign
soft palate
soft photon
softening and swelling of cartilage
softening of brain
Softip diagnostic catheter
soft tissue abnormality
soft tissue calcification
soft tissue contracture
soft tissue contusion
soft tissue defect
soft tissue density structure
soft tissue entrapment
soft tissue interposition
soft tissue mass
soft tissue necrosis

soft tissue ossification
soft tissue osteochondroma
soft tissue radiograph
soft tissue, stippled
soft tissue swelling
soft tissue window
Softouch guiding catheter
Soft-Vu angiographic catheter
Soft-Vu Omni Flush catheter
software (see also *program*)
    DecThreads
    Kodak
    modified vessel image processor
    Neuro Echo
    Neuro Lobe
    Neuro SPGR
    P-LINK
    SPARC
    Starlink
    VERT
    Viewnex
    Voxel-Man
    VoxelView
Solayrès obliquity
soldier's heart syndrome
soldier's patches of pericardium
soldier's spot
soleal line
soleal vein
solenoid surface coil
soleus muscle
solid bolus challenge
solid bone
solid edema of lung
solid lesion, echogenic
solid modeler
solid state manometry catheter
solid state nuclear track detector
solitary cold lesion
solitary lung nodule
solitary mass
solitary pulmonary nodule (SPN)

solitus
    atrial situs
    situs
    visceral situs
Solo catheter with Pro/Pel coating
Solomon syndrome
SoloPass stent and catheter
Solu-Biloptin contrast medium
solution
    Lugol's
    SSKI
SOMA scale
Somatom DR CT scanner
Somatom Plus-S CT Scanner
somatosensory cortex
somatostatin receptor
S1-S5 (five sacral vertebrae)
Sones Cardio-Marker catheter
Sones Hi-Flow catheter
Sones selective coronary arteriography
sonicated albumin microbubbles
sonicated contrast medium
Sonicator portable ultrasound
Sonifer sonicating system
Sonnenberg classification of erosive
    esophagitis
sonoangiogram
Sonocut ultrasonic aspirator
sonogram (see *ultrasound*)
sonographic feature analysis
sonographic Murphy sign
sonographic parameter
sonography (see *ultrasound*)
sonohysterography (SHG)
Sonoline Elegra ultrasound system
sonologist
sonolucent area or zone
sonolucent cystic lesion or mass
sonolucent fluid-filled area
Sonos 500 2.5 MHz ultrasonographic
    transducer
Sorbie calcaneal fracture

sorption kinetics
sorption potential
sorption studies
    Joliot
    radiotracer foil method
Soto USCI balloon
sound beam
sound transmission
S/P (status post)
SPA (single photon absorptiometry)
space
    alveolar dead
    anatomical dead
    antecubital
    apical
    apical air
    axillary
    Baros
    Berger
    Bogros
    Bottcher
    Bowman
    Burns
    capsular
    cartilage
    Chassaignac
    Cloquet
    Colles
    Cotunnius
    C-Y color
    dead
    disk
    Disse
    dorsal subaponeurotic
    dorsal subcutaneous
    echo-free
    epicardial
    epidural
    episcleral
    epitympanic
    extradural
    extrapleural

space *(cont.)*
fifth intercostal
first intercostal
foraminal
fourth intercostal
free pericardial
gingival
Henke
His perivascular
Holzknecht
hyperintense marrow
increased lateral joint
intercellular
intercondylar (ICS) joint
intercostal
intermetatarsal
interpeduncular
interpleural
interstitial
intervertebral disk
intrathecal
intravascular
joint
K-
Kiernan
Kretschmann
Kuhnt
lateral joint
left intercostal (LICS)
Lesgaft
Lesshaft
lung air
Magendie
Malacarne
masticator
Meckel
medial joint
midpalmar
Mohrenheim
narrowing of joint
parapharyngeal
Parona (subtendinous)

space *(cont.)*
patellofemoral joint
peribronchial alveolar
pericardial
perineal
perinephric
perirenal
perisinusoidal
peritoneal
plane of intercostal
pleural
Poirier
Poiseuille
popliteal
posterior septal
presacral
Prussak
pulp
Q
Reinke
retrocardiac
retromammary
retro-orbital
retropancreatic preaortic
retroparotid
retroperitoneal
retrosphenoidal
Retzius
scapholunate
Schwalbe
subarachnoid
subdural
subhepatic
subperitoneal
subtendinous
subumbilical
suprahepatic
supralevator
syndesmotic clear
Tailarach
Tarin
Tenon

space *(cont.)*
  thenar
  tibiocalcaneal
  tissue
  Traube semilunar
  Trautmann triangular
  ventricular
  vesicovaginal
  Virchow-Robin space of the brain
  Waldeyer
  web
  Westberg
  Zang
  zonular
space deficits
Spacemaker balloon dissector
space-occupying lesions
spacing error, raster
spacing, multiple-beam interface
spade-shaped valvotome
Spalding sign
SPAMM sequence
span
  levator
  liver
SPARC software
spare
sparing, arytenoid
sparkling appearance of myocardium
spasm
  artery
  bowel
  bronchial
  catheter-induced coronary artery
  colonic
  coronary artery (CAS)
  coughing
  diffuse arteriolar
  diffuse esophageal (DES)
  hemifacial
  inspiratory
  muscle

spasm *(cont.)*
  muscular
  postbypass
  respiratory
  vascular
  vein
  venous
spastic colon
spastic esophagus
spastic ileus
spatial EPR imaging
spatial mapping
spatial modulation magnetization
spatial peak intensity
spatial presaturation
spatial registration
spatial resolution
spatially selective inversion pulse
specimen, breast core biopsy
speckled pattern
SPECT (single photon emission
    computed tomography)
  acetazolamide-enhanced
  brain perfusion
  dual-head
  dynamic volumetric
  electrocardiogram-gated
  FDG
  ictal
  interictal
  quantitative gated (QGS)
  Tc-99m red blood cell
  Trionix
SPECT brain perfusion scintigraphy
SPECT technetium sestamibi scan
SPECT thallium scintigram
SPECT tomography
SPECT with ^{18}Fl-2-deoxy-D-glucose
  (FDG)
spectography, nuclear magnetic
  resonance (NMR)
spectra (pl. of spectrum)

specular echo
Speedy balloon catheter
Spence, tail of
Spens syndrome
spermatic cord
spermatic vein
SPGR (spoiled gradient-recalled) echo
  sequences
sphenocephaly
sphenoethmoidal encephalocele
sphenoethmoidal suture
sphenoid bone
sphenoid ridge tumors
sphenoid sinus
sphenoid wing
sphenoidal fissure syndrome
sphenoidal sinusitis
spheno-occipital suture
spheno-occipital synchondrosis
spheno-orbital suture
sphenopalatine ganglion
sphenopalatine neuralgia
sphenoparietal suture
sphenopetrosal suture
sphenopharyngeal meningoencephalo-
  cele
sphenosquamous suture
sphenotemporal suture
sphenoturbinal bone
sphenovomerine suture
spherical lesion
spherical map
spherical mass
spherocytosis, hereditary
spheroid-shaped
spheroids, tumor
sphincter
  anal
  antral
  basal
  bicanalicular
  Boyden

sphincter *(cont.)*
  canalicular
  choledochal
  colic
  cricopharyngeal
  duodenal
  duodenojejunal
  external anal
  extrinsic
  first duodenal
  hypertensive lower esophageal
  Hyrtl
  inferior esophageal (IES)
  Lutkens
  Nélaton
  O'Beirne
  Oddi
  pancreatic duct
  pancreaticobiliary
  pharyngoesophageal
  prepyloric
  pyloric
  upper esophageal (UES)
sphingolipidosis
sphingomyelin lipidosis
sphingomyelinase
Sphrintzen velocardiofacial syndrome
sphygmography
sphygmomanometer cuff
spicular density
spicular protrusion
spiculations on colon
spicule of bone
spicules in profile
spider angioma (pl. angiomata)
spidering skeleton
spider-web circulation on angiography
  of glioblastomas
spider nevus (pl. nevi)
spiderweb appearance
spider x-ray view
spike loading

spiky skeletons
spin (pl. spins)
   flowing
   J-coupled
   stationary
   uncoupled
spina bifida
spina bifida occulta (SBO)
spina bifida posterior
spinal abscess, epidural
spinal accessory nerve (eleventh
   cranial nerve)
spinal angiogram
spinal angiolipoma
spinal arthritis
spinal axial loading
spinal axis
spinal block by cord compression
spinal canal narrowing
spinal column
spinal cord
   caliber of
   compression of
   decompression of
   hemisection of
   infarction of the
   laceration of the
   multiple focal lesions of (in
      multiple sclerosis)
   posterolateral sclerosis of
   size of
   tethered
   transection of
spinal cord ependymoma
spinal cord injury (SCI)
spinal cord lesion
spinal cord parenchyma
spinal cord stroke
spinal cord tumor
spinal dural arteriovenous fistula
spinal elements, neoplastic destruction
  of

spinal ependymoma
spinal epidural abscess
spinal epidural hematoma
spinal fixation
spinal fusion
spinal hemiplegia
spinal hydatid cyst
spinal instability
spinal lordosis
spinal roots
   C1-7 (cervical)
   Co. 1 (coccygeal)
   L1-5 (lumbar)
   S1-5 (sacral)
   T1-12 (thoracic)
spinal subarachnoid hemorrhage
spinal subdural hematoma
spinal tuberculosis
spinal videofluoroscopy
spin coupling
spin density, echo
spindle
   aortic
   His
spindle-shaped shadow
spine
   alar
   angulation of
   anterior column of
   anterior maxillary
   anterior superior iliac
   anteroposterior iliac
   cervical (C)
   Charcot
   coccygeal (coccyx)
   dendritic
   dorsal (D)
   functional units of
   iliac
   ischial
   kinetic cervical
   kissing

spine *(cont.)*
  lateral bending views of the
  lumbar (L)
  lumbarized
  lumbosacral (LS)
  maxillary
  mental
  nasal
  poker
  posterior-inferior
  posterior column of
  posterior-inferior
  rotatory loads on
  rugger jersey
  sacral (S)
  static cervical
  thoracic (T)
  thoracolumbar
  trochanteric
spin echo (SE)
spin-echo imaging sequence
spin-echo pulse sequence
spin-label method
spin-lattice relaxation time
spin-lock and magnetization transfer
  imaging
spin-lock imaging
spin-lock induced T1rho weighted
  image
spin-locking, adiabatic off-resonance
spin-lock prepulse
spinocerebellar ataxia
spinocerebellar degeneration
spinoglenoid notch
spinographic angle
spinographic lines
spinography, digitized
spinoreticular tract
spinotectal tract
spinothalamic tract
spinous process
spin-spin relaxation time

spin-warp imaging
SPIO (superparamagnetic iron oxide)
  oral contrast agent
spiral (also spiraling)
spiral appearance
spiral band of Gosset
spiral computed tomography
spiral CT (computed tomography)
  angiography (SCTA)
spiral CT pitch
spiral CT scanner
spiral CT with multiplanar
  reformatting and 3D rendering
spiral dissection
spiral fracture
spiral oblique fracture
spiral pulse sequence
spiral scanning technique
spiral XCT (x-ray computed
  tomography) scanner
spirometric acquisition
spirometrically controlled CT
splanchnic vascular imaging
splanchnic vasculature
splanchnic vessels
splash, succussion
splashing bruit
splayed
splayfoot deformity
splaying of pedicles
spleen
  accessory
  floating
  inflammatory of
  long axis of
  tip of
spleen-to-liver ratio
splenic artery
splenic flexure
splenic lobule
splenic notch
splenic portography

spot compression
spot film
spot-film fluorography
spot images
S-phase fraction
S pouch, ileal
SPP (superparamagnetic particle)
   contrast medium
SPPS (single photon planar
   scintigraphy)
SPR (superior peroneal retinaculum)
sprain
   acute
   chronic
   eversion
sprain fracture
sprain-strain
spread, transfascial
Sprengel deformity
Spring catheter with Pro/Pel coating
Springer fracture
spring-loaded vascular stent
sprinter's fracture
sprodiamide imaging agent
SP6 camera
spur (spurring)
   acromial
   anterior
   bone (or bony)
   calcaneal
   calcific
   degenerative
   heel
   hypertrophic marginal
   impingement
   inferior
   marginal
   Morand
   osteoarthritic
   plantar calcaneal
   posterior
   prominent

spur *(cont.)*
   retrocalcaneal
   traction
   uncovertebral
Squibb catheter
Sr (strontium)
SSD (shaded surface display) algorithms
SSFP (steady state free precession)
SSH (spinal subdural hemorrhage)
SSKI (saturated potassium iodide
   solution)
SSP (slice sensitivity profile)
S-shaped pouch
S-shaped scoliosis
SSQ (sequential scalar quantization)
SSS (subclavian steal syndrome)
stable fracture
stable isotope
stable-state tuberculosis
Stack autoperfusion balloon
stacked foil technique
stacked metaphor workstation
stacked ovoid lesions
stacked scans
stacked tomograms
Stack perfusion coronary dilatation
   catheter
STAE (subsegmental transcatheter
   arterial embolization)
staghorn calculus
staging (see also *grading*)
   Berndt-Harty talar lesion
   distraction-flexion (DFS)
   Ficat avascular necrosis
   Gottschalk
   Greulich and Pyle skeletal
      maturation
   Jackson
   neuroblastoma
   Outerbridge degenerative arthritis
   pre-slip

stagnant loop syndrome
stain, tumor (on cerebral angiography)
stainless steel mesh stent
staircase phenomenon
stairstep air-fluid levels
stairstep artifact
stairstep fracture
stalk
   body
   infundibular
   pituitary
   polyp
   tumor
Stamey-Malecot catheter
standards
   ACR teleradiology standard
   Taveras
   Wilmad reference
standby rate
standing post-void view
standoff
standstill
   atrial
   cardiac
   ventricular
Stand-Up MRI, Fonar
Stanford type B aortic dissection
stannous pyrophosphate
STAR angiography
Starcam camera
star-cancellation test (SCT)
Starling curve
Starlink software
star pattern
STAR registry
STARRT Falloposcopy System
star-shaped vessel lumen
stasis, venous
stasis edema
stasis of blood flow
stasis ulcers
state, chronic constrictive

static 3D FLASH imaging
static image
status post (S/P)
steady state free precession (SSFP)
steal
   arterial
   coronary artery
   subclavian
stealing of cerebral blood by
   subclavian artery
steal phenomenon
STEAM (stimulated echo aquisition
   mode)
STEAM spectroscopy
steep left anterior oblique (LAO) view
steeple sign on chest x-ray
steep Towne projection
steep Trendelenburg position
steerable catheter
steering catheter
steering, electronic independent beam
Steerocath catheter
steganography
stellar nevus
stellate defect
stellate pattern
stellate skull fracture
stellate undepressed fracture
stem
   brain
   bronchus
   reticular formation of the brain
   roundback
   straight
Stener lesion
stenocardia
stenosing ring of left atrium
stenosis
   acquired mitral
   American Heart Association
      classification of
   ampullary

stenosis *(cont.)*
    petrous carotid canal
    post-PTCA
    postangioplasty
    preangioplasty
    pulmonary
    pulmonary artery
    pulmonary valve
    pulmonary vein
    pulmonic (PS)
    pyloric
    rectal
    relative mitral
    renal artery
    rheumatic aortic valvular
    rheumatic mitral
    rheumatic tricuspid
    saphenous vein
    segmental
    senescent aortic
    severe
    silent mitral
    spinal
    stomal
    subaortic
    subclavian artery
    subinfundibular pulmonary
    subpulmonic infundibular
    subvalvar aortic
    supra-aortic
    supraclavicular aortic stenosis
    suprarenal
    supravalvular aortic (SAS, SVAS)
    supravalvular pulmonic
    tapering
    tight
    tracheal
    tricuspid (TS)
    true mitral
    truncal renal artery
    tubular
    tunnel subvalvular aortic

stenosis *(cont.)*
    unicuspid aortic valve
    unilateral carotid
    ureteral
    valvar aortic
    valvular pulmonic
    vertebral artery
stenotic but patent tricuspid valve
stenotic isthmus
stenotic lesion
stenotic valve
Stensen duct
stent (stenting)
    ACS Multilink coronary
    activated balloon expandable
        intravascular
    antegrade ureteral
    balloon-expandable flexible coil
    balloon-expandable intravascular
    balloon-expandable metallic
    beStent balloon-expandable
    biliary
    biodegradable
    CardioCoil self-expanding coronary
    coil vascular
    covered Gianturco
    Dacron-covered
    double pigtail
    EndoCoil biliary
    endoluminal
    EsophaCoil biliary stent
    esophageal
    Gianturco-Rösch Z-stent
    heat-expandable
    helical coil
    iliac artery
    indwelling
    interdigitating coil
    intracoronary
    intravascular
    iridium-192 (^{192}Ir)-loaded
    Medivent vascular

stent *(cont.)*
  nitinol
  nitinol thermal memory
  Palmaz balloon-expandable iliac
  Palmaz-Schatz coronary
  pancreatic duct
  patent
  percutaneous
  pigtail
  polymer-coated drug-eluting
  polyurethane
  porous metallic
  radioisotope
  Reliance urinary control
  renovascular
  Roubin-Gianturco flexible coil
  Schatz-Palmaz tubular mesh
  self-expanding
  Silastic
  spring-loaded vascular
  stainless steel mesh
  straight
  Strecker balloon-expandable
  Strecker tantalum
  T-tube
  tantalum
  thermal memory
  transhepatic biliary
  U-tube
  Ultraflex self-expanding
  ureteral
  Wallstent spring-loaded
  Wiktor
  wire-mesh self-expandable
  zig-zag
stent deployment
stent embolization
stent expansion
stent-graft
  endovascular
  percutaneous endoluminal
    placement of

stentless porcine aortic valve
stent migration
stent-mounted allograft valve
stent-mounted heterograft valve
stent recanalization
stent thrombosis
stent-vessel wall contact
Stenver view
step-down deformity of shoulder
step-off between bone fracture fragments
step-off, orbital rim
stepped-care antihypertensive regimen
stepup (or step-up)
stepwise regression analysis
stercoral ulcer
stercoroma
stereocinefluorography
stereofluoroscopy
stereographic projections
stereogram
stereolithography
stereologic method of volume
  estimation
stereoradiography
stereoscopic view
stereoscopic vision
stereotactic (or stereotaxic)
stereotactic ablation
stereotactic add-on device
stereotactically guided
stereotactic biopsy
stereotactic CT scan
stereotactic data
stereotactic localization
stereotactic method for intracranial
  navigation
stereotactic neurosurgery
stereotactic procedure
stereotactic proton irradiation
stereotactic radiation therapy
stereotactic radiosurgery

stereotactic resection, computer-assisted
stereotactic surface projection (SSP)
stereotaxis
   computer-assisted volumetric
   imaging-based
   volumetric
stereotaxy
sterile
Sterling contrast medium
sternal angle of Louis
sternal border and apex
sternal cartilage
sternal edge
sternal joint
sternal lift
sternal marrow
sternal notch
sternal pleural reflection
sternal splitting
sternal view
Sternberg myocardial insufficiency
sternoclavicular angle
sternoclavicular joint
sternocleidomastoid muscle
sternocostal joint
sternocostal surface of heart
sternohyoid muscle
sternopericardial ligament
sternothyroid muscle
sternum, anterior bowing of
Stertzer brachial guiding catheter
Stieda fracture
Stierlin sign
stiffening
Still disease (juvenile rheumatoid arthritis)
Stiller rib
stimulated echo acquisition mode (STEAM)
stimulated echo artifact
stimulated echo-tagging technique
stimulus-correlated signal

stippled calcification
stippled epiphysis
stippled soft tissue
stippling of lung fields
STIR (short T1 inversion recovery) scan
STIR (Short Tau Inversion Recovery) sequence
stocking-glove distribution
stoma
   abdominal
   bowel
   diverting
   gastrointestinal
   permanent
   prolapsed
   retracted
   Silastic collar-reinforced
stomach
   aberrant umbilical
   antrum of
   bilocular
   canal of
   cardiac
   cascade
   convex border of
   coronary artery of
   cup-and-spill
   distal blind
   distended
   dumping
   greater curvature of
   Holzknecht
   hourglass
   intrathoracic
   leather bottle
   lesser curvature of
   miniature
   Pavlov
   pit of
   riding
   scaphoid

stomach *(cont.)*
- sclerotic
- sour
- thoracic
- trifid
- upset
- upside-down
- water-trap
- waterfall

stomal bag

stone (see also *gallstone*)
- barrel-shaped
- bile duct
- biliary
- biliary tract
- bilirubinate
- black faceted
- bladder
- bosselated
- calcium bilirubinate
- CBD (common bile duct)
- common bile duct
- gall
- gallbladder
- high attenuation
- impacted urethral
- intrahepatic
- intraluminal
- intravesical
- kidney
- lung
- metabolic
- noncalcified
- radiolucent
- renal
- residual
- salivary
- staghorn
- shadowing
- ureteral
- ureteric

stone *(cont.)*
- urinary
- vein
- womb

stone differentiated from tumor
stone formation, vesical
stone manipulation, percutaneous
stop action images
stopcock
stopping power
storage phosphor radiology
storiform pattern
straddle fracture
straight AP pelvic injection
straight chest tube
straight flush percutaneous catheter
straight-line HT (Hough transform)
  mapping
straight ureter
strain
- ligamentous
- lumbosacral spine
- muscle

strain fracture
strain-rate MR imaging
strain-sprain injury
stranding
- fascial
- mesenteric
- soft tissue

strands of increased density on chest x-
  ray
strandy pulmonic infiltrate
strangulated bowel
strangulated hernia
stratigraphy
stray neutron field
streaks of atelectasis on chest film
streaks of increased density
Strecker balloon-expandable stent
Strecker tantalum stent

stress
  adduction (to fingers)
  biomechanical
  mediolateral
  shear
  shearing
  torque
  valgus
  varus
stress and rest images
stress cystogram
stress films
stress fracture
stress gated blood pool cardiac
  examination
stress images (imaging)
stress-induced left ventricular
  dilatation
stress-injected sestamibi-gated SPECT
  with echocardiography
stress management
stress perfusion and rest function by
  sestamibi-gated SPECT
stress radiography
stress-redistribution exam
stress-rest-reinjection examination
stress test
  dipyridamole thallium
  persantine thallium
stress thallium scan
stress thallium-201 myocardial
  imaging
stress ulcer
stricture
  anal
  anastomotic
  annular esophageal
  antral
  benign biliary
  bile duct
  cicatricial
  contractile

stricture *(cont.)*
  esophageal
  irritable
  longitudinal esophageal
  peptic
  pyloric
  recurrent
  spasmodic
  ureteral
  urethral
string guideline
stringlike bands of fibrous tissue
string of beads appearance
string of pearls nuclear arrangement
string of pearls sign
string sign in terminal ileum
strip, primary motor
stripe
  Baillarger
  central intraluminal saturation
  flank
  Gennari
  paraspinal pleural
  paratracheal
  properitoneal flank
  Retzius
  saturation
  vertebral
  Vicq d'Azyr
stripe sign
striping, horizontal
stroke
  cerebrovascular
  hyperacute
  thromboembolic (TE)
stroke distance, Doppler-derived
stroke ejection rate
stroke force
stroke index (SI)
stroke power
stroke scale score
stroke volume (SV)

stroke volume image
stroke volume index (SVI)
stroke volume ratio
stroma
strontium (Sr)
   ^{82}Sr
   ^{89}Sr bracelet
   ^{89}Sr chloride (Metastron) radioactive
     drug
   ^{90}Sr-loaded eye applicator
structural epilepsy
structural weakness of bronchial wall
   supports
structure (pl. structures)
   biliary
   bony
   branching linear
   branching tubular
   calcified density
   central hilar
   cord
   denture-supporting
   elongated
   high-density
   hollow
   intratumoral
   KUB (kidneys, ureters, bladder)
   labyrinthine
   low-contrast
   low-density
   organoid
   osseous
   renal collecting
   ring-like
   satellite
   soft tissue density
   submillimeter
   superior mediastinal
   supraglottic
   tubular
   vascular
structured coil electromagnet

Strümpell-Lorrain disease
Strümpell-Marie disease
strut
   corticocancellous
   optic
   tricuspid valve
   valve outflow
STT (scapho-trapezium-trapezoid)
   joint
studded fissures
study (see *imaging*)
stump
   appendiceal
   cervical
   duodenal
   gastric
   rectal
Sturge-Weber telangiectasia
S2 (serotonin) receptor
styloid process
subacromial bursitis
subadventitial plane
subadventitial tissue
subannular region
subaortic curtain
subaortic glands
subaortic muscle
subaortic stenosis
subapical
subarachnoid cavity
subarachnoid hemorrhage (SAH)
subarachnoid instillation of contrast
   material
subarachnoid metastatic disease
subarachnoid phenol block (SAPB)
   with fluoroscopy
subarachnoid space
subareolar
subarticular cyst
subastragalar dislocation
subatmospheric pressure
sub-band (or subband), wavelet

subcallosal gyrus
subcapital fracture
subcapsular hematoma
subcarina (pl. subcarinae)
subcarinal node
subchondral bone cyst
subchondral bone plate
subchondral microfractures
subchorionic hemorrhage
subclavian aneurysm
subclavian approach for cardiac catheterization
subclavian artery occlusion
subclavian artery steal of cerebral blood
subclavian artery stenosis
subclavian catheter
subclavian loop
subclavian-pulmonary shunt
subclavian steal phenomenon (SSP)
subclavian steal syndrome (SSS)
subclavian vein, blind percutaneous puncture of
subclavian vein catheterization
subclavicular approach
subcollateral gyrus
subcoracoid dislocation of shoulder
subcortical infarct
subcortical ischemic vascular dementia
subcortical intracerebral hemorrhage
subcortical intracranial lesion
subcortical lesion
subcortical tumor
subcostal approach
subcostal artery
subcostal branch
subcostal margin
subcostal nerve
subcostal window
subcu (subcutaneous)
subcutaneous air
subcutaneous array electrode

subcutaneous emphysema
subcutaneous fat line
subcutaneous fracture
subcutaneous hemangioma
subcutaneous injection of contrast artifact
subcutaneous patch
subcutaneous pocket
subcutaneous tissue
subcutaneous tissue gas
subcutaneous tunnel
subcutaneous veins
subcuticular layer
subdeltoid bursal adhesion
subdiaphragmatic abscess
subdural abscess
subdural blood
subdural cavity
subdural clot
subdural effusion
subdural empyema
subdural hematoma
subdural hemorrhage
subdural hygroma
subdural space
subdural window on CT scan
subendocardial infarction (SEI)
subendocardial injury
subendocardial ischemia
subendocardial myocardial infarction
subendocardial necrosis
subendothelial hyalinization
subependymal hemorrhage
subeustachian sinus
subfalcine (subfalcial) herniation
subfascial transposition
subfascially
subfrontal meningioma tumor
subgaleal abscess
subgaleal hematoma
subglenoid dislocation of shoulder
subglottic area

subglottic edema
subhepatic area
subhepatic space
subinfundibular pulmonary stenosis
subintimal cleavage plane
subintimal dissection
sublabral recess
subligamenous disk herniation
sublingual varices
sublux
subluxated
subluxation
 atlanto-axial
 element
 forward
 occult
 patellar
 posterior
 radial head (RHS)
 reduced
 rotary
 tendon
 Volkmann
submandibular ganglion
submandibular triangle
submaxillary
submental vertex view
submillimeter structures
submucosal lesion
submucosal thickening
submucous myoma
suboccipital shortening
suboptimal film due to:
 film quality
 patient cooperation
 positioning
suboptimal results
suboptimal runoff
suboptimal visualization
suboptimally visualized
subpectoral pocket
subperiosteal abscess of frontal sinus

subperiosteal fracture
subperiosteal new bone formation
subperiosteally
subphrenic abscess
subphrenic biloma
subpleural bleb
subpleural curvilinear lines
subpleural dots
subpleural lines
subpubic arch
subpulmonic fluid
subpulmonic infundibular stenosis
subpulmonic obstruction
subrectus placement
subsartorial tunnel
subsegment of lung
subsegmental bibasilar atelectasis
subsegmental bronchus
subsegmental perfusion abnormality
subsegmental transcatheter arterial
 embolization (STAE)
subsegments, right middle lobe
subserosal fibrosis
subserosal layer
subspinous dislocation
substernal angle
substernal goiter
substernal thyroid
substitution bone
substrate, main energy
subtalar articulation
subtalar joint space
subtendinous space
subtentorial lesion
subtotal lesion
subtraction, Epistar
subtraction films
 digital
 manual
 serial
subtraction images
subtraction technique

subtrochanteric fracture
subvalvular aneurysm
subvalvular aortic obstruction
subvalvular aortic stenosis
subxiphoid echocardiography view
subxiphoid implantation
subxiphoid view
sucking pneumothorax
Sucquet-Hoyer anastomosis
Sucquet-Hoyer canal
sucrose dosimeter
sucrose polyester contrast
suction line, aortic vent
Sudbury system
sudden blockage of coronary artery
Sudeck atrophy
SUFE (slipped upper femoral
   epiphysis)
suite, angiography
sulcal skeleton
sulcation
sulcus (pl. sulci)
   angularis
   basilar
   blunted posterior
   cortical
   costal
   Harrison
   atrioventricular
   calcarine
   callosal
   central
   cingulate
   collateral
   dilatation of the
   effacement of
   frontal
   hypothalmic
   lateral occipital
   lips of lateral
   occipitotemporal
   olfactory

sulcus *(cont.)*
   parieto-occipital
   pontomedullary
   postcentral
   posterior interventricular
   precentral
   pulmonary
   rami of lateral
   rolandic
   superior frontal
   superior temporal
   supracallosal
   temporal
   ulnar
   widened (on scan)
sulfobromophthalein (BSP) imaging
   agent
sulfur colloid labeled with Tc 99m
   scan
sulfur colloid, technetium bound to
SULP II catheter
sum-peak method
summation shadow artifact
summing correction
Summit LoDose collimator
summit, ventricular septal
sump catheter
Sun SPARCstation system
Sun workstation
sunburst pattern
sunrise view of patella
sunset view
superabsorbent polymer (SAP) embolic
   material
super scan appearance
superciliary arch
superconducting magnet
superconductor
superdominant left anterior descending
   artery
superfical femoral artery
superficial external pudendal artery

superficial femoral arteries (SFAs)
superficial femoral artery occlusion
superficial femoral vein
superficial lesion
superficial palmar arterial arch
superficial posterior compartment
superficial vein
superimposed
superimposition artifact
superimposition of signals
superincumbent spinal curves
superior border of heart
superior border of rib
superior bronchus
superior caval defect
superior caval obstruction
superior colliculus
superior costotransverse ligament
superior epigastric artery
superior facet
superior frontal gyrus
superior frontal sulcus
superior genicular artery
superior intercostal artery
superior intercostal vein
superior lobe of lung
superior margin of inferior rib
superior marginal defect
superior mediastinal structures
superior mediastinum
superior mesenteric artery (SMA)
superior mesenteric vein (SMV)
superior parietal lobule gyrus
superior pubic ramus
superior pulmonary artery
superior pulmonary vein
superior retraction
superior sagittal sinus
superior segment
superior temporal gyrus
superior temporal sulcus
superior thoracic aperture

superior thyroid artery
superior vena cava obstruction
supernormal conduction
supernormal excitation
supernumerary bone
supernumerary sesamoid bones
superoinferior heart
superolaterally
superomedial portal
superparamagnetic contrast agent
superparamagnetic iron oxide-
    enhanced imaging
superparamagnetic iron oxide (SPIO)
    oral contrast agent
superselective (not supraselective)
superselective angio-CT
superselective angiography
superselective catheterization
superselective intra-arterial
    chemotherapy
supination-adduction fracture
supination-eversion fracture
supine film
supine position
supplemental beam filtration
suppression
    Cytomel (thyroid hormone)
    double-echo three-point Dixon
        method
    fat
    paradoxical
suppressor mesh
suppuration
supra-annular constriction
supra-aortic ridge
supra-aortic stenosis
supracallosal sulcus
supracardiac shunt
supracardiac-type total anomalous
    venous return
supraceliac aorta
supraclavicular aortic stenosis

supraclavicular lymph node
supraclavicular node
supraclavicular region
supraclavicular triangle
supraclinoid internal carotid artery
supracolic compartment
supracollicular spike of cortical bone
supracondylar femoral fracture
supracondylar humerus fracture
supracoronary ridge
supracristal ventricular septal defect
supradiaphragmatic aorta
supraduodenal approach
supraepicondylar
supraepitrochlear
supraglottic larynx
supraglottic structures
suprahepatic caval cuff
suprahepatic space
suprahepatic vena cava
suprainterparietal bone
supralevator space
supraligamentous disk herniation
supramalleolar region
supramarginal gyrus
supranuclear lesion
supraoccipital bone
supraorbital fissure
supraorbital ridges
suprapatellar bursa
suprapatellar plica
suprapatellar pouch
suprapharyngeal bone
suprapubic area
suprarenal aneurysm
suprarenal extension of aneurysm
suprarenal gland
suprarenal stenosis
suprascapular nerve entrapment
"supraselective" (see *superselective*)
suprasellar adenoma
suprasellar aneurysm

suprasellar cistern
suprasellar extension of tumor
suprasellar lesion
suprasellar mass
suprasellar region
suprasellar tumor
supraspinatus nerve
supraspinous ligaments
suprasternal bone
suprasternal bulging
suprasternal notch view on
   echocardiogram
suprasternal window
suprasyndesmotic fixation
supratentorial brain tumor
supratentorial cerebral blood flow
supratentorial primitive neuroectodermal tumor (PNET)
suprathreshold
supratip nasal tip deformity
supratrochlear
supravalvular aortic stenosis (SAS,
   SVAS)
supravalvular aortogram
supravalvular mitral stenosis
supravalvular pulmonic stenosis
supravaterian duodenum
supraventricular crest (SVC)
supravesical obstruction
sural nerve
SureStart feature of Aspire continuous
   imaging
surface
   acromial articular
   anterolateral
   anteromedial
   apposing articular
   articular
   articulating
   arytenoidal articular
   auricular
   axial

suture *(cont.)*
  ethmoidolacrimal
  ethmoidomaxillary
  frontal
  frontoethmoidal
  frontolacrimal
  frontomaxillary
  frontonasal
  frontoparietal
  frontosphenoid
  frontozygomatic
  Gillies
  Gruber
  interparietal
  jugal
  lambdoidal cranial
  mamillary
  metopic
  nonfusion of cranial
  occipital
  occipitomastoid
  occipitoparietal
  occipitosphenoid
  overlapping
  parietal
  parietomastoid
  parieto-occipital
  petrobasilar
  petrosphenobasilar
  petrospheno-occipital
  petrosquamous
  prematurely closed
  radiopaque
  rhabdoid
  sagittal
  sagittal cranial
  sphenoethmoidal
  spheno-occipital
  spheno-orbital
  sphenoparietal
  sphenopetrosal
  sphenosquamous

suture *(cont.)*
  sphenotemporal
  sphenovomerine
  splayed cranial
  spread (cranial sign)
  squamosomastoid
  squamosoparietal
  squamososphenoid
  squamous
  temporal
Sv (sievert) radiation absorbed dose
SV (stroke volume)
SVAS (supravalvular aortic stenosis)
SVC (superior vena cava)
SVC (supraventricular crest)
SVI (stroke volume index)
SvO_2 (venous oxygen saturation)
SVR (systemic vascular resistance)
SVRI (systemic vascular resistance
  index)
swallow
  barium
  dry
  Gastrografin
  ice-water
  water-soluble contrast esophageal
  wet
swallowing artifact
swallowing center
swallowing dysfunction
swallowing function
swallowing mechanism, video
  fluoroscopy of
swallow syncope
swamp-static artifact
Swan-Ganz balloon-flotation catheter
Swan-Ganz thermodilution catheter
swan-neck catheter
swan-neck deformity
swan neck shape of ventricular
  outflow
Swediaur disease

sweep, duodenal
sweeper
Sweet sternal punch
swelling, soft tissue
SWI (stroke work index)
swimmer's view
swinging flashlight test
swirling smokelike echoes
Swiss cheese appearance
Swiss cheese ventricular septal defect
Swissray scanner
swiss roll technique
swivel dislocation (of midfoot)
swollen tissues
Swyer-James unilateral hyperlucency
    of lung
SXA (single-energy x-ray)
    absorptiometer
SXCT (spiral x-ray computed
    tomography)
Sydenham chorea
Syed-Neblett brachytherapy method
sylvian aqueduct syndrome
sylvian candelabra
sylvian fissure
sylvian operculum
sylvian/rolandic junction
Sylvius
    aqueduct of
    cistern of
    fossa of
Syme amputation
symmetrical chest
symmetrical narrowing
symmetrical phased array
symmetric distribution
symmetric pulmonary congestion
symmetry
sympathetic chain
sympathetic denervation
sympathetic ganglia
sympathetic innervation

sympathetic nervous tissue
sympathetic vascular instability
symphysis, pubic
symphysis pubis
symptomatic metastatic spinal cord
    compression
symptomatology
symptom complex
synaptic cleft
synaptic dopamine concentration
synaptic pathways
synchronicity
synchronization device
synchronous carotid arterial pulse
synchrotron, monochromatic
synchrotron radiation
syndactylization of digits
syndactyly
syndrome
Synergy ultrasound system
synkinesis (pl. synkineses)
synostosis
    cervical
    congenital radioulnar
    coronal
    lambdoid
    multiple-suture
    nonsyndromic bicoronal
    nonsyndromic unicoronal
    premature suture
    radiographically firm
    sagittal
    single suture
    terminal
    tibiofibular
synovial cavity
synovial membrane
synovial plica
synovial proliferation
synovial sarcoma of heart
synovial surface
synovial thickening

system *(cont.)*
 directly coupled sample changer
 dominant left coronary artery
 dominant right coronary
 dual-head gamma camera
 Dynarad portable imaging
 Echovar Doppler
 Elscint
 endocavitary applicator
 engorged collecting
 external jugular
 extracranial carotid
 FlimFax teleradiology
 FluoroPlus angiography
 Fonar
 foreign body retrieval
 full-field digital mammography
 Galen teleradiology
 GE (General Electric)
 greater saphenous
 Greenfield vena cava filter
 HDI (high-definition imaging)
    3000 ultrasound
 hepatic ductal
 Hewlett Packard
 high-field
 Hi-Star midfield MRI
 homonuclear spin
 House grading
 HyperPACS
 IBM Speech Server clinical
    reporting
 IMAC
 image analysis
 Imatron
 immunomedics
 Impax PACS
 Instrumentation Laboratory
 internal carotid
 intrahepatic
 Isocam scintillation imaging
 Jackson staging

system *(cont.)*
 Lanier clinical reporting
 lesser saphenous
 Liebel-Flarsheim CT 9000 contrast
    delivery
 lipophilic sequestration
 LymphoScan nuclear imaging
 Magnes biomagnetometer
 Magnetom Open
 Magnetom Vision MR
 Magnex Alpha MR
 Marex MRI
 MEDDARS cardiac catheterization
    analysis
 Medspec MR imaging
 Medweb clinical reporting
 multidetector
 Novacore left ventricular assist
    (LVAS)
 Octreoscan
 OEC Series 9600 cardiac
 1.5T Signa Advantage
 open architecture
 open-configuration MR
 OpenPACS
 OSCAR ultrasonic bone cement
    removal
 OsteoView x-ray
 Ovation Falloposcopy
 Paris
 PenRad mammography clinical
    reporting
 PF-PACS
 Philips
 Picker
 Pinnacle 3 radiation therapy
    planning
 PMT robotic fulcrumless
    tomographic
 polar coordinate
 PortalVision radiation oncology
 PowerVision Ultrasound

system *(cont.)*
    Probe balloon-on-a-wire dilatation
    Profile Mammography
    ProstaScint
    pulmonary venous
    PulseSpray pulsed infusion
    Q-cath catheterization recording
    quadrature surface coil MRI
    radiation therapy planning (RTP)
    radionuclide carrier
    RadNet radiology information
    Redi-Vu teleradiology
    reference coordinate
    renal collecting
    reticuloendothelial
    Retzius
    ring-type imaging
    Rogan teleradiology
    RTP (radiation therapy planning)
    saphenous
    Scanmaster DX
    scanned-slot detector
    scanning beam digital
    scattering
    Schmidt optics
    Scintiview nuclear computer
    Scintron IV (four) nuclear
      computer
    sequestration
    Shape Maker
    Shimadzu
    SICOR (computer-assisted cardiac
      catheter recording)
    Siemens AG
    Signa GEMS MR imaging
    Signal
    Silicon Graphics Reality Engine
    SmartSpot high resolution digital
      imaging
    Sonoline Elegra ultrasound
    Squibb
    STARRT Falloposcopy

system *(cont.)*
    Sudbury
    Summit LoDose collimator
    Sun SPARCstation
    SureStart imaging
    Synergy ultrasound
    thermal dosimetry
    TMS 3-dimensional radiation
      therapy planning
    transluminal lysing
    Triad SPECT imaging
    TRON 3 VACI cardiac imaging
    UltraPACS diagnostic imaging
    UltraSTAR computer-based ultra
      sound reporting
    uPACS picture archiving system
    upper collecting
    USCI Probe balloon-on-a-wire
      dilatation
    Varian brachytherapy
    VARIS radiation oncology
    VasoView balloon dissection
    VAX 4100
    ventricular
    VentTrak monitoring system
    vertebral artery
    Vingmed Sound CFM ultrasound
    Vitrea 3-D
    VoiceRAD clinical reporting
    VoxelView
    Xillix LIFE-GI fluorescence
      endoscopy
    XKnife stereotactic radiosurgery
    x-ray shadow projection
      microtomographic
systematic ultrasound-guided biopsies
systemic anticoagulation with heparin
systemic arterial circulation
systemic arterial oxygen desaturation
systemic arterial vasoconstriction
systemic AV O_2 difference
systemic blood

systemic carnitine deficiency
systemic circulation
systemic diastolic blood pressure (SDBP)
systemic disorder affecting heart function
systemic heparinization
systemic hypoperfusion
systemic inflammatory response syndrome
systemic lupus erythematosus (SLE)
systemic mean arterial pressure (SMAP)
systemic mercury intoxication
systemic oxygen saturation measured after balloon-occluding each collateral
systemic perfusion, diminished
systemic pressure
systemic-pulmonary artery shunt
systemic vascular resistance (SVR)
systemic vascular resistance index (SVRI)
systemic venous hypertension
systemic venous return

systolic acceleration time
systolic and diagnostic gating
systolic anterior motion (SAM) on 2D echocardiogram
systolic blood pressure (SBP)
systolic-diastolic blood pressure
systolic ejection period (SEP)
systolic fractional shortening
systolic gradient
systolic heart failure
systolic hypertension
systolic impulse
systolic mammary souffle
systolic pressure
systolic pressure determination (SLP)
systolic pressure-time index
systolic prolapse of mitral valve leaflet
systolic reserve
systolic retraction of apex
systolic S waves
systolic time interval (STI)
systolic upstroke time
systolic velocity-time integral

T, t

Tc99m or ⁹⁹ᵐTc (see *imaging agent, technetium*)
T condylar fracture
TCP/IP (transmission control protcol/ Internet protocol)
TCS (tethered cord syndrome)
TCT900S helical CT scanner
T/D (thickness-to-diameter of ventricle) ratio
TE (echo delay time)
TE (echo time)
TE (tracheoesophageal) fistula
tear (rupture)
   attritional
   bowstring
   bucket-handle
   cleavage
   dural
   entry
   fishtail
   flap
   full-thickness
   ligament
   Mallory-Weiss
   micro
   parrot-beak
   partial-thickness
   radial
   rotator cuff
   serosal
   tendon (types I-IV)
tearaway sheath
teardrop-shaped flexion-compression fracture
teboroxime cardiac scan for myocardial infarction
teboroxime resting washout (TRW)
TEC (transluminal endarterectomy catheter)
TEC (transluminal extraction catheter)
TECA (technetium albumin) study
Technegas

TechneScan MAG3 (99mTc mertiatide) renal diagnostic imaging
technetium (Tc99m or ⁹⁹ᵐTc) (see *imaging agent*)
Technicare camera
technique (see also *method*)
   acquisition
   Amplatz
   background subtraction
   bayesian
   blended
   brain surface matching
   bread-loaf
   Brown-Roberts-Wells
   bull's-eye
   coronal oblique
   cross-correlation
   cuboid squeeze
   cuboid whip
   cut-film
   deblurring
   deconvolution
   double contrast
   double umbrella
   echo-tagging
   Egan
   EPISTAR perfusion
   equilibrium radionuclide angiocardiography
   esophageal balloon
   exclusion-HPLC
   fast-FLAIR
   field-fitting
   first-pass
   flow mapping
   full bladder
   gated
   gradient echo cine
   Gruentzig PTCA
   half-wedged field
   HARC-C wavelet compression

technique *(cont.)*
  in vivo
  inhalation
  intercomparison measurement
  inverse radiotherapy
  inversion-recovery
  isolation-perfusion
  Judkins
  kissing atherectomy
  kissing balloon
  Leksell
  loading
  low-angle shot (flash)
  low-dose film mammographic
  Markov chain Monte Carlo
  MIDCAB (minimally invasive
    direct coronary artery bypass)
  ML/EM reconstruction
  multimodal image fusion
  multiphasic multislice MRI
  multiplanar
  multislice multiphase spin-echo
    imaging
  multislice spin-echo
  navigator echo motion correction
  NEUGAT (neutron/gamma
    transmission)
  neutron/gamma transmission
    (NEUGAT)
  no-gap
  noncoplanar arc
  noninvasive
  packing, extraction, and calculation
  papillon
  partial saturation
  PASTA (polarity-altered
    spectral-selective acquisition)
  PCICO (pressure-controlled
    intermittent coronary occlusion)
  percutaneous transfemoral
  pharmokinetic
  pressure half-time

technique *(cont.)*
  radiotracer
  region-of-interest imaging
  Riechert-Mundinger
  road-mapping
  robus registration
  scintillation counting
  Seldinger percutaneous
  sequential extraction-radiotracer
  serial cut film
  silhouette
  single-field hyperthermia combined
    with radiation therapy and ultra-
    sound
  single fill/void
  sliding thin-slab, minimum
    intensity projection
  Sones cineangiography
  spin echo
  spin-label
  stacked-foil
  stereotactic or stereotaxic
  stimulated echo-tagging
  subclavian turndown
  subtraction
  tetrahedral interpolation
  three-dimensional (3D)
  tissue characterization
  Todd-Wells
  transcatheter
  transgluteal CT-guided
  trephine
  two-dimensional (2D)
  upgated
  ureteral compression
  volumetric mapping
technology, slip-ring
Tecmag Libra-S16 system
tectal lesion
tectoral ligament
tectospinal tract
TED (thromboembolic disease)

Tedlar bags
TEE (transesophageal echocardi-
    ography) imaging with DTI
teeth
    Hutchinson
    incisor
    milk
    molar
    premolar
    primary
    secondary
    wisdom
TEF (tracheoesophageal fistula)
Teflon ERCP catheter
tegmental tract
tegmentum
    medullary
    midbrain
    pontine
tegmentum of pons
Teichholz ejection fraction in
    echocardiogram
Teichholz equation for left ventricular
    volume
"tek-high-dah" (Tc HIDA) scan
telangiectatic osteosarcoma
telangiectatic vessel
telecobalt
telecom integration
telecurietherapy (radiotherapy)
Telepaque contrast medium
teleradiology videoconferencing
teletherapy, C-60
telos radiographic stress device
temperature, firing
temperature sensors
template irradiation
temporal aliasing
temporal artery
temporal bone fracture
temporal horn
temporal instability artifact

temporal lobe lesion
temporal lobe tumor
temporal-occipital junction
temporal phase delay
temporally
temporo-occipital region
temporomandibular joint (TMJ)
temporoparietal region
temporopontine tract
temporozygomatic region
tendinosis, patellar
tendo (pl. tendines)
tendo Achillis (Achilles tendon)
tendo calcaneus (Achilles tendon)
tendon
    Achilles
    calcaneal
    central (of diaphragm)
    central perineal
    collagen fibrils within
    common
    conjoined
    conjoint
    coronary
    cricoesophageal
    hamstring
    heel (tendo calcaneus)
    membranaceous
    patellar
    peroneal
    rider's
    slipped
    Todaro
    Zinn (common tendinous ring)
tendon rupture
tendon-sheath space infection
tendon sling
tendon tear (types I-IV)
tennis elbow
tennis leg (plantaris rupture)
tennis shoulder
tennis toe

Tennis Racquet angiography catheter
tension pneumothorax
tension-time index (TTI)
tentative diagnosis
tented up
tenth cranial nerve (vagus nerve)
tenting of diaphragm
tentorial edge
tentorial herniation
tentorial meningioma
tentorial notch herniation
TER (therapeutic external radiation)
teratoma
   cystic
   ovarian
   pineal
   sacrococcygeal
   solid
   suprasellar atypical
   testis
terminal
   character cell
   dumb
   X-
terminal air sac
terminal air space
terminal bronchiole
terminal crest
terminal ileum
terminal inversion
terminal reservoir syndrome
terminal thrombosis
termination
   early-phase
   late-phase
Terry-Thomas sign
tertiary collimation
tertiary contraction
tesla (T)
tesla field
test (see *imaging*)

test meal
test-retest precision
testicle
testicular adrenal rest tissue
testicular artery
testicular infarction
testicular torsion
testis (pl. testes)
   appendix
   descended
   ectopic
   efferent ductules of
   infarcted
   rete
   torsion of
   undescended
"tet" (tetralogy) of Fallot
tethered bowel sign
tethered cord
tethered spinal cord
tetrad, Fallot
tetrahedral interpolation technique
tetralogy of Fallot (TOF)
tetrapolar esophageal catheter
texture, echo
texture mapping
texture slice
TFA (thigh-foot angle)
TFA (tibiofemoral angle)
TFC (triangular fibrocartilage)
TFCC (triangular fibrocartilaginous
   complex)
T fracture
TGA (transposition of great arteries)
thalamic fracture of the calcaneus
thalamic infarct
thalamic lesion
thalamocaudate artery
thalamoperforate artery
thalamostriate vein
thalamotegmental involvement

thalamus
thallium (Tl) (see *imaging agent*)
   [201]Tl imaging agent
   [201]Tl myocardial scintigraphy
   [201]Tl stress imaging
thallium SPECT score
thallium-to-scalp ratio
thatched-roof worker's lung
THC (transhepatic cholangiography)
THE (transhepatic embolization)
thebesian circulation
thebesian foramen
thebesian valve
thebesian vein
theca (pl. thecae)
theca externa
theca interna
theca lutein ovarian cyst
thecal sac
thecoperitoneal shunt
thenar eminence
thenar muscle
thenar space abscess
theophylline attenuation
theory
   Beer-Bouguer
   density matrix
   fuzzy set
   Kubelka-Munk
   quantum
therapeutic application of radioactive
   source
therapeutic embolization
therapeutic external radiation (TER)
therapeutic pneumothorax
therapeutic radiation
therapeutic radiology
therapy (see also *radiation therapy*
   adjunctive
   adjuvant radiation
   antineoplastic
   antitubercular

therapy *(cont.)*
   arc
   brachytherapy
   Bragg-peak photon-beam
   brisement
   chemo-
   chemoradiation
   combined-modality radiation
   conformal radiation (CRT)
   conventionally fractionated
      stereotactic radiation
   craniospinal axis radiation
   electron arc
   electron beam
   endoscopic sclerosing
   endovascular
   ethanol
   eye-view 3D-CRT radiation
   fast-neutron
   fibrinolytic
   fluoroscopy-guided subarachnoid
      phenol block (SAPB)
   four-fiber
   fractionated radiation
   fragmentation
   grid
   hyperfractionated radiation
   hypertonic glucose
   hypofractionated
   [192]I high-dose rate single catheter
   immunosuppressive
   indicator dilution
   indomethacin
   interstitial radioactive colloid
   intra-articular radiopharmaceutical
   intracavitary radioactive colloid
   intracoronary thrombolytic
   intraoperative radiation (IORT)
   intravascular radiopharmaceutical
   IORT (intraoperative radiation)
   laser
   megavoltage grid

thin-section (or slice) CT
thin-slice (or section) CT
thin-slice image
thin-walled
third cranial nerve (oculomotor nerve)
third intercondylar tubercle of Parsons
third intercostal space
third left interspace
third order chordae
third portion of duodenum
third space sequestration
third ventricle tumors
30° position
30° right anterior oblique projection
Thixokon contrast medium
thoracentesis, ultrasonic guidance for
thoraces (see *thorax*)
thoracic aortic aneurysm
thoracic aortography
thoracic asymmetry
thoracic cage configuration
thoracic catheter
thoracic cavity
thoracic component of scoliosis
thoracic deformity
thoracic duct
thoracic empyema
thoracic esophagus
thoracic fistula
thoracic gas volumes
thoracic inlet
thoracic inlet (Pancoast) syndrome
thoracic kyphosis, loss of
thoracic outlet syndrome (TOS)
thoracic scoliosis
thoracic spine (T spine)
thoracic stomach
thoracic vertebrae (T1-T12)
thoracic wall
thoracoabdominal aorta
thoracoabdominal aortic aneurysm
thoracoabdominal wall

thoracoepigastric vein
thoracofemoral conversion
thoracolumbar scoliosis
thoracolumbar spine
thoracoport
thorax (pl. thoraces, thoraxes)
   asymmetrical
   bony
   cylindrical
   squared off
   symmetrical
thorax view
Thorel bundle of muscle fibers in
   heart
Thorel pathway
thorium dioxide granuloma
thorium dioxide imaging agent
Thorotrast contrast medium
threatened vessel closure post-PTCA
30 sec./frame time
3:2 block ("three-to-two")
three-axis gradient coil
three-compartment wrist angiography
three-dimensional (3D or 3-D)
   3D anthropometry
   3D connect operation
   3D CRT (conformal radiation
     therapy)
   3D dose profile
   3D echocardiography
   3D freehand ultrasound
   3DFT (three-dimensional Fourier
     transform)
   3DFT GRASS MR imaging
   3DFT magnetic resonance
     angiography
   3DFT-CISS sequence
   3DFT SPGR MR imaging
   3D gadolinium-enhanced magnetic
     resonance angiography for
     aortoiliac inflow
   3D GRE (gradient-recalled-echo)
     MRI

three-dimensional *(cont.)*
  3D H-1 magnetic resonance spectroscopic imaging
  3D helical computerized tomographic angiography (3D helical CTA)
  3D holography
  3D image reconstruction
  3D inflow MR angiography
  3D MRI data sets
  3D magnetic resonance microscopy
  3D magnetic source imaging (MSI)
  3D modeling
  3D MSI (magnetic source imaging)
  3D phase-contrast magnetic resonance angiography
  3D processed ultrafast computerized imaging
  3D-PSIF sequence
  3D spoiled gradient-recalled sequences
  3D stereotaxic surface projections
  3D surface anthropometry
  3D surface digitizer
  3D technique
  3D time-of-flight magnetic resonance (3D TOF MR) angiographic sequences
  3D transesophageal echocardiography
  3D Turbo-FLAIR (fluid-attenuated inversion recovery)
  3D turbo SE imaging
  3D ultrasound
three-head camera
three-head scan
3M scanner
three-part fracture
three-phase bone scintigraphy (TPBS)
three-vessel coronary disease
three-vessel runoff
three-way stopcock

thresher's lung
threshold, malignancy
thresholding method
thrombi (pl. of thrombus)
thromboatherosclerotic process
thromboembolus
thromboembolism
thromboembolization
  catheter-induced
  deep venous
  pulmonary
  venous
thrombolysis
  mechanical
  pharmacomechanical
  pulse-spray
thrombolytic therapy
thrombo-obliterative process
thromboresistance
ThromboScan MRU (molecular recognition units)
thrombosed
thrombosis
  intentional reversible
  syndrome of impending
  therapeutic
thrombostasis
thrombosuction catheter
thrombus
  calcified
  intramural
  mural
thrombus formation
through-and-through fracture
Thruflex PTCA balloon catheter
thumb, gamekeeper's
thumbprints (or thumbprinting) on surface of colon in barium enema
Thurston Holland sign
thymic cyst
thymoma of heart
thymus gland

time *(cont.)*
   myocardial contrast appearance (MCAT)
   perfusion
   pulmonary transit (PTT)
   pulse reappearance
   pyelographic appearance
   radionuclide esophageal dead
   reaction recovery
   real-
   recovery
   relaxation
   repetition (TR)
   resolving
   right ventricle-to-ear
   scan
   short echo
   sinoatrial conduction (SACT)
   sinus node recovery (SNRT)
   small-bowel transit
   spin-lattice proton relaxation
   systolic acceleration
   systolic upstroke
   T1 relaxation
   T2 relaxation
   transit
   venous filling (VFT)
   venous return (VRT)
   ventricular activation (VAT)
   ventricular isovolumic relaxation
time activity curve of contrast agent
time-attenuation curve
time-averaged flow
timed bolus delivery
time-density curve
timed imaging
time-insensitive
time-intensity curve
time-lapse quantitative computed tomography lymphography
time-of-flight (TOF)
time-of-flight angiography
time-of-flight echoplanar imaging
time-of-flight (TOF) magnetic resonance angiography
time-of-flight measurement
time-of-flight (TOF) PET imaging systems
time-out, ventriculoatrial
time-resolved imaging by automatic data segmentation (TRIADS)
time-sensitive
time to peak activity
time to peak contrast (TPC)
time to peak filling rate (TPFR)
TIMI (thrombolysis in myocardial infarction) classification
TIPS (transjugular intrahepatic portosystemic shunt)
tissue
   aberrant
   abnormal
   adventitial
   aerated
   areolar
   bony
   cartilaginous
   cavernous
   chondroid
   chorionic
   collagenous
   connective
   cortical
   crushed
   damaged
   dartoic
   dead
   degenerated
   dense
   destruction of
   ectopic
   exuberant
   fatty
   fibroadipose

tissue *(cont.)*
   fibroareolar
   fibrocartilaginous
   fibrofatty
   fibroglandular
   fibromuscular
   fibrosing
   fibrotic
   fibrous
   fibrous scar
   fibrovascular
   gangrenous
   gelatinous
   glandular
   granulation
   grumous
   hyperplastic
   hypertrophic
   interlobular
   isointense soft
   joint
   lipomatous-like
   lymph node
   lymphatic
   lymphoid
   lymphoreticular
   mesenchymal
   mesenteric
   muscle
   muscular
   necrotic
   neoplastic
   nodal
   noncritical soft
   nonviable
   osseous
   ossification of soft
   parenchymal
   periarticular
   proliferation of fibrous
   regeneration of
   scar

tissue *(cont.)*
   soft
   subadventitial
   subcutaneous
   synovial
   taenia
   tendon
   tuberculosis granulation
   underlying
tissue-based T2 relaxation
tissue-borne
tissue characterization technique
tissue contrast
tissue deficit compensator
tissue density
tissue Doppler imaging
tissue inhomogeneity factors
tissue mass
tissue migration
tissue outflow valve
tissue perfusion
tissue sequelae
tissue slice
tissue veil
tissue viability
titanium capsule
titanium plate
Tl (thallium)
TLC (triple-lumen catheter)
TLD (thermoluminescent dosimeter)
   rod
TLI (total lymphoid irradiation)
T loop (vectorcardiography)
TMA (true metatarsus adductus)
TME (trapezium-metacarpal
   eburnation)
TMJ (temporomandibular joint)
   syndrome
TMS three-dimensional radiation
   therapy planning system
TMST (treadmill stress test)
TNM classification of carcinoma

Todaro, triangle of
Todd cirrhosis
TOF (tetralogy of Fallot)
TOF (time-of-flight) magnetic
  resonance angiography
TOF PET (time-of-flight positron
  emission tomography)
Tolosa-Hunt syndrome
toluene scintillator
Tomocat contrast medium
tomogram (see *imaging*)
tomographic cut
tomographic section
tomographic slice
tomography (see *imaging*)
tomomyelography
tomoscanner, Philips T-60
tomoscintigraphy
T1 (longitudinal or spin-lattice
    relaxation time) constant
  T1 pulse sequence
  T1 relaxation time
  T1 weighted coronal image
  T1-weighted fat-suppressed images
    (T1FS)
  T1-weighted image (short TR/TE)
  T1-weighted sagittal image
T (thoracic)
T1-T12 (twelve thoracic vertebrae)
TONE (tilted optimized nonsaturating
  excitation)
tongue and trough bone
tongue of tissue
tongue-type fracture
tonsil, herniated cerebellar
tonus
toothpaste shadow
top normal limits in size
tophaceous gout
tophus (pl. tophi) formation
topical water-soluble contrast media
topodermatography

topogram (see *topography*)
topograph
topographic identification
topographic measurement
topography
  balloon
    scintigraphic balloon
  vessel
  x-ray
Torcon NB selective angiographic
  catheter
Tornwaldt cyst in nasopharynx
torr pressure
torsed appendage
torsion fracture
torsion of fracture fragment
torsional abnormalities
torsional alignment
torsional impaction force
torsional stress
torso phased-array coil (TPAC)
tortuosity and elongation
tortuosity precluding catheter passage
tortuous emptying
torus fracture
TOS (thoracic outlet syndrome)
Toshiba Aspire CI (continuous imaging)
Toshiba CT scanner
Toshiba echocardiograph machine
Toshiba helical CT scanner
Toshiba MR scanner
Toshiba 900S helical CT scanner
Toshiba 900S/XII scanner
Toshiba TCT-80 CT scanner
Toshiba Xpress scanner
Toshiba Xpress SX helical CT
  scanner
Toshiba Xvision scanner
total anomalous pulmonary venous
  drainage (TAPVD)
total atrial refractory period (TARP)

total body irradiation
total body scanning
Total-Cross PTA catheter
total fracture
total lymphoid irradiation (TLI)
Towne projection in skull x-rays
Towne view
toxic adenoma
toxic nodular goiter
toxicity, flutamide-associated liver
TPAC (torso phased-array coil)
TPBS (three-phase bone scintigraphy)
TPC (time to peak contrast)
TPFR (time to peak filling rate)
Tpot, flow cytometry
TPR (total peripheral resistance)
TPR (total pulmonary resistance)
TR (repetition time)
TR (tricuspid regurgitation)
TR/TE (repetition time/echo time),
    long (T2-weighted image)
    short (T1-weighted image)
trabecula (pl. trabeculae)
trabecular bone
trabecular pattern
trabeculated atrium
trabeculated outline
trabeculation, endocardial
trace (see *imaging agent*)
trace amount of radiopharmaceutical
trace element distribution
tracer accumulation
tracer activity
tracer bolus
tracer dose
tracer, neutron-rich biomedical
tracer uptake
trachea
    annular ligament of
    carina of
    scabbard
tracheal anastomosis

tracheal bifurcation
tracheal deviation
tracheal displacement
tracheal ring
tracheal shift
tracheal stenosis
tracheobronchial fistula
tracheobronchial foreign body
tracheobronchial tree
tracheoesophageal fistula (TEF)
tracheomalacia
tracing, vessel-
track cone length
Tracker catheter
track etching
tracking
    bolus
        magnetic resonance needle
        real-time biplanar needle
        real-time magnetic resonance
            imaging
tracking limit
tract
    alimentary
    ascending
    atriohisian
    Bekhterev
    biliary
    Bruce and Muir
    bulbar
    Burdach
    central tegmental
    cerebellorubral
    cerebellorubrospinal
    cerebellospinal
    cerebellotegmental
    cerebellothalamic
    comma tract of Schultze
    conariohypophyseal
    corticobulbar
    corticopontine
    corticorubral

tract *(cont.)*
    corticospinal
    corticotectal
    crossed pyramidal
    cuneocerebellar
    Deiters
    dentatothalamic
    descending
    digestive
    direct pyramidal
    dorsolateral
    extracorticospinal
    extrapyramidal
    fastigiobulbar
    fistulous
    Flechsig
    flow
    frontopontine
    frontotemporal
    gastrointestinal (GI)
    geniculocalcarine
    geniculostriate
    genital
    genitourinary
    GI (gastrointestinal)
    Goll
    Gombault-Philippe
    Gowers
    habenulopeduncular
    Helweg
    hepatic outflow
    hypothalamicohypophysial
    ileal inflow
    intermediolateral
    internodal
    intersegmental
    interstitiospinal
    intestinal
    intrahepatic biliary
    Lissauer
    long
    Lowenthal

tract *(cont.)*
    lower
    Maissiat
    mammilopeduncular
    mammilotegmental
    mammilothalamic
    Marchi
    mesencephalic
    Meynert
    Monakow
    motor
    Muir and Bruce
    nigrostriate
    occipitopontine
    pancreaticobiliary
    paraventriculohypophysial
    parietopontine
    patent needle
    peduncular
    Philippe-Gombault
    pilonidal
    posterior spinocerebellar
    pulmonary conduit outflow
    pulmonary outflow
    pyramidal
    respiratory
    reticulospinal
    rubrobulbar
    rubroreticular
    Schultze comma
    Schutz
    semilunar
    sensory
    septomarginal
    sinus
    spinal
    spinocerebellar
    spinocervical
    spinocervicothalamic
    spinothalamic
    Spitzka-Lissauer
    strionigral

tract *(cont.)*
  sulcomarginal
  tectobulbar
  tectocerebellar
  tegmental
  tegmentospinal
  temporopontine
  testobulbar
  thalamo-olivary
  transverse
  triangular
  trigeminal nerve
  trigeminothalamic
  tuberohypophysial
  upper
  upper gastrointestinal (UGI)
  urinary
  uveal
  ventral amygdalofugal
  vestibulocerebellar
  Vicq d'Azyr
tract embolization
traction diverticulum
tragus
train, fast SE
tram track pattern on x-ray in
  Sturge-Weber syndrome
tramline cortical calcification
tramlines shadow
transabdominal scanning
transaortic radiofrequency ablation
transapical endocardial ablation
transarterial embolization
transaxial CT scan
transaxial images
transaxial maximum-intensity
  projection (MIP)
transaxial slice
transaxillary lateral view
transbronchial lung biopsy
transbronchial needle aspiration
  (TBNA)

transcapitate fracture
transcatheter ablation
transcatheter arterial chemo-
  embolization
transcatheter arterial embolization
  (TAE)
transcatheter filter placement
transcatheter introduction of
  intravascular stent
transcatheter oily chemoembolization
transcatheter therapy
  embolization
  infusion
transcatheter variceal embolization
transcervical balloon tuboplasty (TBT)
transcervical catheterization of fallopian tube
transcervical fracture
transchondral talar fracture
transchoroidal approach
transclival approach
transcondylar axis (TCA)
transcondylar fracture
transcranial color-coded duplex
  sonography
transcranial color-coded real-time
  sonography
transcranial Doppler (TCD)
  ultrasound (sonography)
transcutaneous extraction catheter
  atherectomy
transducer, sector
  Acuson linear array
  broadband
  catheter-borne
  epicardial Doppler flow
  linear
  M-mode
  magnetic resonance imaging-guided
    focused ultrasound
transect, transected
transection

transependymal uptake of tracer
transepiphyseal fracture
transesophageal Doppler color flow
  imaging
transesophageal echocardiography
  (TEE)
transesophageal imaging
transesophageal transducer
transfemoral arteriogram
transfer
  energy
  magnetization
  rapid image
  saturation
  ultrafast video
transfer mode, asynchronous (ATM)
transferrin receptor
transform
  cosine
  fast Fourier
  Fourier
  K-L
transformation matrix
transgluteal CT-guided technique
transhamate fracture
transhepatic cholangiography
transhepatic embolization (THE)
transient ischemic attack (TIA)
transient shunt obstruction
transillumination
transit, bolus
transit time
transition zone
transitional rhythm
transitional vertebra
transjugular cholangiogram
transjugular intrahepatic portosystemic
  shunt (TIPS)
translation-invariant filter
translocation of coronary arteries
translucency, first-trimester nuchal

translucent depression in interatrial
  septum
translumbar aortogram
translumbar aortography
transluminal angioplasty, percutaneous
  (PTA)
transluminal atherectomy
transluminal balloon angioplasty
transluminal coronary angioplasty
transluminal coronary artery
  angioplasty complex
transluminal dilatation
transluminal endatherectomy catheter
  (TEC)
transluminal extraction catheter (TEC)
transluminal lysing system
transluminally placed stented graft
transmalleolar axis (TMA)-thigh angle
transmedial plane
transmesenteric plication
transmetatarsal amputation (TMA)
transmission block
transmission control protocol/Internet
  protocol (TCP/IP)
transmission CT
transmission data
transmission dosimetry
transmission scan
transmitral flow
transmitral gradient
transmitted carotid artery pulsations
transmural cryoablation
transmural fibrosis
transmural match
transmural myocardial infarction
transmural steal
transmutation
transmyocardial perfusion pressure
transnasal endoluminal ultrasonography
  of GI tract
transnasally

transoral
transorally
transparent rendering
transpedicular decompression
transphyseal
transplant (or transplantation)
transport
  forward
  reverse
transporter, dopamine
transposed aorta
transposition
  atrial
  carotid-subclavian
  congenitally corrected
  corrected great arteries
  gastric
  great vessel
  Jatene
transposition cipher
transposition of great arteries (TGA)
    (great vessels)
  complete
  corrected (CTGA)
  partial (of great vessels)
transpulmonary echo ultrasound
  reflectors
transpulmonary pressure (PTP)
transpulmonic gradient
transradial styloid perilunate
  dislocation
transradiancy
transradiant air
transradiant zone
transrectal echography
transrectal ultrasound (TRUS)
transscaphoid perilunate dislocation
transsection, spinal cord
transseptal angiocardiography
transseptal left heart catheterization
transseptal perforation
transseptal puncture

transseptal radiofrequency ablation
transsyndesmotic screw fixation
transtentorial herniation
transtentorial
transtentorially
transthoracic echocardiography (TTE)
transthoracic imaging
transthoracic needle aspiration,
    ultrasound-guided
transthoracic needle biopsy (TNB)
transthoracic three-dimensional
    echocardiography
transtriquetral fracture-dislocation
transudate
transudation
transudation of fluid
transudative pericardial fluid
transurethral ultrasound-guided laser-
    induced prostatectomy (TULIP)
transurethral
transurethrally
transvaginal echography
transvaginal oocyte retrieval
transvaginal sonography
transvaginal ultrasound (TVS)
transvaginal uterine cervical dilation
    with fluoroscopic guidance
transvalvar (or transvalvular) gradient
transvenous implantation
transverse arch
transverse colon
transverse cord lesion
transverse diameter
transverse fracture
transverse heart
transverse hypoplasia
transverse ligaments of atlas
transverse magnetization
transverse orientation
transverse pelvic diameter
transverse plane
transverse plane forces

transverse presentation
transverse process
transverse relaxation rate
transverse section
transverse slice
transverse sinus
transverse ultrasound
trapeziometacarpal joint
trapezioscaphoid joint
trapeziotrapezoid joint
trapezium (greater multangular) bone
trapezius muscle
trapezoid (lesser multangular) bone
trapezoid bone of Henle
trapezoid bone of Lyser
trapezoid ligament
Trapper catheter exchange
trapping, air
trapping of radioisotope
Traube aortic regurgitation sign
Traube semilunar space
trauma
  acoustic
  birth
  blunt
  multiple
  penetrating
  physical
traumatic aneurysm
traumatic avulsion
traumatic brain injury (TBI)
traumatic dislocation
traumatic disruption
traumatic emphysema
traumatic infarct
traumatic intracranial aneurysm
traumatic meningeal hemorrhage
traumatic pneumothorax
traumatic pseudoaneurysm
traumatic rupture
traumatic spondylolisthesis (grades 1-4)
traumatic spondylolysis

traumatic thrombus
traumatogenic occlusion
traversing the fracture
Treacher Collins syndrome
treadmill exercise stress test
treadmill exercise test (TET)
treadmill inclination, incremental
  increases in
treadmill slope
treadmill speed, incremental
  increases in
treadmill stress test (TMST)
treatment energy
treatment port
tree
  arterial
  biliary
  bronchial
  coronary artery
  hepatobiliary
  iliocaval
  intrahepatic biliary
  lower extremity arterial
  tracheobronchial
tree artifact
tree-in-bud (TIB) pattern
tree-in-winter appearance
tree-like airway structure
tree-shaped spot on radiograph
trefoil balloon catheter
Treitz hernia
Treitz ligament
trend-correction
Trendelenburg position
Trevor disease
TRH (thyrotropin releasing hormone)
  stimulation test
T_4RIA (thyroxine radioisotope assay)
triad
  acute compression
  Charcot
  Dieulafoy

triad *(cont.)*
  hepatic
  portal
  Saint
  Whipple
TRIADS (time-resolved imaging by
  automatic data segmentation)
Triad SPECT imaging system
triangle
  anal
  aponeurotic
  auricular
  axillary
  Burger scalene
  Calot
  cardiohepatic
  carotid
  cephalic
  cervical
  clavipectoral
  Codman
  crural
  cystohepatic
  deltoideopectoral
  digastric
  Einthoven
  facial
  femoral
  Garland
  Gerhardt
  Grynfeltt
  Henke
  Hesselbach
  iliofemoral
  inguinal
  insular
  internal jugular
  Koch
  Korányi-Grocco
  Labbé
  Langenbeck
  Lesgaft

triangle *(cont.)*
  Livingston
  lumbocostoabdominal
  mesenteric
  paramedian
  Pawlik
  posterior
  scalene
  Scarpa
  submandibular
  supraclavicular
  Todaro
  urogenital
  vertebrocostal
  Ward
triangular area of dullness
triangular bone
triangular defect
triangular external ankle fixation
triangular fibrocartilage (TFC)
triangular fibrocartilage complex
  (TFCC)
triangular ligament
triangulation of Carrel
tributary (pl. tributaries)
trichinous embolism
tricuspid aortic valve
trifid stomach
triflanged nail
trifoil balloon
trifurcation of artery
trigeminal cavernous fistula
trigeminal cavity
trigeminal hemangioma
trigeminal nerve (fifth cranial nerve)
trigeminal pattern
trigeminy
triggering ventricular contraction
trigonal hypertrophy
trigone
  angles of
  collateral

trigone *(cont.)*
   deltoideopectoral
   fibrous
   Henke
   hypertrophied
   hypoglossal
   inguinal
   lateral ventricle
   Lieutaud
   Müller
   Pawlik
   vertebrocostal
Triguide guide catheter
triisocyanide ^{99m}Tc imaging agent
trilaminar appearance
trilayer appearance
trileaflet
trilinear interpolation
trimalleolar fracture
Trionix camera
Trionix scanner
Trionix SPECT
triphasic spiral CT
triplane fracture
triple-dose gadolinium imaging
triple-head SPECT with FDG
triple-lumen central venous catheter
triple label
triple match
triple resonance NMR probe circuit
triple ripple
triplet beat
tripod position
tripolar electrode catheter
triquetral bone
triquetral fracture
triquetrohamate joint
triquetrohamate ligament
triquetrolunate dislocation
triradiate cartilage
trisacryl gelatin microspheres
tristimulus values

trochanter
   greater
   lesser
trochlear nerve (fourth cranial nerve)
trochlear notch
trochlear process
Troisier node
TRON 3 VACI cardiac imaging
   system
trophedema
trophic fracture
trophoblastic material
true channel
true conjugate
true lumen
truncal artery
truncal renal artery stenosis
truncal valve
truncated NMR probe
truncation band artifact
truncus arteriosus
   embryonic
   persistent
trunk
   articulations of
   atrioventricular (AV)
   bifurcation of
   brachiocephalic
   bronchomediastinal
   bronchomediastinal lymph
   celiac
   cordlike
   costocervical
   joints of
   lumbosacral
   lymph
   nerve
   posterior vagal
   thyrocervical
   vagal
Trunkey fracture classification system
TRUS (transrectal ultrasound)

Tru-Scint AD imaging agent
Tru-Trac high-pressure PTA balloon
TRW (teboroxime) resting washout
TS (tricuspid stenosis)
T-shaped fracture
TSH (thyroid-stimulating hormone)
    TSH-dependent functioning nodule
    TSH stimulation test
T spine (thoracic spine)
TSPP (technetium stannous pyrophos-phate) rectilinear bone scan
TTC (T-tube cholangiogram)
TTE (transthoracic echocardiography)
T3 resin uptake test
TTS (tarsal tunnel syndrome)
T-tube cholangiogram
T tubogram
T2 (transverse or spin-spin relaxation time) constant
    T2 pulse sequence
    T2 QMRI (T2 quantitative MRI)
    T2 relaxation time
    T2 shortening
    T2 star relaxation
    T2 time constant
    T2 weighted image (long TR/TE)
    T2 weighted spin-echo image
tubal insufflation
tubal pregnancy
tubal ring
tube
    anode
    auditory
    bilateral pleural
    blocked shunt
    bronchial
    calices (calyces)
    capillary
    cathode-ray
    Chaoul voltage x-ray
    chest
    collecting

tube *(cont.)*
    corneal
    cuffed endotracheal
    digestive
    double-lumen endobronchial
    endobronchial
    endotracheal (ET)
    enterolysis
    Eppendorf
    ET (endotracheal)
    eustachian
    fallopian
    feeding
    fenestrated
    J-shaped
    large-caliber
    muscular
    nasogastric (NG)
    nasotracheal
    neural
    NG (nasogastric)
    obstructed shunt
    oroendotracheal
    orogastric
    pharyngotympanic
    pickup
    pleural
    polyethylene
    right-angle chest
    separator
    Shiner radiopaque
    shunt
    solid-phase extraction
    stomach
    straight chest
    suction
    T-
    T self-retaining drainage
    tracheal
    uterine
    water-seal chest
    x-ray

tube current
tube drainage
tube geometry module of VIDA
tube position rotation
tuber cinereum
tubercle
  accessory
  acoustic
  adductor
  amygdaloid
  articular
  auricular
  calcaneal
  carotid
  Chaput
  conoid
  corniculate
  costal
  crown
  cuneiform
  darwinian
  dental
  dissection
  epiglottic
  fibrous
  genial
  genital
  Gerdy
  Ghon
  greater
  iliac
  intercondylar
  lesser
  Lister
  Parsons
  prominent
  pubic
  rib
  scalene
  sella turcica
  tibial

tubercle bacillus
tubercular empyema
tuberculoma
tuberculosis (TB)
  bone
  disseminated
  exudative
  fulminant
  genitourinary
  hematogenous
  inhalation
  meningeal
  miliary
  postprimary
  primary
  pulmonary
  renal
tuberosity (pl. tuberosities)
  bicipital
  calcaneal
  coracoid
  costal
  deltoid
  femoral
  greater
  iliac
  infraglenoid
  ischial
  lesser
  navicular
  omental
  radial
  tibial
  ulnar
tuberous sclerosis
tubogram
tuboplasty, balloon
tubular bone
tubular lesion
tubular magnet
tubular stenosis

tubular structure
tubule
  collecting
  connecting
  convoluted
  dental
  dentinal
  discharging
  distal convoluted
  proximal convoluted
  renal
  seminiferous
  straight
  tortuous
tuft fracture
tulip sheath
TULIP (transurethral ultrasound-
  guided laser-induced prostatectomy)
tumor
  apple core
  Askin
  benign
  Brenner
  carcinoid
  cavernous
  chondrogenic
  chordoma
  chromophobe adenoma
  clivus meningioma
  CNS (central nervous system)
  colloid cyst
  craniopharyngioma
  cutaneous
  cystic
  deep-seated
  discrete
  dumbbell
  echogenic
  embryonal
  ependymoma
  epidermoid
  Ewing

tumor *(cont.)*
  extension of
  extracompartmental
  extramedullary
  fatty
  fibroadenoma
  fibroid
  finger of
  focal
  ganglion
  globular
  gross
  highly vascular
  hourglass
  hypoechogenic
  intra-axial brain
  intracompartmental
  intracranial
  intradural
  intramedullary
  invasive
  Krukenberg
  lobulated
  locally invasive
  lymphoid
  main
  malignant
  metastatic
  microadenoma
  napkin ring
  nonechogenic
  non-neoplastic
  Pancoast
  papilloma
  pedunculated
  phyllodes
  pilocytic
  pinealoma
  pontine glioma
  poorly circumscribed
  poorly differentiated
  Pott puffy

tumor *(cont.)*
  primary
  prolactin-secreting adenoma
  pseudo-
  pseudomalignant
  radiosensitive
  RIF-1
  scirrhous
  secondary
  seeding of
  sessile
  smooth muscle
  solid
  spread of
  subcortical
  submucosal
  subserosal
  vascular
  Warthin (adenolymphoma)
  well-circumscribed
  Wharton (cystadenoma)
  Wilms
tumor-bearing bone
tumor bed
tumor blush on cerebral angiography
tumor boundary
tumor capillary permeability
tumor cleavage plane
tumor embolism
tumor embolization
tumor extirpation
tumorlike shadow
tumor marker
tumor mass
tumor matrix
tumor osteoid
tumor recurrence
tumor staining on cerebral
  angiography
tumor-to-normal brain ratio
tumor vascularity
tumor volume

tumor volumetry
tungsten eye shield
tungsten target
tunica adventitia
tunica intima
tunica media
tunica propria
tuning unit, reflectometer
tunnel
  carpal
  cubital
  retropancreatic
  tarsal
tunnel view
turbid effusion
turbinate bone
Turbo-FLAIR imaging
Turbo-FLASH sequence
turbo SE sequences
turbulence
turbulent flow
turbulent signal
turcica, sella
turf-toe
Turkish sabre syndrome
Turner marginal gyrus
turning-point morphology (TPM)
turricephaly
TV (tricuspid valve)
TV-interlaced (TVI)
T vector
TVS (transvaginal ultrasound)
twelfth cranial nerve (hypoglossal
  nerve)
twig
  cutaneous
  muscular
twinkling artifact
twin-to-twin transfusion syndrome
  (TTTS)
twin trunk
2-nitroimidazole nucleoside analog

24-bit image
270 MHz VT multinuclear spectrometer
two-channel phased array RF receiver
coil system
2D (see *two-dimensional*)
two-dimensional (2D or 2-D)
2D B-mode ultrasound machine
2D color-coded imaging of blood
flow
2D echocardiography (sector scan)
2D format
2D Fourier imaging
2D Fourier transform (2DFT)
2DFT (two-dimensional Fourier
transform)
2D GRE dynamic protocol
2D J-resolved 1H MR spectroscopy

two-dimensional *(cont.)*
2D portal image registration
2D pulsatility index mapping
2D resistance index mapping
2D sector scan
2D spatially selective radiofrequency (RF) pulses
two-frame gated imaging
two-part fracture
two-phase computed tomographic
imaging
two-phase helical computed
tomography
two-vessel runoff
two-view chest x-ray
Tygon catheter
tympanic bone
type I, II, and III dens fracture
tyropanoate sodium contrast medium

U, u

U (uranium)
UBM (ultrasound backscatter
  microscopy)
UC (ulcerative colitis)
UCG (ultrasonic cardiography)
UCL (ulnar collateral ligament)
UCLA imaging protocol
UEs (upper extremities)
UES (upper esophageal sphincter)
UFCT (ultrafast computed tomography)
UGI (upper gastrointestinal) series
UGI SBF (upper GI series with
  small-bowel follow-through)
Uhl syndrome
UHMM (ultra-high magnification
  mammography)
UJ (uncovertebral joint)
ulcer (ulceration)
  acid peptic
  active duodenal
  acute peptic
  amebic
  anastomotic
  anterior wall antral
  antral
  aortic

ulcer *(cont.)*
  arteriolar ischemic
  atheromatous
  atherosclerotic aortic
  Barrett
  bear claw
  benign
  bleeding
  bulbar peptic
  chronic
  chronic peptic
  collar button
  colonic mucosal
  craterlike
  Cruveilhier
  Curling
  Cushing
  Cushing-Rokitansky
  duodenal
  esophageal
  flask-shaped
  focal
  gastric
  gastrointestinal
  giant peptic
  greater curvature
  healing

UltraLite flow-directed microcatheter
ultra-low profile fixed-wire balloon
    dilatation catheter
Ultramark 4 ultrasound
Ultramark 8 transducer
Ultramark 9 scanner
UltraPACS diagnostic imaging system
ultrasmall superparamagnetic iron
    oxide (USPIO) imaging agent
ultrasonically activated scalpel
ultrasonic aortography
ultrasonic aspiration
ultrasonic assessment
ultrasonic cardiogram
ultrasonic cardiography (UCG)
ultrasonic guidance for interstitial
    radioelement application
ultrasonic guidance for intrauterine
    fetal transfusion
ultrasonic guidance for placement of
    radiation therapy fields
ultrasonic knife, UltraCision
ultrasonic lithotripsy
ultrasonic nebulizer (USN)
ultrasonic scalpel
ultrasonic tomographic image
ultrasonographic catheter
ultrasonographic images,
    cross-sectional
ultrasonography
ultrasound (US)
    abdominal
    ACM (automated cardiac flow
      measurement)
    Acuson
    ADR
    AI 5200 diagnostic
    Aloka linear
    Aloke sector
    A-mode
    Aspen digital
    ATL real-time

ultrasound *(cont.)*
    BladderManager
    BladderScan
    B-mode
    breast
    Bruel-Kjaer
    color-coded duplex
    color-coded real-time
    color Doppler
    color duplex
    color power transcranial Doppler
    compression
    contact B-scan
    continuous wave
    contrast-enhanced
    cranial
    CUSALap
    diagnostic
    diagnostic range
    Diasonics
    diathermy
    DIMAQ integrated
    Doppler
    duplex
    duplex B-mode
    duplex carotid
    duplex Dopper
    duplex pulsed-Doppler
    DUST (dynamic ultrasound of
      shoulder)
    Echo-Gen enhanced
    endoanal
    endorectal
    endoscopic (EUS)
    endovaginal
    endovascular
    EUS (endoscopic ultrasonography)
    fatty meal (FMS)
    fetal
    5 MHz
    freehand interventional
    frequency domain imaging (FDI)

ultrasound *(cont.)*
full-bladder
gallbladder
gastrointestinal endoscopic
GI (gastrointestinal) endoscopic
graded compression
gray-scale
Hewlett-Packard
high-frequency therapeutic
high-intensity focused (HIFU)
high-resolution
Hitachi
immersion B-scan
intracaval endovascular (ICEUS)
intracavitary prostate
intracoronary
intraoperative
intraportal endovascular
intrarectal
intravascular (IVUS)
Irex Exemplar
laparoscopic (LUS)
laparoscopic contact (LCU)
laparoscopic intracorporeal (LICU)
low-intensity pulsed
M-mode
MUSTPAC (medical ultrasound 3D portable, with advanced communications)
neonatal adrenal
NeuroSector
noninvasive
obstetric
Olympus endoscopic
pancreaticobiliary (or pancreatic-biliary)
pelvic
Pentax EUP-EC124 ultrasound gastroscope
Pentax-Hitachi FG32UA endosonographic system
photoacoustic

ultrasound *(cont.)*
power Doppler
PowerVision
pulsed
pulsed Doppler
real-time
rectal endoscopic
renal
RT 3200 Advantage
RT 6800
sagitta
Siemens Sonoline Elegral
SieScape
single-field hyperthermia combined with radiation therapy and
Sonicator portable
Synergy
three-dimensional (3D) freehand
two-dimensional (2D) B-mode
transcranial color-coded duplex
transcranial Doppler (TCD)
transnasal endoluminal
transrectal (TRUS)
transthoracic
transvaginal (TVS)
transverse
TRUS (transrectal ultrasound)
Ultramark 4
VingMed
ultrasound backscatter microscopy (UBM)
ultrasound diffraction tomography
ultrasound echocardiography
ultrasound-enhanced stylet, INRAD HiLiter
ultrasound for foreign body detection
ultrasound gel
ultrasound-guided percutaneous interstitial laser ablation
ultrasound-guided stereotactic biopsy
ultrasound-guided transthoracic needle aspiration

ultrasound-guided TULIP (transurethral laser-induced prostatectomy)
ultrasound hyperthermia treatment
ultrasound imaging technology
ultrasound monitoring
ultrasound pad
ultrasound probe, Olympus UM-1W
   transendoscopic
ultrasound scanning, high-resolution
ultrasound system (see *ultrasound*)
ultrasound venography
UltraSTAR computer-based ultrasound
   reporting system
ultrastructural abnormality
Ultravist (iopromide) imaging agent
UM 4 real-time sector scanner
umbilical artery
umbilical catheter
umbilical cord
   three-vessel
   two-vessel
umbilical hernia
UMI catheter
unattached fractions
unbuttoning of device
uncalcified pleural plaque
uncal gyrus
uncal herniation syndrome
uncertainty principle
unciform bone
uncinate aura
uncinate gyrus
uncinate process of pancreas
uncinate region of temporal lobe
uncommitted metaphyseal lesion
uncommon pneumoconioses
uncomplicated myocardial infarction
uncontrolled bronchospasm
uncoupled spins
uncovertebral joint (UJ)
uncovertebral spurring

uncus, arachnoid of
uncus corporis
undercorrection
underdetection
underdrive termination
under fluoroscopic guidance
underinflation of lung
underloading, ventricular
underperfused
underperfusion
under-scan method/projection
undersurface
underventilation
undifferentiated nasopharyngeal
   carcinoma (UCNT)
undisplaced fracture
undulant impulse
undulating contour
undulating course
unenhanced magnetic resonance
   imaging scan
unfused physis
unguicular tuberosity
unicameral bone cyst
unicameral brain
unicommissural aortic valve
unicommissural valve
unicompartmental knee prosthesis
unicorn
unicornuate uterus
unicoronal synostosis
unicortical screw
unicusp with central raphe
unicuspid aortic valve
unidirectional lead configuration
unifascicular block
unifocal
unifocalization
uniform attenuation coefficient
uniform loading
uniform resource locator (URL)
uniform sensitivity

unshunted hydrocephalus
unstable angina
unstable fracture
unsuppressed exam
untether
untethered
ununited (nonunited) fracture
U-1100 UV-Vis spectrophotometer
(also U-2001, U-2010, U-3000,
U-3010, U-3300, U-3310)
U1-NA cephalometric measurement
up-regulation, radiation-induced
uPACS picture archiving system
updraft therapy
UPJ (ureteropelvic junction)
upper airway obstruction, foreign
body
upper collecting system
upper gastrointestinal series
upper GI (gastrointestinal) series
upper GI with small bowel follow-
through
upper-limb cardiovascular syndrome
upper limits of normal
upper lobe vein prominence
upper lung field
upper mantle radiotherapy
upper pole collecting system
upper pole moiety
upper pole ureter
upper rate interval
upper respiratory tract disease
upright chest film
upright PA (posteroanterior) film
upright post-void view
upright view
UP7 film
Upshaw-Schulman syndrome
upstairs-downstairs heart
upstream blood
upstroke, carotid pulse
upstroke phase of cardiac action
potentials

uptake (of organ)
contrast
diffuse
dye
fluorescein
focal
heterogeneous
localized
observed maximal
predicted maximal
radioiodine
radioisotope
radiotracer
tracer
uniform
uptake and excretion
uptake and retention
uptake in radionuclide scan
upward and backward dislocation
upward retraction
uranium (U)
^{235}U (uranium-235)
uremia
uremic pneumonitis
ureter
atonic
circumcaval
dilatation of
dilated
ectopic
intravesical
kinked
moderately dilated
orthotopic
postcaval
retrocaval
retroiliac
rigid
straight
tortuosity of
ureteral achalasia
ureteral bud, accessory

V, v

V (lung volume)
V (ventricular)
VA (ventriculoatrial)
   VA conduction
   VA interval
V-angle, femoral torsion
VABES (vasoablative endothelial
   sarcoma)
vacuum cleft
vacuum disk
vacuum, facet joint
vacuum joint phenomenon
vagina
   anterior fornix of
   azygos artery of
   double
   fornix of
   vestibule of
vaginal cone irradiation
vaginal ligament of hand
vaginogram
vagus (tenth cranial) nerve
vagus trunk
valgus
   adolescent hallux
   hallux (HV)

valgus *(cont.)*
   hindfoot
   metatarsus
   pes
   talipes
valgus carrying angle
valgus deformity
valgus foot
valgus fracture, impacted
valgus heel
valgus tilt
vallecula cerebelli
valley-to-peak dose rate
Valsalva maneuver
value
   attenuation
   bright pixel
   comparative
   CT attenuation
   dark pixel
value flips
   negative predictive
   P
   positive predictive
   predictive
   tristimulus

valve plane
valve pockets
valve replacement
valve scarring
valve strut
valve thickening and scarring
valve tip
valviform
valvular aortic insufficiency
valvular aortic stenosis
valvular apparatus
valvular atresia
valvular cardiac defect
valvular damage
valvular disease
valvular dysfunction
valvular heart disease
valvular incompetence
valvular opening
valvular orifice
valvular pneumothorax
valvular pulmonic stenosis
valvular regurgitant lesion
valvular regurgitation
valvular stenosis
VAN (vein, artery, nerve)
vanishing lung syndrome (on x-ray)
Vaquez disease
variability
   anatomic
   beat-to-beat
   interpretive
   peak flow
variable-angle uniform signal
   excitation (VUSE)
variable energy
variable flip angle excitation
variable murmur
variable response rate
Varian Associates 11.7T (500
   MHz)/51 mm bore spectrometer
Varian brachytherapy system

Varian LINAC (linear accelerator)
Varian NMR spectrometer
variance images
variant
   anatomic
   labral
   ossification
variant angina pectoris
variation
   area/hemidiameter
   BO field
   exposure
   normal anatomic
   positional
variation in density
variceal column
variceal hemorrhage
variceal sclerotherapy
varices (pl. of varix)
varicocele, idiopathic
varicography
varicose aneurysm
varicose bronchiectasis
varicose vein
varicosity (pl. varicosities)
Variflex catheter
VARIS radiation oncology system
varix (pl. varices)
varum, genu
varus
   metatarsus
   rearfoot
   subtalar
   talipes
   tibial
varus angle
varus deformity
varus heel
varus metatarsophalangeal (MTP)
   angle
varus tilt
VAS (vestibular aqueduct syndrome)

Vas-Cath catheter for percutaneous
    thromboarterectomy
Vas-Cath PTA balloon catheter
Vascoray imaging agent
vascular access
vascular accident
vascular anastomosis
vascular anomaly
vascular atrophy
vascular attachments
vascular bed, pulmonary
vascular blush (on carotid
    angiography)
vascular bud
vascular bundle
vascular catastrophe
vascular channels, aberrant
vascular cirrhosis
vascular compromise
vascular congestion
vascular cord damage
vascular disease, peripheral
vascular ectasia
vascular encasement
vascular engorgement
vascular enhancement
vascular flasks
vascular flow imaging
vascular graft
vascular hamartoma
vascular hemangioma
vascular heterograft
vascular hydraulic conductivity
vascular impedance
vascular insult
vascular invasion
vascular lumen
vascular malformation
vascular markings
vascular network
vascular obstruction

vascular occlusive disease
vascular patency
vascular pedicle
vascular phase
vascular plexus
vascular protrusion
vascular redistribution
vascular reserve
vascular resistance
vascular ring
vascular segmentation and extraction
vascular sling
vascular spasm
vascular supply
vascular syndrome
vascular systemic resistance
vascular tone
vascular tuft
vascular wall
vascular xenograft
vascularity
vasculature
vasculitic lesion
vasoconstriction
vasodepressive
vasodepressor reaction (VDR)
vasodilate
vasodilation
vasodilatation
vasography
vasopressor
vasoreactivity, pulmonary
vasospasm
vasospastic vessel
vasovagal phenomenon
VasoView balloon dissection system
vastus lateralis muscle
vastus medialis advancement (VMA)
vastus medialis muscle
vastus medialis obliquus (VMO)
VAT (vaso-occlusive angiotherapy)

VAT (ventricular activation time)
Vater
   ampulla of
   papilla of
VATER (acronym for vertebral or
   vascular defects, anorectal malfor-
   mation, tracheoesophageal fistula,
   and radial, ray, or renal anomaly)
Vater diverticulum
vaterian segment
VATS (video-assisted thoracic
   surgery)
vault
   cranial
   plantar
   rectal
VAX 4100 system
VBI (vertebrobasilar insufficiency)
VC (vital capacity)
VCB (ventricular capture beat)
VCF (ventricular contractility function)
VCG (vectorcardiogram)
VCO_2 (venous CO_2 production)
VCUG (vesicoureterogram)
VCUG (voiding cystourethrogram)
VD (valvular disease)
VDI (venous distensibility index)
VDR (vasodepressor reaction)
VDS (ventral derotating spinal)
VEA (ventricular ectopic activity)
VEB (ventricular ectopic beat)
vector
   expression
   mean cardiac
vectocardiogram
vectorcardiography
   Frank
   frontal plane
   sagittal plane
   spatial
   transverse plane
  vector loop

vegetation of valve
vein (pl. veins)
   accessory cephalic
   accessory hemiazygos
   accessory saphenous
   accessory vertebral
   accompanying
   anal
   anastomosing
   anastomotic
   aneurysmal
   angular
   anonymous
   antebrachial
   antecubital
   anterior cardiac
   anterior jugular
   anterior terminal (ATV)
   appendicular
   aqueous
   arciform
   arcuate
   arterial
   ascending lumbar
   auditory
   auricular
   autogenous
   axillary
   azygos
   basal
   basal vein of Rosenthal (BVR)
   basilic
   basivertebral
   Boyd perforating
   brachial
   brachiocephalic
   bronchial
   bulb of
   cannulated central
   capacious
   capillary
   cardiac

vein *(cont.)*
  cardinal
  cavernous
  central
  cephalic
  cerebral
  cervical
  choroid
  ciliary
  circumflex
  colic
  common basal
  common cardinal
  common facial
  communicating
  companion
  condylar emissary
  congenital stenosis of
  conjunctival
  coronary
  costoaxillary
  cutaneous
  cystic
  deep
  digital
  dilated
  diploic
  distended
  Dodd perforating group of
  dorsispinal
  duodenal
  embryonic umbilical
  emissary
  engorged
  epigastric
  episcleral
  esophageal
  ethmoidal
  external jugular
  external pudendal
  facial
  familial varicose

vein *(cont.)*
  feeder
  femoral
  fibular
  flat neck
  frontal
  gastric
  gastroepiploic
  great cardiac
  great cerebral vein of Galen
  great saphenous
  harvested
  hemiazygos
  hepatic
  ileocolic
  iliofemoral
  inferior pulmonary
  inferior rectal
  inferior thyroid
  infradiaphragmatic
  innominate
  intercostal
  internal cerebral (ICV)
  internal jugular
  internal thoracic
  intussusception of
  jugular
  Labbé
  labial
  leaking
  left hepatic
  lesser saphenous
  lobe of azygos
  marginal
  Marshall
  median antebrachial
  medullary
  meningeal
  mesenteric
  middle cardiac
  middle rectal
  nodularity

ventricular pressure, right
ventricular pseudoperfusion beats
ventricular puncture
ventricular rate
ventricular reflux
ventricular refractoriness
ventricular refractory period
ventricular repolarization
ventricular reservoir
ventricular response
ventricular right-handedness
ventricular segmental contraction
ventricular sensed (VS) event
ventricular septal (VS)
ventricular septal aneurysm
ventricular septal defect (VSD), Swiss
  cheese
ventricular septal summit
ventricular shift
ventricular single and double
  extrastimulation
ventricular size
ventricular space
ventricular span
ventricular standstill
ventricular status
ventricular stiffness
ventricular synchrony
ventricular system
ventricular systole
ventricular tachycardia (VT, V tach)
ventricular transposition
ventricular wall motion
ventricularization of pressure
ventriculoarterial conduit
ventriculoarterial connections
ventriculoarterial discordance
ventriculoatrial (VA) conduction
ventriculoatrial effective refractory
  period
ventriculoatrial time-out

ventriculogram
  axial left anterior oblique
  bicycle exercise radionuclide
  biplane
  bubble
  digital subtraction
  dipyridamole thallium
  exercise radionuclide
  first-pass radionuclide
  gated blood pool
  gated nuclear
  gated radionuclide
  intraoperative
  LAO (left anterior oblique)
    projection
  left (LVG)
  metrizamide
  radionuclide (RNV)
  RAO (right anterior oblique)
    projection
  retrograde left
  single plane left
  ventriculography
  xenon 133 (^{133}Xe)
ventriculogram
ventriculography
ventriculoinfundibular fold
ventriculomegaly
ventriculoperitoneal (VP)
ventriculoradial dysplasia
ventriculovenous shunt
ventriculus cordis
ventriculus terminalis
Venturi effect
venule (pl. venules)
Verbatim balloon catheter
verge, anal
vergence, downward
vermian medulloblastoma
vermian veins
vermicular appendage

vermicular appendix
vermiform process
vermis
  cerebellar
  folium
vernix membrane
VERP (ventricular effective refractory
  period)
vertebra (pl. vertebrae)
  arch of
  articular process of
  basilar
  caudal
  cervical (C1 through C7)
  coccygeal
  codfish
  cranial
  displaced
  dorsal (D)
  facet surface of
  false
  fractured
  fused
  last normal (LNV)
  lumbar (L1 through L5)
  midbody of
  olisthetic
  pear-shaped
  sacral (S1 through S5)
  scalloping of
  subluxed
  thoracic (T1 through T12)
  transitional
  transverse process of
  true
  wedging of olisthetic
vertebral ankylosis
vertebral arterial dissection
vertebral artery occlusion
vertebral artery syndrome
vertebral artery system
vertebral-basilar artery syndrome

vertebral-basilar ischemia
vertebral basilar insufficiency
vertebral body collapse
vertebral body endplate
vertebral collapse
vertebral column
vertebral endplate
vertebral pleural reflection
vertebral scalloping
vertebral segmentation anomaly
vertebral steal phenomenon
vertebral stripe
vertebral vein
vertebral venous plexus
vertebra plana fracture
vertebrobasilar circulation
vertebrobasilar disease
vertebrobasilar distribution stroke
vertebrobasilar insufficiency (VBI)
vertebrobasilar ischemia
vertebrobasilar occlusion
vertebrobasilar system
vertebrocostal rib
vertebrophrenic angle
vertebrosternal rib
vertex, cube
vertex presentation
Vertex camera
vertex (pl. vertices)
vertical fracture
vertical heart
vertical-long axial (VLA) images
vertical long-axis slice
vertical plane
vertical shear fracture
vertical talus
VERT software
vesalianum of vertebral body
vesical (adj.)
vesical calculus, radiopaque
vesical distention
vesical injury

view *(cont.)*
   lateral oblique
   lateral tilt stress ankle
   Laurin x-ray
   Law
   left anterior oblique (LAO)
   limited
   long axial oblique
   long axis
   long-axis parasternal
   lordotic
   Low-Beers
   Mayer
   mediolateral
   mediolateral oblique
   Merchant
   mortise
   multiplanar reformatting (MPR)
   navicular
   Neer lateral
   Neer transscapular
   nonstanding lateral oblique
   nonweightbearing
   notch
   oblique
   occipital
   odontoid
   open-mouth
   optimally positioned
   orthogonal
   outlet
   over couch
   overhead
   overhead oblique
   Owen
   PA (posteroanterior)
   parasternal long-axis
   parasternal short-axis
   patellar skyline
   Pillar
   plain
   planar

view *(cont.)*
   plantar axial
   plantarflexion
   plantarflexion stress
   portable
   postvoid
   postevacuation
   postoperative
   preliminary
   preoperative
   prereduction
   prone
   prone lateral
   push-pull ankle stress
   push-pull hip
   RAO (right anterior oblique)
   ray-sum
   recumbent
   retromammary space
   Rhees
   right anterior oblique (RAO)
   right lateral decubitus
   right ventricular inflow
   routine magnification
   Schatzki
   Schüller
   scout
   selective coronary arteriography
   serendipity
   short-axis
   short-axis parasternal
   single breath
   sitting-up
   skijump
   skyline
   spider
   spot
   standing
   standing dorsoplantar
   standing lateral
   standing post-void

Virchow perivascular space
Virchow psammoma
Virchow-Robin space
Virchow sentinel node
Virchow thrombosis triad
Virchow triad
Virchow-Troisier node
virtual angioscopy
virtual bronchoscopy
virtual colonsocopy
virtual endoscopy
virtual reality imaging
virtual reality simulator
virtual reality viewbox
virus
viscera (pl. of viscus)
   abdominal
   abdominopelvic
   hollow
   intra-abdominal
   intraperitoneal
   pelvic
visceral angiogram
visceral cholesterol embolization
   syndrome
visceral embolus
visceral layer
visceral pericardium
visceral peritoneum
visceral pleura
visceral pleurisy
visceral situs solitus
visceromegaly
visceroptosis
viscid
viscous (adj.)
viscus (pl. viscera)
   hollow
   perforated
   strangulated
VISI (volarflexed intercalated segment
   instability) deformity

visible anterior motion
Visible Human Project (VHP)
Vision camera
Vision MRI scanner
Vision Ten V-scan scanner
Vistec x-ray detectable sponge
visual cortex
visual
visualization
   delayed
   inadequate
   optimal
   poor
   suboptimal
visualization and quantification
vital capacity (VC)
Vitalcor venous catheter
vitelline duct
Viterbi decoding
Vitrea 3-D system
VJ (ventriculojugular) shunt
VLA (vertical-long axial) images
VMO (vastus medialis obliquus)
vocal cords
   true
   false
VOD (veno-occlusive disease)
Voda catheter
VoiceRAD clinical reporting system
void (verb)
void
   flow
   signal
void determination
voiding cystogram
voiding cystourethrogram (VCUG)
voiding sequence
voiding study
volar angulation
volar capsule
volar carpal ligament
volarly

W, w

wafer of endocardium
wagon wheel fracture
Wagstaffe fracture
waist (of anatomical structure)
Walcher position
Waldenström disease
Waldeyer fascia
wall
  abdominal
  aneurysmal
  anterior abdominal
  anterolateral
  apical
  axial
  bladder
  body
  bowel
  carotid
  cavity
  chest
  cyst
  cystic
  gallbladder
  inferior
  inferoapical
  intestinal
  left anterior chest wall

wall *(cont.)*
  luminal
  midabdominal
  nasal cavity
  posterior
  posterior abdominal
  posterolateral
  septal
  stomach
  thickened gallbladder
  thoracic
  vaginal
  variceal
  ventricular
wall akinesis
Wallenberg lateral medullary
  syndrome
wall filter
wall hypokinesis
wall motion study
wall motion abnormalities (WMA)
wall shear stress
wall thickening
wall thickness
wallerian degeneration
Wallstent
wand, programmer

Wanderer microcatheter
Ward triangle
warm nodule
washboard effect on myelography in
    cervical spondylosis
wash-in phase
washout
    delayed
    lung
    nitrogen
    teboroxime resting (TRW)
washout curve
washout gradient
washout kinetics
washout phase
washout view
Wassel classification of thumb
    polydactyly
wasting
    muscle
    muscle fiber
wasting syndrome
Watanabe classification of discoid
    meniscus
water
    doped
    purified (contrast)
water bath
water bolus
water-contrast computed tomography
water density
waterfall stomach
Waterhouse-Friderichsen syndrome
water path
water perfusable tissue index
water range
water retention
water selective SE imaging sequence
water signal on magnetic resonance
    imaging scan
watershed infarct (infarction)
water-soluble contrast media

Waters projection
Waterston groove
Waters view
Watson-Jones classification of spinal
    fractures
wave
    abdominal fluid
    fluid
    peristaltic
    primary peristaltic
    secondary
    secondary peristaltic
    tertiary
waveform, segmental renal artery
waveforms, gradient
wavelength
    de Broglie
    readout
wavelet compression
wavelet-encoded
wavelet scalar quantization (WSQ)
wavelet sub-band (or subband)
WBCS (white blood cell scintigraphy)
    with indium-111 (^{111}In)
weak carotid upstroke
weak signal
weaver's bottom
web
    duodenal
    esophageal
    fibrous
    finger
    hepatic
    intestinal
    laryngeal
    postcricoid
    terminal
    thumb
    venous
Web browser (World Wide Web in
    teleradiology)
Weber C fracture

Weber, circle of
Weber-Osler-Rendu syndrome
web space
wedge
   dynamic
   match-line
   mediastinal
wedge bonds
wedge compression fracture
wedged beam
wedged hepatic venography
wedge factors
wedge flexion-compression fracture
wedge fracture
wedge isodose angle
wedge-shaped mass
wedge position, pulmonary capillary
wedge pressure
wedge-shaped vertebra
wedge-pair beam
wedge-shaped density
wedge-shaped lobe
wedge-shaped zone
wedging deformity
wedging of olisthetic vertebra
wedging of vertebral interspace
weeping willow appearance on
   venogram
weeping willow view
Wegener granulomatosis
weight, estimated fetal
weight loading, axial
weightbearing (also weight-bearing)
weightbearing dome of acetabulum
weightbearing rotational injury
weightbearing films
weighted spin-echo column (MRI)
weighting, human visual sensitivity
Weil disease or syndrome (Adolf
   Weil)
Weill sign of pneumonia in infant
   (Edmond Weill)

Weinberg-Himelfarb syndrome
Weingarten syndrome
Weisenburg syndrome
Weiss-Baker syndrome
Weitbrecht ligament
welder's lung
well-inflated lung
well-preserved ejection fraction
well-type ionization chamber
Wenckebach AV (atrioventricular)
   block
Wenckebach phenomenon
Werner syndrome
Wernicke-Korsakoff syndrome
Wernicke region
Westermark sign
Westphal-Strumpell disease
wet lung syndrome
wet pleurisy
wet reading of x-ray film
wet swallow (on esophageal
   manometry)
Wexler catheter
wheelchair artifact
whettle bone
whiplash injury
Whipple disease
whirlpool sign
Whitacre spinal needle
Whitaker test
white-appearing blood pool
white blood cell scintigraphy (WBCS)
   with indium-111
white cerebellum sign
white clot syndrome
white commissure of spinal cord
white echo writing
Whitehead deformity
White leg-length view
white light pattern projector
white lung syndrome
white matter infarct

white matter signal hyperintensity
white metastasis
white noise
white-out of lungs
white point
white noise artifact
whitlow, melanotic
whole blood monoclonal antibody
whole body 29FDG scanning
whole body imaging with magnified
 views
whole brain mean CBF
whole-body imaging
whole-body 1.5T Siemens Vision
 MRI scanner
whole-body PET scan
whole-body 3T MRI system scanner
whole-brain radiation therapy
whorl, coccygeal
whorled appearance
WHVP (wedged hepatic venous
 pressure)
Wiberg, CE angle of
Wiberg classification of patellar types
wide-beam scanning
wide-mouth sac
wide pulse
wide window setting
widened heart shadow
widened mediastinum
widened sulci
widened teardrop distance
widened thoracic outlet
widening
 ankle mortise
 crural cistern
 growth plate
 interpedicular distance
 interspinous
 joint
 mediastinal
widespread metastases

width
 collimation
 isodose
 pulse
 window
Wiener MRI filter
Wiktor stent
Wilcoxon signed-rank test
Wilkins classification of radial
 fracture
Williams-Beuren syndrome
Williams-Campbell syndrome
Williamson sign
Willis
 antrum of
 arterial circle of
 artery of
 circle of
Willis pancreas
Willis pouch
willow fracture
Wilmad reference standards
Wilms tumor
Wilson cloud chamber
Wilson disease
Wilson-Mikity syndrome
winding, zero-pitch solenoidal
window
 acquisition
 acoustic
 aorticopulmonary
 apical
 bone
 brain
 cortical
 esophageal
 gastric
 parasternal
 pericardial
 pulmonary parenchymal
 soft tissue
 subcostal

window *(cont.)*
  subdural
  suprasternal
window width
window ductus
window/level settings
window settings
windowing, intensity
windsock aneurysm
windup injury
wing
  iliac
  sphenoidal
winged scapula
Winiwarter-Buerger disease
Winiwarter-Manteuffel-Buerger
  disease
Winprint imaging laser printer
Winquist-Hansen classification of
  femoral fracture
Winslow, foramen of
Winslow pancreas
Winston-Lutz for LINAC-based
  radiosurgery
Winter-King-Moe scoliosis
Wintrich sign
wire
  calibrated guide
  encircling
  figure-of-8
  guide
  Ilizarov
  interfragment
  intravascular guide
  lead
  monitoring
wire fixation
wire localization
wire-related defect
Wirsung duct
Wishard catheter
Wiskott-Aldrich syndrome

wispy connection
Wits cephalometric measurement
WMA (wall motion abnormalities)
Wolf-Hirschhorn syndrome
Wolfe mammographic parenchymal
  patterns
Wolff law (bone structure)
Wolff-Chaikoff effect
Wolff-Parkinson-White (WPW)
  syndrome
Wolin meniscoid lesion
Wolman xanthomatosis
womb
woody mass
woolsorter's inhalation disease
word segmentation algorithm
workstation
  imaging
  ISG medical imaging
  MacSpect real-time NMR
  Radstation radiology
  Shebele physician reporting
  stacked-metaphor
  Sun
  Unix/X11
workup (n.), work up (v.)
wormian bone
wound
  exit
  gunshot (GSW)
  missile
  penetrating
  perforating
  puncture
  stab
WPW (Wolff-Parkinson-White) syndrome
wrap-around ghosting artifact
wrestler's elbow
wrinkle artifact
wrinkled pleura
Wrisberg cardiac ganglion

Wrisberg, intermediate nerve of
Wrisberg ligament
wrist
  gymnast's
  palmar
  SLAC (scapholunate arthritic
    collapse)
  volar
  Volz

wrist capsule
wristdrop
wryneck (torticollis)
W-shaped ileal pouch
WSQ (wavelet scalar quantization)
Wyburn-Mason arteriovenous
  malformation

X, x

x-ray detector, Si (Li)
x-ray film jacket
x-ray in plaster (XIP)
x-ray out of plaster (XOP)
x-ray sensitive vidicon
x-ray topography

X-terminal
X trough
X, Y, and Z coordinates for target
 lesion
xylenol orange
Xylocaine

Y, y

Y (yttrium)
YAG (yttrium, aluminum, garnet)
  laser
Yb (ytterbium)
Y bone plate
Y configuration, inverted
Yergason test of shoulder subluxation
Y fracture
yield comparison
yoke
yokelike

yolk sac (YS) diameter
Y plate
YS (yolk sac)
Y-shaped distortion
Y-T fracture
Y trough
ytterbium (Yb)
  ^{169}Yb (Yb-169) brachytherapy
yttrium radioactive source
yttrium-90 microspheres
Y view

Z, z

Zahn
   lines of
   pockets of
Zang space
Z axis
Z-dependent computed tomography
Z disk
zebra artifact
Zeek syndrome
Zellweger syndrome
Zener diode
Zenker diverticulum
Zenker pouch
zero-field splitting
zero-fill artifact
zero-pitch solenoidal winding
zeugmatography, Fourier
   transformation
Z interpolation algorithms
Zickel fracture classification system
Ziegler syndrome
Zielke derotation level
zinc, irradiated
Zinn, tendon of
zipper artifact
ZK44012 contrast medium

Z-line of esophagus
Zlotsky-Ballard classification of
   acromioclavicular injury
Z-Med balloon catheter
Zollinger-Ellison syndrome (ZES)
zonal gastritis
zone
   fracture
   Rolando
   slow conduction (ZSC)
   sonolucent
   Westphal
z point pressure
ZSC (zone of slow conduction)
Zucker catheter
Zuckerkandl bodies
Zuckerkandl convolution
ZY plane
zygapophyseal articulation
zygapophyseal joint
zygoma
zygomatic arch
zygomatic bone
zygomatic process
zygomaticomalar area
zygomaticomaxillary fracture